Advanced Techniques in Canine and
Feline Neurosurgery

Advanced Techniques in Canine and Feline Neurosurgery

Edited by

Andy Shores

Clinical Professor and Chief, Neurosurgery and Neurology
Mississippi State University College of Veterinary Medicine
The Veterinary Specialty Center
Mississippi State, Starkville, MS, USA

Brigitte A. Brisson

Professor of Small Animal Surgery
Department of Clinical Studies
Ontario Veterinary College
University of Guelph
Guelph, Ontario, Canada

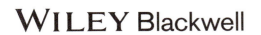 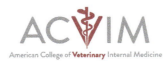 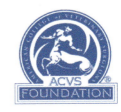

This edition first published 2023
© 2023 John Wiley & Sons, Inc.

All rights reserved. No part of this publication may be reproduced, stored in a retrieval system, or transmitted, in any form or by any means, electronic, mechanical, photocopying, recording or otherwise, except as permitted by law. Advice on how to obtain permission to reuse material from this title is available at http://www.wiley.com/go/permissions.

The right of Andy Shores and Brigitte A. Brisson to be identified as the authors of the editorial material in this work has been asserted in accordance with law.

Registered Office
John Wiley & Sons, Inc., 111 River Street, Hoboken, NJ 07030, USA

For details of our global editorial offices, customer services, and more information about Wiley products visit us at www.wiley.com.

Wiley also publishes its books in a variety of electronic formats and by print-on-demand. Some content that appears in standard print versions of this book may not be available in other formats.

Trademarks: Wiley and the Wiley logo are trademarks or registered trademarks of John Wiley & Sons, Inc. and/or its affiliates in the United States and other countries and may not be used without written permission. All other trademarks are the property of their respective owners. John Wiley & Sons, Inc. is not associated with any product or vendor mentioned in this book.

Limit of Liability/Disclaimer of Warranty

The contents of this work are intended to further general scientific research, understanding, and discussion only and are not intended and should not be relied upon as recommending or promoting scientific method, diagnosis, or treatment by physicians for any particular patient. In view of ongoing research, equipment modifications, changes in governmental regulations, and the constant flow of information relating to the use of medicines, equipment, and devices, the reader is urged to review and evaluate the information provided in the package insert or instructions for each medicine, equipment, or device for, among other things, any changes in the instructions or indication of usage and for added warnings and precautions. While the publisher and authors have used their best efforts in preparing this work, they make no representations or warranties with respect to the accuracy or completeness of the contents of this work and specifically disclaim all warranties, including without limitation any implied warranties of merchantability or fitness for a particular purpose. No warranty may be created or extended by sales representatives, written sales materials or promotional statements for this work. The fact that an organization, website, or product is referred to in this work as a citation and/or potential source of further information does not mean that the publisher and authors endorse the information or services the organization, website, or product may provide or recommendations it may make. This work is sold with the understanding that the publisher is not engaged in rendering professional services. The advice and strategies contained herein may not be suitable for your situation. You should consult with a specialist where appropriate. Further, readers should be aware that websites listed in this work may have changed or disappeared between when this work was written and when it is read. Neither the publisher nor authors shall be liable for any loss of profit or any other commercial damages, including but not limited to special, incidental, consequential, or other damages.

Library of Congress Cataloging-in-Publication Data applied for:

ISBN 9781119790426 (hardback)

Cover Design: Wiley
Cover Images: Courtesy of Andy Shores

Set in 9.5/12.5pt STIXTwoText by Straive, Chennai, India.

SKY10042641_021023

To all those professionals and paraprofessionals, devoted to the supportive care and rehabilitation of the small animal neurosurgical patients. We deal with many complex and challenging procedures and the care of these patients requires a team of individuals with a heart.
To my colleagues who have supported my efforts in completion of this volume.
To my family that means the world to me with special recognition of the new addition,
Derek Alejandro Shores – you are a blessing.

Andy Shores

To my girls, Julia and Éloïse – watching you grow into strong, confident young women is the best gift a parent could ask for. I love you to the moon and back. Always and forever. No matter what.
To my husband – thank you for your continued love and support. I couldn't do it without you.
To my dad –thank you for pushing me to do what I love and to always strive for being the best I can be. I miss you every day.
To my residents – stay thirsty for new knowledge and continue to grow the excellent neurosurgical skills you have developed throughout your training.

Brigitte A. Brisson

Contents

List of Contributors *xvii*
ACVS Foreword *xix*
ACVIM Foreword *xxi*
Preface *xxiii*
About the Companion Website *xxv*

1 A History of Veterinary Neurosurgery: 1900–2000 *1*
Don Sorjonen
Introduction *1*
Advances in Imaging Techniques *1*
Advances in Spinal Procedures *2*
   Thoracolumbar (T1–S1) *2*
   Cervical (C1–C7) *5*
Advances in Intracranial Procedures *8*
Epilogue *11*
References *12*

2 Applications of 3D Printing in Veterinary Neurosurgery *17*
Fred Wininger
Steps of the 3D Printing Process *18*
   Acquisition *18*
   Thresholding *18*
   Segmentation *18*
   File Format Creation *19*
   Manifold Manipulation *19*
   Anatomic Modeling *19*
   Printing *20*
Current Spinal Applications *20*
Customized Tools *20*
Current Brain Applications *21*
Future Applications of 3D Printing in Veterinary Neurosurgery *23*
References *23*

3 Postoperative Radiation Therapy of Intracranial Tumors *25*
M. W. Nolan
Introduction *25*
Overview of Radiation Therapy *25*

viii | Contents

Radiobiology *25*
  DNA as The Target for Radiation *25*
  Normal Tissue Injury *26*
  Rationale for Radiation Fractionation *26*
Radiation Physics and Treatment Planning *28*
  Beam Energy Selection *28*
  Dose Calculations *28*
  Target Localization Strategies *29*
  Delivery Systems *31*
  Plan Evaluation *32*
Specific Tumor Types *33*
  Meningioma *33*
    Clinical Data *33*
    Radiotherapeutic Techniques *34*
  Glial Tumors *34*
    Clinical Data *34*
    Radiotherapeutic Techniques *35*
  Choroid Plexus Tumors *35*
    Clinical Data *35*
    Radiotherapeutic Techniques *35*
  Spinal Tumors *35*
    Clinical Data *35*
    Radiotherapeutic Techniques *36*
Stereotactic Radiosurgery and Stereotactic Radiation Therapy *36*
References *37*

4 Practice and Principles of Neuroanesthesia for Imaging and Neurosurgery *39*
Claudio C. Natalini
Introduction *39*
Increases in ICP *39*
  Clinical Signs *39*
  Dynamics *39*
  Cerebral Perfusion and Anesthesia *40*
  The Cushing Reflex and Anesthesia *40*
  Increases in ICP During Anesthesia *41*
  ICP and Contrast Myelography *42*
  Hydrocephalus *42*
Neurologic Monitoring: Monitoring Brain State During Anesthesia *42*
  Modalities of Neurologic Monitoring *42*
    Electroencephalogram EEG *42*
    Sensory-Evoked Responses (SERs) and Somatosensory-Evoked Potentials (SSEPs) *42*
  Glycemic Control *42*
Monitoring Nociception *42*
Other Modalities *43*
Sedation versus General Anesthesia for Imaging *43*
  Regional Anesthesia for Laminectomy, Hemilaminectomy, and Vertebral Fractures *43*
  Anesthesia Protocol for Intracranial Surgery *43*
References *44*

Part I   Spinal Procedures *45*

5   Cervical Ventral Slot Decompression   *47*
Andy Shores and Allison Mooney
Cervical IVD Syndrome   *47*
  History   *47*
  Clinical Signs   *47*
  Radiographic Signs   *48*
  Advanced Imaging   *49*
Indications for Surgery   *50*
Ventral Approach to the Cervical Spine   *50*
Decompression of the Cervical Spinal Cord   *54*
  Ventral Slot Method   *54*
  Perioperative and Postoperative Care   *58*
References   *58*

6   Thoracolumbar Decompression: Hemilaminectomy and Mini-Hemilaminectomy (Pediculectomy)   *59*
Brigitte A. Brisson
Indications   *59*
Procedures   *59*
Technique: Surgical Approach for Mini-Hemilaminectomy (Video 6.1)   *60*
  Dorsolateral Approach [14–17] (Video 6.2)   *60*
  Variation   *61*
  Recommended Variation   *61*
Technique: Mini-Hemilaminectomy Procedure   *63*
Technique: Surgical Approach for Hemilaminectomy   *64*
Technique: Hemilaminectomy Procedure   *65*
Removal of Disk Material: Mini-Hemilaminectomy and Hemilaminectomy   *66*
Closure   *67*
Complications   *67*
Postoperative Care   *68*
References   *68*

7   Thoracolumbar Disk Fenestration   *70*
Brigitte A. Brisson
Indications   *70*
Technique – Surgical Approach   *71*
  Variations   *72*
Technique – Fenestration Procedure (Video 7.1)   *72*
  Blade Fenestration   *73*
  Power Fenestration   *73*
  Other Requirements   *75*
  Closure   *75*
Complications   *75*
Postoperative Care   *76*
References   *76*

x | Contents

8 Percutaneous Laser Disk Ablation *78*
Danielle Dugat
Introduction *78*
Laser Ablation *78*
Candidate Selection *79*
Procedure Description *80*
Procedure Complications and Recurrence *82*
Diagnostic Evaluation of PLDA *83*
Conclusion *84*
References *84*

9 The Cranial Thoracic Spine: Approach via Dorsolateral Hemilaminectomy *86*
Yael Merbl and Annie Vivian Chen-Allen
Indications *86*
Surgical Anatomy *87*
Patient Positioning *87*
Surgical Technique *88*
Postoperative Care *89*
References *90*

10 Principles in Surgical Management of Locked Cervical Facets in Dogs *91*
Andy Shores and Ryan Gibson
Introduction *91*
Unilateral Locked Cervical Facets in Humans *91*
Clinical Presentation *91*
Surgical Techniques *92*
Postoperative Care *94*
Summary/Conclusions *94*
References *95*

11 Spinal Stabilization: Cervical Vertebral Column *96*
Bianca F. Hettlich
Introduction *96*
Preoperative Planning *96*
Anatomical Considerations *96*
Implant Selection *97*
Positioning and Approach *97*
Vertebral Distraction *98*
Diskectomy *99*
Intervertebral Spacer *99*
Indication for Additional Decompression *101*
Surgical Stabilization *101*
  Monocortical Screw/PMMA Fixation *101*
  Vertebral Body Plates *102*
  Other Techniques *104*
  Stabilization of Multiple Spaces *105*
Postoperative Assessment *105*
Complications *106*
References *107*

12 Stabilization of the Thoracolumbar Spine *109*

Simon T. Kornberg and Brigitte A. Brisson

Preoperative Planning *109*
  Decompression with Stabilization *111*
Technique *111*
  Implant Selection *111*
Thoracolumbar Spine *114*
  Positioning and Approach *114*
  Implant Selection *114*
  Spinal Stapling/Segmental Fixation *116*
Lumbosacral Spine *118*
  Anatomy *118*
  Positioning and Approach *118*
  Reduction *119*
  Implant Selection *119*
Postoperative Imaging *120*
Complications *120*
Aftercare *122*
Acknowledgments *122*
References *122*

13 Surgical Management of Congenital Spinal Anomalies *124*

Sheila Carrera-Justiz and Gabriel Garcia

Diagnostics *124*
Treatment *125*
Prognosis *126*
Future Directions *127*
Summary *127*
References *127*

14 Lumbosacral Decompression and Foraminotomy Techniques *129*

Stef H. Y. Lim and Michaela Beasley

Pathophysiology and Anatomy *129*
  L7–S1 Foramina Anatomy *129*
Diagnosis *130*
  History and Clinical Signs *130*
  Physical Examination Findings *130*
  Orthopedic Examination Findings *130*
  Neurologic Examination Findings *131*
  Radiography *131*
  Myelography (Contrast Study) *132*
  Computed Tomography (CT) *132*
  Magnetic Resonance Imaging (MRI) *133*
  Force Plate Analysis *134*
  Electrodiagnostics *134*
Treatment: Conservative and Medical Therapy *134*
Surgery *134*
  Dorsal Laminectomy *135*
    Patient Preparation and Positioning *135*
    Surgical Technique *135*

xii | Contents

Foraminotomy *136*
Facetectomy *137*
Distraction, Fusion, and Stabilization *137*
Pins and PMMA *137*
SOP Plating *137*
Surgical Technique *138*
Pedicle Screw and Rod Fixation (PSRF) *138*
Minimally-Invasive Transilial Vertebral (MTV) Blocking *138*
Postoperative Management *139*
References *139*

15 Surgical Management of Spinal Nerve Root Tumors *143*
Ane Uriarte
Introduction *143*
Clinical Presentations *143*
Meningioma *143*
Peripheral Nerve Sheath Tumors *143*
Diagnosis *144*
Imaging *144*
Spinal Meningioma MRI *144*
PNST MRI *144*
Electrodiagnostics *147*
Cytology/Histology *147*
Meningiomas *147*
PNST *147*
Surgery of PNST Within the Spinal Nerves *148*
Cervical Approach *148*
Positioning *148*
Lateral Surgical Approach to Caudal Cervical Foramen After Amputation *148*
Dorsal Surgical Approach for Cervical Hemilaminectomy *149*
Respiratory Compromise in Cervical Myelopathies *149*
Lumbar Approach *150*
Approach to the L7–S1 Foramen *150*
Postoperative Care *150*
Prognosis *151*
Radiation Therapy *151*
References *151*

16 Surgical Management of Craniocervical Junction Anomalies *153*
Sofia Cerda-Gonzalez
Indications *153*
Surgical Anatomy *154*
Patient Preparation and Positioning *155*
Surgical Technique *156*
Outcomes *159*
References *159*

17 Ventral Approach to the Cervicothoracic Spine *161*
Isidro Mateo
Introduction *161*
Surgical Anatomy [10–12] *161*
Muscles *161*

Contents | xiii

Vessels *163*
Nerves *163*
Viscera *163*
Surgical Technique [10, 12] *163*
Clinical Results *165*
Conclusion *167*
References *167*

Part II Intracranial Procedures *169*

18 Intraoperative Ultrasound in Intracranial Surgery *171*
Alison M. Lee, Chris Tollefson and Andy Shores
Introduction *171*
Artifacts in Imaging *172*
Accuracy of Intraoperative Ultrasound *173*
Scanning Procedure and Equipment *173*
Appearance of Tumor on Ultrasound *175*
Ultrasound Guided Procedures *177*
Conclusion *177*
References *177*

19 Brain Biopsy Techniques *179*
John Rossmeisl and Annie Chen
Introduction *179*
Indications and Contraindications *179*
Frame-based Stereotactic Brain Biopsy (SBBfb) *179*
SBBfb Technique *181*
Preoperative Evaluation *181*
Headframe Placement and Acquisition of Stereotactic Images *181*
SBBfb Planning *181*
SBBfb Procedure *183*
Postoperative Care and Adverse Events *184*
Processing of Brain Biopsy Specimens *184*
Frameless Stereotactic Brain Biopsy (SBBfl) *185*
SBBfl Technique *185*
Attachment of the Fiducial Markers *185*
Acquisition of Magnetic Resonance Images *186*
Registration Procedure *186*
Trajectory Planning *187*
Brain Biopsy *187*
Biopsy Sample Processing *187*
Conclusion *187*
References *188*

20 Surgical Management of Sellar Masses *190*
Tina Owen, Annie Chen-Allen and Linda Martin
Introduction *190*
Case Selection *191*
Preoperative Work up *192*
Neurologic Exam *192*
Preoperative Testing and Diagnostics *193*

xiv | Contents

Endocrine Testing 193
Brain Imaging 193
Imaging of Pituitary Masses 194
Imaging of Non-Pituitary Sellar Masses 195
Surgery 196
Anatomy 196
Localization 196
Positioning 197
Approach 197
Surgical Outcome 198
In Hospital Care 200
Postoperative Management and Monitoring 200
Postoperative Complications 200
Endocrine and Metabolic Complications 200
Respiratory Complications 203
Neurologic Complications 204
Procedural Related Complications 204
Long term Follow Up 205
References 206

21 Surgical Management and Intraoperative Strategies for Tumors of the Skull *211*
Jonathan F. McAnulty
Osteosarcoma and Multilobular Osteochrondrosarcoma of the Cranium 211
Diagnosis and Characterization 212
Surgical Planning and Treatment 212
Exposure 212
Challenges in Skull Tumor Resection 214
Parietal Calvarial and Dorsal Frontal Bone Lesions 214
Frontal Bone within the Orbit and Sphenoid Bone Lesions 215
Occipital Bone Lesions 215
MRI Assessment of Blood Flow to the Transverse Sinuses 216
Slow Occlusion of Flow from the DSS to the Transverse Sinus Using a Balloon Catheter 217
Extension of Tumor to the tentorium Cerebelli 218
Zygomatic Arch and Ramus of the Mandible 218
Complications and Risks 219
Cranioplasty 220
References 221

22 Surgical Management of Intracranial Meningiomas *223*
R. Timothy Bentley
Introduction 223
Anatomy 223
Transfrontal Craniotomy (Bilateral Transfrontal Craniotomy) 225
Technique 225
Closure 227
Modifications 228
The Falx Cerebri and the Dorsal Sagittal Sinus (DSS) 229
Rostrotentorial Craniectomy/Craniotomy (Lateral Craniectomy/Craniotomy) 231
Technique 232
Closure: Craniectomy vs Craniotomy 233
Combined Rostrotentorial–Transfrontal Approach 234
Suboccipital Craniectomy (See Also Chapter 24 Surgery of Caudal Fossa Tumors) 235

Technique *235*

Closure *236*

Meningioma Resection and Instrumentation *236*

Simpson Classification of Meningioma Resection in Humans (Table 22.2) *237*

Substitutes for Resected Dura Mater *237*

Complications and Mitigation Strategies *239*

References *239*

23 Lateral Ventricular Fenestration *241*

Andy Shores

Introduction *241*

Rationale *241*

Technique *242*

Potential Complications *243*

Discussion *243*

References *248*

24 Surgery of the Caudal Fossa *249*

Beverly K. Sturges

Anatomy *249*

Indications for Surgery *250*

Preoperative Assessment and Anesthetic Management *251*

Surgical Positioning *251*

Surgical Approach(es) to the Caudal Fossa *252*

Midline Occipital Approach [3–5] *252*

Extended Lateral Approach with Occlusion of The Transverse Sinus [3, 6] *255*

Lateral Approach to The Cerebellum in Cats [8] *258*

Closing and Reconstruction *258*

Postoperative Care *259*

Complications *260*

References *261*

25 Transzygomatic Approach to Ventrolateral Craniotomy/Craniectomy *262*

Martin Young and Sandy Chen

Introduction *262*

Patient Positioning/Preparation *262*

Surgical Procedure *263*

References *266*

Index *269*

List of Contributors

Michaela Beasley, ACVIM
Mississippi State University
Mississippi State, Mississippi, USA

R. Timothy Bentley, ACVIM
Purdue University
West Lafayette, Indiana, USA

Brigitte A. Brisson, ACVS
University of Guelph
Guelph, Ontario, Canada

Sheila Carrera-Justiz, ACVIM
University of Florida
Gainesville, Florida, USA

Sofia Cerda-Gonzalez, ACVIM
MedVet Chicago
Chicago, Illinois, USA

Sandy Chen
Bush Veterinary Neurology Service
Springfield, Virginia, USA

Annie Vivian Chen-Allen, ACVIM
Washington State University
Pullman, Washington, USA

Danielle Dugat, ACVS
Oklahoma State University
Stillwater, Oklahoma, USA

Gabriel Garcia, ACVIM
University of Florida
Gainesville, Florida, USA

Ryan Gibson, ACVIM
Auburn University
Auburn, AL, USA

B. F. Hettlich, ACVS
University of Bern
Bern, Switzerland

Simon T. Kornberg, ACVIM
Southeast Veterinary Neurology
Miami, Florida, USA

Alison M. Lee, ACVR
Mississippi State University
Starkville, Mississippi, USA

Stef H. Y. Lim
Bush Veterinary Neurology Service
Leesburg, Virginia, USA

Linda Martin, ECC
Washington State University
Pullman, Washington, USA

Isidro Mateo, ECVN
Neurology and Neurosurgery Department
Hospital Veterinario VETSIA,
Leganés, Madrid, Spain

Jonathan F. McAnulty, ACVS
University of Wisconsin-Madison
Madison, Wisconsin, USA

Yael Merbl, ECVN
Washington State University
Pullman, Washington, USA

Allison Mooney, ACVIM
Allison Mooney, ACVIM
WestVet, Boise, Idaho, USA

Claudio C. Natalini, ACVAA
Mississippi State University
Starkville, Mississippi, USA

M. W. Nolan, ACVR
North Carolina State University
Raleigh, North Carolina, USA

Tina Owen, ACVS
Washington State University
Pullman, Washington, USA

John Rossmeisl, ACVIM
Virginia Tech, Blacksburg
Virginia, USA

Andy Shores, ACVIM
Mississippi State University
Mississippi State, Mississippi, USA

Don Sorjonen, ACVIM
Auburn University College of Veterinary Medicine
Auburn, Alabama, USA

Beverly K. Sturges, ACVIM
University of California
Davis, California, USA

Chris Tollefson, ACVR
Cornell University
Ithaca, New York, USA

Fred Wininger, ACVIM
CARE Charlotte Animal Referral and Emergency
Charlotte, North Carolina,
USA

Ane Uriarte, ECVN, EBVS
European Specialist in Veterinary Neurology
Head of Neurology at Southfields Veterinary Specialist,
UK

Martin Young, ACVIM
Bush Veterinary Neurology Service
Richmond, Virgina, USA

ACVS Foreword

The American College of Veterinary Surgeons Foundation is pleased to present *Advanced Techniques in Canine and Feline Neurosurgery* in the book series entitled *Advances in Veterinary Surgery*.

The ACVS Foundation is an independently charted philanthropic organization that supports the advancement of surgical care of all animals through funding of educational and research opportunities for veterinary surgical residents and board-certified veterinary surgeons.

Our collaboration with Wiley Publishing Company brings unique contributions that can benefit and enhance the learning process to all interested in veterinary surgery.

One of the key missions of the ACVS Foundation is to promote innovative education for residents in training and diplomates. This book underscores our intent, focusing on achievements made by scientists, their latest key findings, along with new techniques made possible by state-of-the-art equipment. This book will inspire, inform, and provide direction for residents in training as well as surgeons already employing neurosurgical procedures in their practices.

Advanced Techniques in Canine and Feline Neurosurgery is edited by Drs. Andy Shores and Brigitte Brisson. I'd like to congratulate and thank them for helping to move this fast-growing field forward. They have chosen an international group of strong contributing authors to cover canine and feline neurosurgical skills, equipment, techniques, and procedures. I am sure you will find this reference extremely valuable.

The ACVS Foundation is proud to collaborate with Wiley in this important series and is honored to present this newest book in the *Advances in Veterinary Surgery* series.

R. Reid Hanson, DVM, ACVS, ACVECC
Chair, Board of Trustees
ACVS Foundation

ACVIM Foreword

It is my pleasure on behalf of the ACVIM to introduce the book, *Advanced Techniques in Canine and Feline Neurosurgery*, edited by Drs. Andy Shores and Brigitte Brisson. The content provided includes basic and advanced knowledge of veterinary neurosurgery shared by many who are ACVS, ACVIM, and ECVN trained. The information is practical and focuses on techniques that are directly applicable and relevant to practice of neurosurgery. Veterinary neurosurgery continues to grow and certainly has reached an area of expertise in our profession. Our veterinary patients must have access to neurosurgeons who are experts in the most current surgical techniques.

The neurosurgical topics are comprehensive and bring forth new techniques and technologies in performing spinal and intracranial procedures. Neurosurgery will be forever evolving as we adopt human neurosurgical principles and procedures into veterinary medicine. Of special note is the chapter on the history of neurosurgery. Many have paved the way to our learning and understanding of veterinary neurosurgery and let us not forget those who led us in our neurosurgical training. Trainees and their mentors will utilize this textbook as a comprehensive guide, which provides accurate and concise information of neurosurgery. The videos on the website also are a valuable resource and innovative way to demonstrate techniques and procedures. This dynamic resource enables visual learning on another scale.

My colleagues who have contributed to this textbook are to be commended on their efforts especially during a pandemic that posed many challenges. It is because of their time and talents, and those of our fellow ACVIM Diplomates, that ACVIM is able to continually advance our mission to be the trusted leader in veterinary education, discovery, and medical excellence.

Joan R. Coates, DVM, MS, DACVIM (Neurology)
ACVIM Neurology Specialty President

Preface

The interest of many and the many advancements in the field of veterinary neurosurgery prompted the development of this book. And while some routine or standard approaches are included in these chapters, much of the content is devoted to advanced techniques being performed by many of the top veterinary neurosurgeons in the world. Some are ACVS trained, some are ACVIM (Neurology) or ECVN trained, but we share the same vocation: veterinary neurosurgery. Veterinary neurosurgery continues to grow and certainly has reached a point of being a very important subspecialty in our profession. The hours of training and devotion to this discipline by my fellow neurosurgeons is noteworthy and certainly deserving of formal recognition for what it has become – its own entity. And while I do not expect a major change in my lifetime, I sincerely hope this work will foster the continued development of our subspecialty by the many fine individuals currently engaged and for those to come. As such, I believe formal recognition should and will come with time: the ABVS should give strong consideration to the development of a separate specialty or a sub-pecialty.

This book contains many spinal and intracranial procedures, several of those (such as the surgical management of sellar masses) are on the cutting edge of our discipline. I am very grateful for the many hours my colleagues have put into these works and they are well deserving of my heartfelt thanks. In the midst of a pandemic, these colleagues came through with outstanding works.

I trust the readers will benefit from the content and especially from the number of accompanying videos on the website.

I sincerely appreciate the tremendous effort put forth by my colleagues that contributed to this volume.

Andy Shores
Mississippi State, MS, USA 2023

About the Companion Website

This book is accompanied by a companion website.

 http://www.wiley.com/go/shores/advanced

The website features procedural videos.

Video 3.1 Radiation therapy in a 7-year-old spayed female dog, 3 weeks following surgical resection of a choroid plexus carcinoma.
Video 4.1 Balanced anesthetic protocol procedure for a 17-year-old female/spayed cat for craniectomy to remove a large intracranial mass.
Video 5.1 The ventral midline surgical approach to the cervical spine.
Video 5.2 Ventral slot decompression of a cervical disk extrusion.
Video 6.1 Pediculectomy performed at T13-L1 through a dorsolateral approach on the left side (entire procedure).
Video 6.2 Modified dorsolateral surgical approach for pediculectomy.
Video 6.3 Following the initial approach through a dorsolateral incision, the spinal musculature is elevated using a periosteal elevator to identify the appropriate site for pediculectomy at T13-L1 on the left.
Video 6.4 An air drill is used to create a pediculectomy for removal of herniated disc material from the spinal canal.
Video 6.5 After drilling through cortical, medullary and inner cortical bone, the spinal canal is entered by removing the remaining, thin inner periosteum using an iris spatula or 90 degree bent needle and #11 blade.
Video 6.6 Using a bent iris spatula to retrieve herniated disc material from the spinal canal. The spatula is manipulated from craniodorsal and dorsocaudal toward the mid section of the pediculectomy ventrally to avoid pushing disc away from the pediculectomy window.
Video 6.7 Surgical closure of the modified dorsolateral approach used for pediculectomy.
Video 7.1 Blade fenestration performed at T13-L1 on the left following a pediculectomy procedure.
Video 8.1 Video showing the positioning the patient, placement of needles using fluoroscopy and application of the laser to perform the fenestrations.
Video 9.1 A live surgical video of the approach to the cranial thoracic spine with instructive narration.
Video 13.1 Video depicting a pre-operative and post-operative videos of a patient that underwent surgical management of a congenital spinal anomaly using the biological *in situ* technique.
Video 14.1 Video of Lumbosacral Decompression and Foraminotomy Techniques.
Video 14.2 Video demonstrating the sciatic nerve entrapment test exam in a dog.
Video 15.1 Removal of lumbar PNST / Limb sparing technique.
Video 15.2 Removal of cervical PNST / with limb amputation.

xxvi | *About the Companion Website*

Video 17.1 Video showing the integrity of the mediastinum in a cadaveric model in which median manubriotomy has been performed and 200 ml of air injected into the thoracic cavity through a catheter. The video shows an expansion of the pleura without any evident leak in the cranial mediastinum.

Video 18.1 This video depicts the use of intraoperative ultrasound in the removal of a supratentorial mass in a canine patient.

Video 19.1 Video demonstrating a brain biopsy procedure using the BrainsightTM Frameless Stereotactic Biopsy Device.

Video 20.1 Video depicting a transshphenoidal hypophysectomy in an 8 year-old female/spayed mixed breed dog.

Video 21.1 Guidelines for surgical management of tumors of the Canine Skull.

Video 22.1 This video demonstrates the Purdue Diamond transfrontal craniotomy.

Video 22.2 Exposure of the olfactory bulbs using the Purdue Diamond frontal craniotomy approach.

Video 22.3 Video of the removal of a cerebellar meningioma using traction in a cat through a suboccipital craniectomy.

Video 23.1 Lateral ventricular fenestration.

Video 24.1 This video depicts a 4th Ventricular Mass Excision via Occipital Craniectomy in a live patient.

Video 25.1 Demonstration of the Transzygomatic Approach in a Cadaver.

1

A History of Veterinary Neurosurgery: 1900–2000

Don Sorjonen

Auburn University College of Veterinary Medicine, Auburn, Alabama, USA

Introduction

Any treatise of merit regarding the history of veterinary neurosurgery must include, as a preamble, a brief history of veterinary medicine [1, 2]. Early writings suggest that the practice of veterinary medicine was born from human necessity. Diseases that afflicted domestic animals were also a threat to a principal source of food and transportation for humans. Consequently, most of the notable early practices of veterinary medicine focused on diseases of cattle, sheep, and horses. Economic losses from animal plagues (example, rinderpest, anthrax, blackleg) were so consequential that in 1762 the first college of veterinary medicine was created in Lyons, France. Between 1762 and 1862, 17 additional schools of veterinary medicine were established throughout Europe, England, and Scotland; in the United States, the New York College of Veterinary Surgeons was established in 1857. It is through the growth and maturation of the worldwide veterinary schools that veterinary neurosurgery was born. This review considers the historical events that promoted advances in veterinary neurosurgery from its inception through the end of the twentieth century. Although attempts have been made to faithfully include every contribution to the advancement of veterinary neurosurgery, with any work of this time expanse some contributions may have been missed.

Advances in Imaging Techniques

It is worth noting that seminal advances in human neurosurgery are typically credited with the development of cerebral localization theory, antiseptic/aseptic technique, and anesthesia [3]. While these are important tenets, they were developed before the inception of the specialized practice of veterinary neurosurgery; consequently, they have been largely adopted en bloc from human medicine. Important advances in veterinary neurosurgery more commonly followed advances in diagnostic imaging techniques of the central nervous system (CNS). In fact, with the development of radiographic techniques that offered more exquisite anatomic detail came neurosurgical techniques that offered more positive outcomes. This relationship is best illustrated by the progress made in veterinary neurosurgery following the advent of computed tomography (CT) and magnetic resonance imaging (MRI) of CNS tissues.

Obtaining diagnostic imaging is foundational to any successful surgery of the CNS. While articles regarding veterinary radiology first appeared in 1896 [4], just one year after the discovery of x-ray, routine use of radiographs to confirm a clinical diagnosis of pathology of the CNS of animals did not occur for nearly a half century later [5]. Initially, conventional radiological images were the only technique available for veterinary neurosurgeons to confirm a neurological lesion. However, because of the relatively small size of the offending pathology and the isodense nature of CNS tissue, researchers sought new techniques that offered better tissue discernment. In Sweden (1951), Olsson [6] reported on myelography as part of a more comprehensive monograph on disk disease. In 1953, Hoerlein [7] at Auburn University, published a report evaluating several aqueous- and oil-based iodized contrast media for myelography. Many of these early contrast media were subsequently abandoned because of poor flow qualities and various sequelae from toxicity like seizures, general muscular fasciculation, cord malacia, fibrotic leptomeningitis, and death [8, 9]. The continued quest for improved diagnostic quality imaging lead to studies utilizing epidurography [7, 10, 11] diskography [12] and venography [13]. In the 1970s, clinical trials

---

Advanced Techniques in Canine and Feline Neurosurgery, First Edition. Edited by Andy Shores and Brigitte A. Brisson.
© 2023 John Wiley & Sons, Inc. Published 2023 by John Wiley & Sons, Inc.
Companion site: www.wiley.com/go/shores/advanced

in humans using the non-ionic, biologically inert contrast agent metrizamide (Amipaque®) were reported [14]. Metrizamide and other non-ionic contrast medias were also found to be of value for the confirmation of various spinal cord diseases in veterinary patients and were used extensively until the advent of diagnostic CT and MRI.

Advances in imaging techniques of the skull and brain of animals followed a pattern similar to spinal studies. Early reports utilizing plain film radiographs of the skull emphasized the importance of head position to achieve precise symmetry [5], the most essential criterion for interpretation of brain and skull radiographs [15]. While these early radiographic methods were typically adequate to confirm bony lesions, they were inadequate to confirm most intracranial forms of pathology. Several early investigators [16–19] experimented with various head positions, contrast agents, and injection techniques for cerebral angiography and venography; however, these images were difficult to interpret because of imprecise head positioning and consistent variations in vessel patterns. In 1961, Hoerlein and Petty [20] and Cobb [21] published articles describing pneumoencephalography in dogs. Again, positioning difficulties and filing artifacts made clinical application uncommon. In his 1961 article, Hoerlein [20] reported the result of injection of air or opaque medium into one or both lateral ventricles and concluded that "ventriculography in clinical practice is of value in demonstrating either unilateral or bilateral ventricular dropsy as well as a space-occupying lesions."

All of the neuroradiographic techniques previously discussed are restricted by their invasive nature, inconsistent reproducibility, limited visualization of the pathologic lesion, and undesirable morbidity and mortality. Before the 1980s most veterinary neurosurgeons experienced frustration dealing with these restrictions. To the relief of the veterinary neurosurgeon and to the benefit of the animal patient and their owners, a remedy to the earlier restrictions was found in CT and MRI technology. The principles of computed tomography were first elucidated by Hounsfield in 1973 [22] and the first clinical report of CT application in veterinary medicine was published in 1980 by Marineck and Young [23] followed in 1981 by LeCouter et al. [24]. Interestingly, both reports involved canine patients with neoplasia of the CNS. Although the theory of nuclear magnetic resonance (NMR) was first advanced in the 1950s [25], MRI technology became clinically relevant in the 1970s following the development of a mechanism of encoding spatial information from NMR data [26]. Veterinary reports involving MRI studies of the canine head and brain first appeared in the 1980s [27, 28] with clinical reports of spinal disease occurring in the 1990s [29].

Advances in Spinal Procedures

Thoracolumbar (T1–S1)

The vast majority of the veterinary publications that chronicle surgery of the thoracolumbar spine involved degenerative disk disease. However, Olsson [6] and Vaughn [30], both notable early authors, regarded both hemilaminectomy and laminectomy too hazardous a surgical procedure to be recommended as a treatment for disk protrusion in the dog. These authors observed dogs with spinal cord injury from a ruptured disk could recover without surgery and theorized it imprudent to risk a potential permanent surgically induced spinal cord damage in dog that may recover without surgery. In 1951, Olsson recommended a dorsolateral approach for disk fenestration but not "intervention into the vertebral canal" for dogs with disk protrusion, ascribing the reduced risk of injury to the nerves and spinal cord and prophylaxis as benefits of fenestration. After Olsson's report, multiple fenestration procedures were proposed for the dog. In 1971 Leonard [31] proposed ventral fenestration; in 1969 Ross [32] and in 1965 Northway [33] each proposed ventrolateral fenestration; in 1968 Hoerlein [34], in 1975 Flo [35] and in 1973 Yturraspe [36] proposed dorsolateral fenestration; in 1968 Seemann [37] proposed a lateral muscle separation approaches for disk fenestration and in 1976 Braund et al. [38] proposed a lateral approach for both spinal decompression and disk fenestration.

Numerous neurosurgeons differed with Olsson and Vaughn regarding the prohibition of spinal cord decompressive procedures for disk disease. Although reports of disk protrusion creating neurologic disability in dogs was recognized as early as 1913 [39], the introduction of myelography in the early 1950s heralded the use of hemilaminectomy and laminectomy for the treatment of intervertebral disk protrusion. In 1951, Greene [10] at Alabama Polytechnic Institute (later Auburn University) described a dorsolateral approach for a hemilaminectomy (Figure 1.1). Also, in 1951, Redding [40] at the University of California Davis published a laminectomy technique that he originally developed at Ohio State University (Figure 1.2). In 1956, Hoerlein [41] at Auburn University reported the benefits of dorsolateral hemilaminectomy with prophylactic fenestration that he originally worked on at Cornell (Figure 1.3). Interestingly, by the mid-1950s, Greene et al., all surgical pioneers, were actively engaged in the field of neurology and neurosurgery at Auburn University. In 1976 [42] and again in 1977 [43], Swaim at Auburn University published on the use of bilateral hemilaminectomy for extensive spinal cord decompression (Figure 1.4).

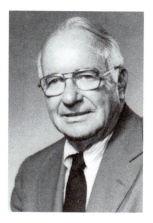

Figure 1.1 Dr James (1978) – Dr Greene was Dean of the Auburn University College of Veterinary Medicine at the time of this photo. He is credited with first describing the dorsolateral approach for a hemilaminectomy in the dog. *Source:* Photo courtesy of *The Auburn Speculum* – 1978.

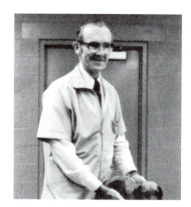

Figure 1.3 Dr Hoerlein, shown here in a photo from 1977. In 1952, Dr Hoerlein described the treatment of canine intervertebral disk disease using the hemilaminectomy. He made several pioneering contributions to the field of veterinary neurosurgery, including his groundbreaking textbooks on canine neurology. *Source:* Photo courtesy of *The Auburn Speculum* – 1977.

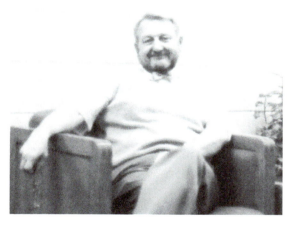

Figure 1.2 Dr Redding is pictured here in 1977 as a professor at the Auburn University College of Veterinary Medicine. Dr Redding published his technique for the dorsal laminectomy in 1951. *Source:* Photo courtesy of *The Auburn Speculum* – 1977.

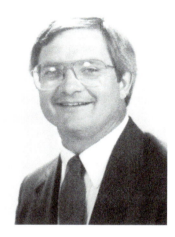

Figure 1.4 Dr Steven F. Swaim, shown here in a 1985 photo as director of the Scott-Ritchey Research Centre. Earlier in his career, Dr Swaim made many significant contributions to veterinary neurosurgery, including his description of the ventral slot technique for cervical intervertebral disk disease in dogs in 1973. *Source:* Photo courtesy of the Auburn University Library System.

Some workers saw a benefit to dorsal laminectomy as a treatment for spinal cord compression. In 1962, Funkquist [44] at the Royal Veterinary College in Stockholm, Sweden published a comprehensive volume on dorsal decompressive laminectomy. She prescribed an extensive thoracolumbar laminectomy (method A) for the treatment of disk protrusion that involved removal of both dorsal arches to a level equal to approximately one-half the height of the spinal cord. However, this technique most often resulted in a secondary cicatrix compression of the spinal cord at the surgical site. In method B, Funkquist proposed a modification of her method A where the compact bone of the dorsolateral portion of the dorsal arch, including the articular process, remained intact. This modification helped to prevent the unwanted sequela of dorsoventral compression of the spinal cord from cicatrix formation. In 1975, Trotter (Figure 1.5) and de Lahunta [45] at Cornell University, proposed a modified deep dorsal laminectomy as a remedy to the postoperative cicatrix sequela noted with the Funkquist method A technique. Trotter's technique removed the laminae and pedicles to the level of the vertebral body resulting in a spinal cord laid bare at the surgical site. Trotter contended that the deep dorsal laminectomy technique was "superior for the excision of intra- and extradural neoplasm within the vertebral canal in the thoracic, thoracolumbar, and lumbar regions of the vertebral column." Trotter also

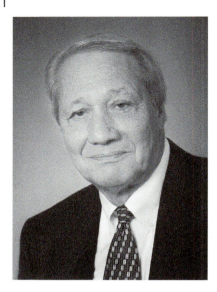

Figure 1.5 Dr Eric developed the modified deep dorsal laminectomy in the dog and published a 10-year review of surgical correction of caudal cervical vertebral malarticulation-malformation in Great Danes and Doberman Pinchers. *Source:* Photo courtesy of Dr. Eric Trotter.

commended the deep dorsal technique for the management of dogs with massive disk extrusion in the thoracolumbar and lumbar regions [45]. In 1981, Prata [46] at the Animal Medical Center New York (AMCNY) strongly advocated for the dorsal laminectomy as the treatment of choice in dogs with peracute and chronic disk disease. Prata recommended a laminectomy over two vertebral bodies with bilateral facetectomy and foraminotomy at the site of disk extrusion. In addition, bilateral pediculectomy was performed to facilitate removal of extruded disk material. Hoerlein [47] contended that laminectomy surgery was not indicated for disk protrusions because of the need for excessive spinal cord manipulation, risk of postoperative vertebral instability, excessive muscle dissection, and difficulty in performing a prophylactic disk fenestration. These two competing philosophies resulted in a north(east) versus south(east) debate regarding the best treatment for disk protrusions that continued into the 1990s. From then, the prevailing wisdom among veterinary neurosurgeons has favored hemilaminectomy as the treatment of choice for the management of dogs with thoracolumbar intervertebral disk disease [48].

In 1953, Hoerlein [49] reported on the successful use of a spinal plate applied dorsally to the spinous processes to correct a fracture of the fourth lumbar vertebra. In 1956, Hoerlein [50] published a comprehensive article on immobilization techniques for fractures and dislocations of the thoracolumbar spine. These procedures included placement of vertebral body plates for immobilization and bone grafts for fusion; application of bone plates with various fasteners to the spinous processes and ventral vertebral surfaces (Auburn Spinal Plates, Richards Manufacturing Co., Memphis TN); wiring the spinous processes together and placement of vinylidene fluoride resin plates (Lubra plates, Lubra Co., Fort Collins, CO) using a series of bolts fastened with nuts and applied to the spinous processes through the interspinous ligament. Swaim [51] modified Hoerlein's body plating technique and Gage at Auburn University devised a cross-body pinning technique [52] and a "stapling" technique for small dogs [53]. One of the earliest reports of methyl methacrylate (MMA) for repair of a spinal fractures was reported by Rouse and Miller [54] in 1975. Subsequently, numerous authors have advocated for the use of MMA combined with pins or screws applied to numerous areas of the spine to stabilize fractures/luxations and other causes of vertebral instability [55, 56].

In 1972, Brasmer and Lumb [57] and in 1975, Yturraspe et al. [58] reported on experimental techniques for spondylectomy of L2 which was replaced with a vertebral prosthesis and stabilized with dorsal spinous plating. These procedures were indicated in cases of gross vertebra infection, neoplasia, or severe trauma. Also in 1972, Knecht (Figure 1.6) reported results for hemilaminectomies in 99 dogs with thoracolumbar disk extrusions [59].

The location and anatomical peculiarities of L7 present unique challenges to the neurosurgeon; consequently, unique surgical techniques have been suggested to repair fractures or dislocations that occur at L7. In 1966, Northway [60] published a technique for para-anal insertion of an intramedullary pin through the bodies of the sacrum and L7 to L4. In 1975, Slocum and Rudy [61] published a report using a transilial intramedullary pin for

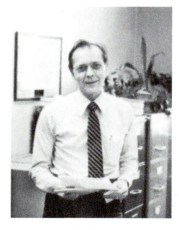

Figure 1.6 Dr Charles (pictured here in 1984 at Auburn University) reported on 99 cases of thoracolumbar IVD extrusions in dogs in 1972. *Source:* Photo courtesy of *The Auburn Speculum* – 1984.

stabilizing L7 dislocations. Dulisch and Nichols at Michigan State University [62] modified the transilial technique by combining plastic plates affixed to the spinous processes rostral to the fracture-dislocation with two transilial pins that pass through holes in the plates. To mitigate pin migration, Ullman and Boudrieau [63] at Tufts University used crossed transilial Steinmann pins connected by double Kirschner clamps. McAnulty et al. [64] at the University of Pennsylvania proposed a modified segmental spinal instrumentation technique utilizing multiple Steinmann pins on either side of the spinous processes. The pins were initially advanced through the ilial wing and then bent 90° and wired to the articular processes and dorsal spinous processes rostral to the fracture site. Shores et al. [65] at Michigan State University combined Kirschner-Ehmer external fixator apparatus with internal dorsal spinal plate fixation for the repair of caudal lumbar fractures. This technique provided rigid fixation of the fracture site, allowed decompression procedure, and could be used in dogs with fractures of the spinous and articular processes.

Compared to the thoracolumbar spine, the lumbosacral (LS) region has other unique pathologic distinctions. The L7–S1 disk space must accommodate the biomechanical forces attendant to the relative mobile L7 vertebra and the nearly immobile sacral vertebra. These forces typically converge at the intervertebral disk, the diarthrodial joint, and associated soft tissues. Over time, these forces can result in degenerative changes in the disk, joint capsule, ligamentum flavum, and diarthrodial joint producing stenosis that compresses the associated neural elements. Before the advent of CT and MRI, clinicians could only confirm LS pathology with plain film radiographs, myelography, epidurography, or interosseous venography; regrettably, radiographic findings in these cases were usually inconclusive. Consequently, most of the early surgical procedures were devised as all-purpose procedures designed to decompress the nervous tissues and to stabilize the LS joint. In 1978, Oliver et al. at the University of Georgia [66] proposed that the LS region pathology was akin to the malarticulation-malformation pathology noted in the caudal cervical region of Doberman Pinschers and described a dorsal laminectomy for decompression of the cauda equine and removal of disk prolapse and attendant fibrous adhesions. A foraminotomy was prescribed for L7 nerve root entrapment. Tarvin and Prata [67] at the AMCNY endorsed a dorsal laminectomy and bilateral facetectomies/foraminotomies for LS stenosis. Slocum and Devine [68] advocated distraction of the LS joint with a pin fixation technique that incorporated a corticocancellous bone graft harvested from the wings of the ilia for management of cauda equina compression.

Over time, advances in imaging technology promoted refinement of most spinal techniques but most notably for the management of intervertebral disk disease. Workers strived to develop procedures that were less invasive and removed less bone, thus preserving vertebral stability and improving postoperative recovery as compared to laminectomy and hemilaminectomy. These modifications included accessing the spinal canal by creating an opening in the pedicle, the vertical segment of bone that emanates from the body of the vertebra; such an operation has been termed a pediculectomy. When the pedicle and articular process is removed, the operation has been termed a mini-hemilaminectomy. In 1976, Braund et al. [38] in Sydney and Auburn devised a lateral muscular approach to the thoracolumbar spine with removal of the bony pedicle and accessory process without involvement of the articular process or lamina. In 1986, Bietto and Thatcher [69] at the AMCNY, published a modification of Braund's lateral technique that accesses the spine utilizing a dorsolateral muscle separation approach. In 1997, McCartney [70] described a partial pediculectomy technique that allows access to the ventral aspect of the spinal canal with preservation of accessory process and the diarthrodial joint. In the appropriate cases, this procedure provides adequate access for retrieving ventrally or laterally displaced disk material while reducing surgical morbidity.

Cervical (C1–C7)

Cervical disk disease is a well-recognized clinical condition of dogs. In the 1950s workers [6, 71] suggested that the treatment of choice to manage dogs with cervical pain from intervertebral disk disease was a ventral disk fenestration. In cases involving motor deficits, more aggressive techniques were suggested. In 1962, Funkquist [72] published a dorsal laminectomy technique for cervical disk protrusion in the dog. Also in 1962, Hoerlein [73] reported on dorsal cervical laminectomy and hemilaminectomy surgical techniques. Although initially these dorsal decompressive approaches were considered methods of choice to manage dogs with cervical disk disease, the intensive immediate postoperative care attendant to recovery demanded a less invasive technique. The ventral decompression procedure is far less traumatic and achieves decompression by removal of the offending disk mass. In 1971, Popovich [74] at Walter Reed Army institute of Research modified Cloward's [75] fusion technique for surgical management of cervical disk disease in humans with a ventral trephination centered over the disk space and vertebral body fusion using a slightly oversized autogenous bone dowel placed in the trephination hole. In 1973, Swaim [76] reported on a ventral midline spondylectomy and diskectomy (slot technique) that he developed while at Auburn University. Swaim's technique did not employ a bone graft. Also, in 1973, Prata and Stoll [77], concerned about the need to stabilize the surgical site, employed Swaim's technique with the addition of an autogenous iliac bone graft.

Although the ventral approach was considered preferential to the dorsal approach for the management of most cases of cervical disk disease, a dispute occurred among neurosurgeons regarding the need to stabilize the surgical site. In 1976, Gilpin [78] reported on three different ventral slot techniques in normal dogs. In Gilpin's experiment, three dogs received a contiguous slot that extended over two intervertebral disk spaces and one-third of a vertebral width; three dogs received a slot that extended over one intervertebral disk space and the full-width of the ventral vertebral body; and three dogs received a contiguous slot that extended over two intervertebral disk spaces and the full-width of the ventral vertebral body. All dogs had a normal recovery save two of three dogs in the third group that experienced mild postoperative pain. Gilpin's work provided a sound and secure basis of support for Swaim's technique as the treatment of choice for the management of cervical disk disease in the dog. In 1991, Goring et al. [79] at the University of Florida modified the traditional ventral slot for treating Doberman Pinschers with cervical vertebral instability by laterally expanding the slot boundary adjacent to the spinal canal, creating a decompression window that resembles an inverted cone. These authors suggest that this modification allows for a more expansive decompression at the site of disk compression while minimizing collapse of the disk space that could lead to postoperative nerve root entrapment.

However, in some animals, the offending disk pathology requires the neurosurgeon to provide an expansive decompression of the spinal cord. In 1963, Pettit and Whittaker [80] at Washington State University published a dorsal approach for a hemilaminectomy as a means to manage a dog with a cervical disk protrusion. In 1973, Parker [81] at the University of Illinois reported on a dorsal approach to the cervicothoracic junction for the purpose of a dorsal laminectomy. In 1983, Felts and Prata [82] at the AMCNY published on the dorsal approach for hemilaminectomy and facetectomy for intraforaminal and lateral disk extrusions. 1992, Lipsitz and Bailey [83] at the University of California described a hemilaminectomy/facetectomy that extended from the base of the spinous process to near the floor of the spinal canal. These authors recommended this approach for decompression and removal of lateral masses and for nerve root exploration; sites less accessible by either the ventral or dorsal cervical approach.

Atlantoaxial instability/subluxation (AIS) is a relatively common disorder noted largely in young toy-breed dogs but can occur in larger dogs and can be associated with trauma in any animal. Initially, dorsal exposure of the occiput, axis, and atlas was the surgical approach recommended for remedy of AIS. In 1967, Geary et al. [84] at Cornell University, and in 1970, Gage and Smallwood [85] at Texas A&M University (Figure 1.7), described a dorsal approach used to tether the atlas to the axis with a single strand of orthopedic wire passed under the atlas then looped back over the top of the atlas and tied to its mate that has been inserted into a hole drilled in the spine of the axis; a hemilaminectomy was recommended in cases that required spinal cord decompression. Geary's original technique has been modified by various workers. In 1973, Oliver and Lewis [86] at Purdue University proposed using a loop of wire passed ventral to the atlas that when cut and tied individually through two holes in the axis formed a "saddle type" configuration. In 1977, Chambers et al. [87] at the University of Georgia recommended replacing wire with non-metallic suture material because of the high frequency of postoperative wire breakage and the difficulty of passing large gauge wire in the relatively small epidural space that exists under the atlas of small dogs. In 1979, Renegar and Stoll [88] at the University of Missouri, described incorporating MMA with the dorsal wire technique in a dog where wires placed earlier had cut through the dorsal arch of the atlas. In 1980, LeCouter et al. [89] at the University of Guelph advocated for using the nuchal ligament as a means of securing the spinous process of the axis to the dorsal arch of the atlas. These authors used this technique with success in one of two toy-breeds with AIS and two larger dogs with fracture of the axis. In 1984, Kishigami [90] in Osaka, Japan developed a custom-made tension band retractor with a lip that fitted under the

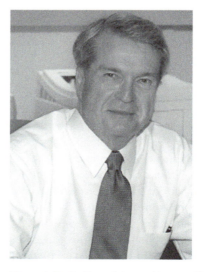

Figure 1.7 Dr Dean (pictured here at Texas A&M University in 2016). Dr Gage and Hoerlein published several papers describing techniques to repair spinal fractures and luxations.

rostral arch of the atlas and two legs that extended caudally on either side of the axis which accepted a wire suture that was crisscrossed through holes in the axis. The author reported success in one cat and four dogs with AIS. In 1996, Jeffery [91] at the Animal Health Trust, Newmarket, Suffolk, used Steinmann pins inserted through one side of the spine of the axis into the wing of the atlas on the opposite side. This crossing configuration was used in conjunction with a cancellous bone graft and MMA fixation.

Numerous postoperative complications have been reported when utilizing any of the various iterations of the dorsal repair for ASI. To redress these concerns, Sorjonen and Shires [92] at Auburn University reported on a ventral surgical technique for decompression, fixation, and fusion of atlantoaxial instability. Their technique accomplished spinal cord decompression by odontoidectomy and boney alignment, with pin fixation for stabilization and cancellous bone graft for fusion. The ventral technique has also been recommended by various workers [93–95] with modifications that include lag screw fixation [93], Steinmann pins and MMA fixation [94], bone plating, and cannulated screw fixation with cancellous graft fusion [95].

Caudal vertebral malformation-malarticulation syndrome (CVMMS) is a condition that affects both large- and small-breed dogs. In 1971, de Lahunta [96] at Cornell University described the neurologic, radiographic, and pathologic features in young rapidly growing Great Dane dogs and suggested naming the syndrome *Wobbler* because of the ataxic and paretic gait common to these dogs. Since then, Wobbler Syndrome has been reported by numerous names (cervical vertebral instability, cervical spondylomyelopathy, cervical spondylolisthesis, and cervical spondylopathy) and purported surgical remedies. In 1972, Gage and Hall [97] reported a successful repair of C6–7 subluxation with a hemilaminectomy for decompression and Auburn spinal plate for fixation. In 1973, Dueland et al. [98] at the University of Saskatchewan reported on a dorsal laminectomy with bone graft and articular wiring technique. Also in 1973, Gage and Hoerlein [99] advocated fenestration with interbody lag screw stabilization. In 1975, Swaim [100] evaluated four techniques for cervical spinal fixation in dogs with mid- and caudal-cervical vertebral instability and concluded that bilateral screws through the articular processes provided the most solid fixation. In 1976, Trotter et al. [101] published a comprehensive 10-year review of cases at Cornell University and concluded that no one surgical technique could be recommended for all cases. They proposed a dorsal laminectomy for stenotic cranial orifice of a vertebral foramen or with a stable malarticulation; a laminectomy with arthrodesis for stenotic cranial orifice and an unstable malarticulation or unstable malarticulation alone; and ventral decompression with

fusion for prominent craniodorsal projection of the vertebral body, with or without unstable malarticulation. In 1985, Lincoln and Pettit [102] at Washington State University reported on 17 large dogs treated solely with disk fenestration and concluded that disk fenestration alone provided inadequate treatment for CVMMS. Following Lincoln's report, in 1988, Ellison et al. [103] at the University of Florida reported on a distraction-fusion technique designed to help resolve the inadequacies of standalone fenestration. Ellison technique utilized a cancellous bone graft for fusion and cancellous bone screws and MMA for stabilization. In 1989, Bruecker et al. [104] at Colorado State University reported on a modification of Ellison's technique using Steinmann pins and MMA. In 1990, McKee et al [105] at the University of Melbourne reported on the use of two orthopedic washers inserted into the disk space for distraction and a cancellous bone screw advanced from the cranial vertebra through the intradiskal washers and into the caudal vertebra for fusion. In 1991, Goring et al. [79] introduced the inverted cone decompression technique to provide maximal spinal cord decompression with reduced intra- and postoperative morbidity. In 1991, Lyman [106] published a report originally presented in 1987, proposing a dorsal laminectomy that extends from C5 through C7. Lyman stated that his "continuous dorsal laminectomy procedure offers the best chance for definitive management and long-term survival with a good quality of life in Doberman Pinschers with CVMMS."

The abundance of surgical options for repair of CVMMS suggest that one remedy cannot be applied to all cases. While most neurosurgeons select their technique based on the needs of the animal patient, cervical distraction and stabilization has become increasingly popular for the treatment of CVMMS.

Cervical fractures and dislocations occur less frequently than thoracolumbar fractures/dislocations [107]; perhaps a benefit of the more robust cervical musculature or greater mobility of the cervical vertebrae [108]. The atlantoaxial region is the most common reported site of fracture/dislocation pathology. In 1958, Hoerlein [109] reported a successful repair of a fractured axis using a plate on the spinous process. In 1968, Gage [108] reported on a repair of a fractured atlas, axis, and odontoid process using a hemilaminectomy for decompression and wiring of the atlantoaxial joint for stabilization. In 1969, Gendreau and Cawley [110] at the University of Guelph reported the successful repair of a fracture of the axis in two dogs using two plates affixed to either side of the ventral midline of C2. In 1979, Rouse [111], concerned about screw penetration into the spinal canal when used to affix a ventral body plate, reported on the repair of the axis using Steinmann pins that were placed tangential to the spinal canal then stabilized using MMA. In 1986, Basinger et al. [112] at the University of Georgia reported on the entrapment of the cranial articular process of C6 over the caudal articular process of C5 resulting from a dog fight in two poodles. Cervical vertebral hyperflexion with rotation was proposed as a mechanism for the pathology. The subluxation was mechanically reduced and stabilized using two lag screws through the articular processes. In 1997, Boudrieau [113] at Tufts University reported on the successful repair of axis fractures in three dogs using the Scoville-Haverfield laminectomy retractor for fracture reduction and a screw-MMA construct for stabilization. Interestingly, in 1999, Hawthorne et al. [114] at Purdue University, concerned about an observation of high perioperative mortality associated with cervical spinal surgery in dogs with cervical fractures, advocated for cage rest with external support in animals with cervical fractures (unstable or displaced) unless the neurological signs are progressive.

Advances in Intracranial Procedures

Intracranial surgery is the sector of veterinary neurosurgery that has profited the most from advances in imaging technology. Prior to the advent of CT and MRI imaging, brain surgery was relegated to experimental studies and to animals with pathologic conditions that could be determined without the aid of sophisticated radiological techniques. Consequently, early veterinary surgery textbooks were limited to descriptions of pathology like skull fractures that could be confirmed by routine radiological techniques [115, 116]. Remarkably, some bold early workers relied on knowledge of neuroanatomy and neurophysiology to develop new intracranial surgical procedures. In 1956, Andersson [117] at Veterinarhogskolan, Stockholm, Sweden reported the successful treatment of canine distemper with prefrontal lobectomy. In 1972, Redding [118] at Auburn University and Allen et al. [119] at Cornell University reported successful management of aggression in dogs with prefrontal lobotomy. In 1982, Hart [120] at the University of California reported on the successful use of olfactory tractotomy in cats using a frontal sinus approach. In all cases, these authors used easily palpable external landmarks to guide their entrance into the cranial vault. Hydrocephalus is another clinical condition that early neurosurgeons were able to manage after confirming their diagnosis by plain film radiographs, angiograms, and contrast ventriculograms. In 1966 Few [121] and in 1968 Gage and Hoerlein [122], both at Auburn University, reported on the successful treatment of hydrocephalus in dogs with a ventriculoatrial shunt (Holter ventriculo-caval shunt valve, type B, Holter Co, Bridgeport, PA). In 1956,

Markowitz and Archibald [123] at the University of Ontario, in 1961 Alvarez-Buylla et al. [124] at the University of Colima, Henry et al. [125] at Louisiana State University, and in 1988 Niebauer and Evans [126] at the University of Pennsylvania all reported on various approaches for hypophysectomy in the dog. Markowitz, Alvarez-Buylla, and Henry relied on the intrasphenoid suture, the emissary vein, and the hamulate process as intraoperative anatomic landmarks to help determine the correct site to create the ostectomy that facilitated the hypophysectomy. Niebauer utilized three witness screws placed in the sphenoid bone followed by a cranial sinus venogram to outline the cavernous sinus that surrounded the hypophysis. All four authors recorded successful hypophysectomies utilizing their techniques. Meij [127] in 1998, at Utrecht University, was the first to utilize CT to enable accurate assessment of the pituitary size and location relative to intraoperative anatomic landmarks.

Finally, one extraordinary case report deserves attention. In 1965, Oliver [128] at Auburn University published a report of an emergency rostrotentorial craniotomy in a Boxer dog with seizures. The only available preoperative workup was a partial neurologic examination; based on a slow direct and consensual pupillary light response in the right eye, a right-sided craniotomy was performed. At surgery, two 4 by 2 mm abnormalities were noted, one on the surface in the occipital region and the other in the frontal area. A liquid-like material was suctioned from both lesions. Subsequently, exposure of the left cerebrum in a similar operative manner as the right showed no abnormal findings. The dog was discharged on the twelfth postoperative day. Oliver's report serves to illustrates the boldness of some early veterinary neurosurgeons.

In the vast majority of clinical cases with intracranial pathology, an accurate antemortem lesion localization is a prerequisite for a successful surgical outcome. Following the development of cerebral arteriography, ventriculography, and pneumoencephalography in the early 1960s, some veterinary neurosurgeons were incentivized to develop intracranial procedures that could offer a surgical remedy for animals with various intracranial pathologies not amendable to medical treatment. These early reports focused on surgical approaches to the brain and were a distillation of intracranial procedure used in human with similar brain pathology. In 1963, Hoerlein et al. [129] published the first comprehensive report on brain surgery in the dog. In their treatise, the authors addressed pre- and postoperative animal husbandry requirements, management of brain edema with various hypertonic solutions, the value of intraoperative hypothermia, anticonvulsants for seizures, preoperative sedative medications, cerebral spinal fluid withdrawal to relieve intracranial pressure (ICP), proper selection of anesthetic agents, proper patient positioning, and provided an extensive list of surgical equipment needed for successful intracranial surgery. Unilateral and bilateral dorsal craniotomy and a cerebellar approach were described in detail. While these approaches were performed largely in experimental dogs, the authors had the foresight to envision their use in animals with brain hemorrhages, abscesses, meningiomas, cysts, and skull fractures. In 1968, Oliver [130] reported on five surgical approaches that were developed as part of his master's study at Auburn University (Figure 1.8). Oliver proposed a lateral rostrotentorial craniotomy for access to the parietal lobe, occipital lobe, lateral ventricle, and pituitary gland; bilateral rostrotentorial craniotomy for access to both sides of the cerebrum and the third ventricle; suboccipital caudotentorial craniotomy for access to the cerebellum and fourth ventricle; rostrotentorial-caudotentorial craniotomy for access to the anterior cerebellum; and an oral approach to the pituitary gland, pons, and medulla and a ventral cervical approach to the pons and medulla. A total of 50 craniotomies were performed of which 41 dogs survived from 11 to 322 days. In 1972, Parker [131] published a technique for transfrontal craniotomy. The report emphasized the importance of a watertight dural seal and the need to replace and stabilize the outer table of the frontal bone in such a way as to avoid compression of the frontal cerebral cortex. By 1973, reports describing approaches to the canine brain were no longer considered peculiar. Swaim [132] described the use of cutting burs, spherical burs, an oscillating saw, and a craniotome to create bone flaps for rostrotentorial, caudotentorial, and paracranial approaches. In 1977, de Wet et al. [133] at Ohio State University presented information regarding the relationship of intracranial brain structures to the various types of skulls in dogs to serve as a quick anatomical reference prior to or during brain surgery. In 1982, de Wet [134] published a comprehensive work that included instrumentation, preoperative, operative, and postoperative details for a radical transfrontal craniotomy to access the rostral cranial fossa in dogs.

In the decade following the work of Hoerlein et al. and others describing approaches to the brain of dogs, reports of successful surgical application of these techniques to manage intracranial pathology began to emerge. In 1971, Parker and Cunningham [135] reported the successful surgical removal of an epileptogenic focus caused by an Aspergillus infection of the frontal sinus and frontal cortex by a transfrontal craniotomy. In 1972, Bagedda [136] at the University of Sassari published a report detailing the successful management of a depressed skull fracture in a puppy by a rostrotentorial craniotomy. Both reports confirmed the lesion localization by plain film radiographs. However, in the 1980s and 1990s, following the advent of CT and MR imaging in veterinary medicine, workers had accrued sufficient surgical expertise and case material regarding brain surgery to publish retrospective reviews. In 1987, Kostolich and Dulisch [137] at Tufts University reported on transfrontal craniotomy in four dogs with meningiomas of the olfactory bulb. In 1991, Niebauer et al. [137] reported an evaluation of craniotomy procedures in 26 dogs and 5 cats. These authors stated that "owing to the advent of refined diagnostic tools, brain surgery in pet animals has become more practical" and "these new tools have made available for surgery a fair number of dogs and cats, with intracranial neoplasia, that otherwise would have undergone palliative treatment (corticosteroids, phenobarbital) alone or would have been euthanatized." Similarly, in 1993, Jeffery and Brearley [138] reported on the successful surgical treatment of brain tumors in 10 dogs and concluded that "successful control of canine meningioma can be achieved by surgery plus radiotherapy" but cautioned that "the optimal therapy for intra-axial tumors has also yet to be determined."

To attend to the surgical management concerns regarding dogs with intra-axial brain tumors, in 1993, Sorjonen et al. [139] investigated a radical cerebral cortical resection in 10 normal dogs. Their hypothesis was that despite earlier reports, descriptions of surgical landmarks, techniques for manipulation of intracranial tissue, and postsurgical results following resection of a large volume of cerebral tissue that is often associated with the removal of large and deep-seated neoplasia were largely incomplete. Results of the study indicated that radical cerebral cortical resection was feasible and offered a viable alternative to palliative medical treatment or euthanasia in dogs with large or deep-seated brain tumors.

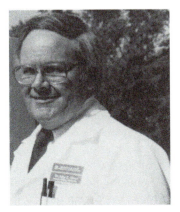

Figure 1.8 Dr John is considered the pioneer of canine intracranial surgery. Most of our current surgical approaches to the brain are based on his original work published in 1968.
Source: Picture courtesy of UGA Library Systems and Dr Marc Kent.

The 1990s were also witness to advances in diagnostic techniques and intracranial instrumentation. The increasing availability of CT technology promoted the opportunity to harvest pathologic tissue from animals with brain diseases for the purpose of distinguishing various types of pathologic conditions and to help stage brain tumors. In 1990, Harari et al. [140] at Washington State University evaluated a CT-guided, free-hand needle biopsy of brain tumors in eight dogs. Although the technique was deemed safe and easy to perform, it yielded diagnostic samples in only two dogs. In 1993, Thomas et al. [141] at Auburn University, evaluated an ultrasound-guided brain biopsy technique of the cingulate gyrus and head of the caudate nucleus in 10 normal dogs. Postmortem examination indicated that the biopsy specimen was obtained from the desired site in 9 dogs (90%) and the tissue specimen was suitable for histologic examination in all 10 dogs (100%). In 1999, Koblik et al. [142] at the University of California, reported the results of a CT-guided stereotactic brain biopsy technique in 50 dogs using a commercially available device (Pelorus Mark III Stereotactic System, Ohio Medical Instrument Company, Cincinnati, OH). A definitive diagnosis was made in 22 dogs by histologic examination of tissue obtained by surgical resection or at necropsy. The definitive diagnosis was in agreement with the stereotactic biopsy diagnosis in 20 (91%) dogs. Morbidity associated with the biopsy procedure was reported to be minimal. The authors concluded that CT-guided biopsy procedure can provide an accurate pathologic diagnosis of brain lesions detected by CT or MR neuroimaging.

A natural upshot of improvements in the antemortem diagnosis of intracranial pathology is the development of instrumentation that reduces the morbidity and mortality associated with brain surgery. In 1991, Shores [143] at Michigan State University, described the technique of brain tumor removal using the Cavitron ultrasonic aspirator (CUSA, Valley Lab, Inc., Stamford, CT) in three dogs. In 1993, Feder et al. [144] at Oklahoma State University described the use of a neodymium: yttrium-aluminum-garnet (Nd:YAG) laser (MediLas2®: Medizintechnik Gmbh, Munich, Germany) to aid in the removal of a large, invasive meningioma in a Boxer dog. In both reports, the authors commended use of these instruments based on a decrease in peritumoral tissue damage as compared to traditional dissection/suction techniques.

Advances in diagnostic techniques and intracranial instrumentation prompted workers to investigate regions of the brain previously considered inaccessible. One long-held belief was that any violation of the dural sinus system during brain surgery would invariably result in substantial brain swelling and death of the animal patient [130]. In 1995, Bagley et al. [145] at Washington State University reported on the results of longitudinal division of the corpus callosum in six normal dogs. These authors proposed this procedure as an adjunct for intractable seizures. A bilateral rostrotentorial craniectomy was performed and the dorsal sagittal sinus was manipulated in an effort to remove the overlying cranium and perform the callosotomy. Elevation in ICP was not noted. The authors concluded that surgical division of the corpus callosum is a safe procedure in dogs. In 1996, Pluhar et al. [146] at Washington State University reported on the changes in ICP following acute unilateral transverse sinus occlusion in six normal dogs. This study was undertaken to validate or invalidate earlier concerns regarding the reluctance of many veterinary neurosurgeons to avoid violation of the transverse sinus. Such reluctance has resulted in an inability to adequately expose the lateral cerebellomedullary pontine area, thus limiting the effectiveness of surgery in that region. The authors reported that ICP did not rise after unilateral transverse sinus occlusion and proffered the idea that the transverse sinus could safely be occluded to increase surgical exposure to the caudal fossa of the brain. As a clinical follow-up to their 1996 study, in 1997, Bagley et al. [147] safely removed the bone overlying the transverse sinus after performing a combined lateral rostrotentorial and suboccipital craniectomy. Bone wax was then placed in the remaining bony canal of the transverse sinus. These authors successfully performed this procedure in seven dogs with space-occupying disease; six located in the cerebellopontine angle and one in the caudal medulla. In 1998, Bagley [148] reported the results of a multicenter study of trigeminal nerve-sheath tumor in 10 dogs. Three dogs received surgery and for one of the cases surgery was described as a lateral rostrotentorial craniectomy that was extended ventrally to expose the trigeminal nerve and tumor, which was explored and excised near its origin in the brain stem. In one dog with subtotal excision of the nerve-sheath tumor, gene therapy was administered. Death or euthanasia resulted in all dogs not receiving surgery; consequently, these authors concluded that "aggressive local treatment, with surgery or possibly radiation therapy, may be necessary to arrest the progression of this tumor." In 2000, Glass et al. [149] at the University of Pennsylvania modified surgical techniques first reported by other workers [134, 135, 150] to approach both the frontal lobe and olfactory bulb in five dogs with seizures. Their technique, a modified bilateral transfrontal sinus approach, provided clear visualization of olfactory bulb, cribriform plate, and the frontal lobe as far caudal as the cruciate sulcus. These authors reported resolution of seizure activity in all five dogs.

Reports of intracranial surgery are not as common in cats as in dogs with the vast majority of reports involving brain tumors. Similar to the pattern in dogs, the occurrence of reports involving intracranial pathology in cats began to increase in the 1970s and continued to increase into the 1990s. Prior and up to 1960, reports of intracranial pathology in cats were largely relegated to textbooks of veterinary pathology [151, 152]. In 1961, Luginbuhl [153] at the University of Bern reported that one or more meningiomas were found in 8 of 155 cat brains examined at necropsy. Although this author addressed the prevalence of meningioma in these cats, the paucity of published reports and the small sample size of this report disallowed him from any conclusions regarding incidence, significance, and types of meningiomas which occur in cats. However, in the ensuing years, this information regarding meningioma in cats became apparent. In 1979, Nafe [154] at the AMCNY, reported on 36 cases of meningiomas in cats; surgery was not performed on any cat. In 1984, Lawson et al. [155] at the AMCNY reported on the diagnosis and surgical treatment of cerebral meningioma in 10 cats. Interestingly, the diagnosis was confirmed by hyperostotic bone noted in skull radiographs in nine cats. A rostrotentorial craniectomy of varying extent was performed in all cats. The tumors were debulked or removed en bloc when possible. In three cats with falx meningiomas, the craniectomy was made to cross the midline without disruption of the dorsal sagittal sinus. In the two cats with tumors involving the sphenoid wing, brain retraction was performed to access the floor of the calvarium. One cat died of brain herniation and nine cats were released to home by postoperative day five. An uptick in case reports of brain tumors in cats, coincident with the advent of CT and MRI, occurred in the 1990s. In 1991, Niebauer et al. [137] at the University of Pennsylvania, in 1993 Gallagher et al. [156] at Tufts University, and in 1994 Gordon et al. [157] at the AMCNY all reported a series of intracranial meningiomas in cats treated with surgery. Surgical techniques similar to those employed in dogs were used and varied based on lesion localization. In general, meningiomas in cats are more likely to be firm compared to the friable meningiomas in dogs allowing a greater opportunity for en-bloc tumor removal in cats. Compared to dogs, cats are more likely to have multiple sites of meningioma in the brain and can often experience life threating postoperative anemia.

Whereas meningioma is the most common brain tumor of cats, surgical management of tumors affecting the hypophysis and ependyma have been reported. In 1993, Abrams-Ogg et al. [158] at the University of Guelph reported on a cat with a large pituitary mass noted in MRI. These authors performed a transsphenoidal approach to the hypophysis as described by Niebauer and Evans [126]. A cryoprobe was applied to the pituitary mass and two freeze–thaw cycles were performed. The histopathological diagnosis of the pituitary tumor was an acidophilic adenoma. The cat was euthanized 15 months postoperative for aggressive behavior. Necropsy revealed no evidence of the pituitary tumor. The aggression was attributed to changes in the hippocampus and temporal cortex, a sequela to a postoperative hypoglycemic events. The authors concluded that transsphenoidal hypophysectomy was feasible in the cat and cryosurgery was beneficial. In 1999, Simpson, et al. [159] at the University of Sydney, reported the surgical removal of an ependymoma from the third ventricle of a cat. These authors performed a rostrotentorial craniectomy to expose the brain. A longitudinal incision in the ectomarginal gyrus allowed exposure of the lateral ventricle through which the third ventricle was accessed. A friable grey mass was removed from the lumen of the third ventricle. A histopathological diagnosis of ependymoma was rendered. This cat made an unremarkable recovery. The authors concluded that "ependymoma should be considered together with meningiomas as intracranial tumours amendable to surgical intervention, even when situated in the relatively inaccessible third ventricle."

Epilogue

The twentieth century stands witness to a multitude of remarkable advances in both the art and science of veterinary neurosurgery. From reports of early workers using largely logic and intuition to guide their decisions for surgery, to more contemporary workers with an armamentarium of advanced imaging and diagnostic modalities to predicate surgical goals, one unifying concept emerges: to provide the best care for the animal patient with neurologic disease. One has to believe that the concern for the wellbeing of the animal patient and the boldness necessary to establish newer neurosurgical techniques is not unique to earlier neurosurgeons but instead is common among individuals driven by compassion to be of help. These human characteristics, well established among veterinarians, together with the continuing advancement in diagnostic techniques and the availability of newer surgical instrumentation, will serve to provide the opportunity for ever improving animal care in the twenty-first century.

References

1. Guthrie, E. (1939), History of veterinary medicine. In: *Iowa State University Veterinarian*, vol. 2, 6–10. Ames, IA: Iowa State Press.
2. RCVS (2010). Global veterinary medicine timeline. https://knowledge.rcvs.org.uk/heritage-and-history/history-of-the-veterinary-profession/global-veterinary-medicine-timeline/ (accessed 21 April 2022).
3. Greenblatt, S.H., Dagi, T.F., and Epstein, M.H. (ed.) (1997). *A History of Neurosurgery*, 625. Park Ridge, IL: The American Association of Neurological Surgeons.
4. Tufts University (2013). A brief history of radiologic time. www.tuftsyourdog.com/doghealthandmedicine/a-brief-history-of-radiologic-time/ (accessed 21 April 2022).
5. Carlson, W.D. (1967). *Veterinary Radiology*, 2e, 275. Philadelphia, PA: Lea & Febiger.
6. Olsson, S.E. (1951). On disk protrusion in the dog (enchondiosis intervertebralis). *Acta Orthop. Scand. Suppl.* 8: 1–49.
7. Hoerlein, B.F. (1953). Various contrast media in canine myelography. *J. Am. Vet. Med. Assoc.* 123: 311–315.
8. Bartles, J.E., Hoerlein, B.F., and Boring, B.S. (1978). Neuroradiology. In: *Canine Neurology*, 3e (ed. B.F. Hoerlein), 103–133. Philadelphia, PA: WB Saunders.
9. Wilson, J.W., Bahr, R.J., Leipold, H.W., and Guffy, M.M. (1976). Acute leptomeningeal reaction to the subarachnoid injection of ethyl iodophenyl undecylate in dogs. *J. Am. Vet. Med. Assoc.* 169: 415–419.
10. Greene, J.E. (1951). Surgical intervention for paraplegia due to herniation of the nucleus pulposus. *North Am. Vet.* 32: 411–412.
11. Klide, A.M., Steinberg, S.A., and Pond, M.J. (1967). Epiduralograms in dogs: the use and advantages of the diagnostic procedure. *J. Amer. Vet. Radiol.* 8: 39–42.
12. Garrick, J.G. and Sullivan, C.R. (1961). A technic of performing diskography in dogs. *Proc. Mayo. Clin.* 39: 270–275.
13. Conrad, C.R. (1975). Radiographic examination of the central nervous system. In: *Textbook of Veterinary Internal Medicine: Diseases of the Dog and Cat* (ed. S.J. Ettinger), 351–355. Philadelphia, PA: WB Saunders.
14. Holtermann, H. (1973). Metrizamide. *Acta Radiol. Suppl.* 335: 1–4.
15. Douglas, S.W. and Williamson, H.D. (1963). *Principals of Veterinary Radiology*, 177–184. Baltimore, MD.
16. James, C.W. and Hoerlein, B.F. (1960). Cerebral angiography in the dog. *Vet. Med.* 55: 45–49.
17. James, C.W. (1963). Radiographic anatomy of the cerebral arterial system of the dog. Master thesis. Auburn University, Auburn, AL.
18. Whiteleather, J.E. and DeSaussuer, R.I. (1956). New contrast medium (Hypaque) for cerebral angiography. *Radiology* 67: 537–541.
19. Dorn, A.S. (1968). Cerebral angiography in the dog. Thesis (MS). Auburn University, Auburn, AL.
20. Hoerlein, B.F. and Petty, M.F. (1961). Contrast encephalography and ventriculography in the dog-preliminary studies. *Am. J. Vet. Res.* 22: 1041–1046.
21. Cobb, L.M. (1960). Pneumoencephalography in the dog. *Can. Vet. J.* 1: 444–449.
22. Hounsfield, G.N. (1973). Computerized transverse axial scanning (tomography). 1. Description of system. *Br. J. Radiol.* 46: 1016–1022.
23. Marineck, B. and Young, S.W. (1980). Computed-tomography of spontaneous canine neoplasms. *Vet. Radiol.* 21: 181–184.
24. LeCouter, R.A., Fike, J.R., Cann, C.E., and Pedroia, V.G. (1981). Computed-tomography of brain-tumors in the caudal fossa of the dog. *Vet. Radiol.* 22: 244–251.
25. Hawn, E.L. (1950). Spin echoes. *Phys. Rev.* 80: 580–594.
26. Lautebar, P.C. (1973). Image formation by induced local interactions: examples of employing nuclear magnetic resonance. *Nature* 242: 190–191.
27. Goldstein, E.J., Burnett, K.R., Wolf, G.L. et al. (1985). Contrast enhanced spontaneous animal CNS tumors with gadolinium DTPA: a correlation of MRI with x-ray CT. *Physiol. Chem. Phys. Med. NMR* 17: 113–122.
28. Kraft, S.L., Gavin, P.R., Wendling, L.R., and Reddy, V.K. (1989). Canine brain anatomy on magnetic resonance images. *Vet. Radiol. Ultrasound* 30: 147–158.
29. Kärkkäinen, M., Punto, L.U., and Tulamo, R.M. (1993). Magnetic resonance imaging of canine degenerative lumbar spine disease. *Vet. Radiol. Ultrasound* 34: 399–404.
30. Vaughan, L.C. (1968). Studies on intervertebral disk protrusion in the dog. I. Etiology and pathogenesis. II. Diagnosis of the disease. III. Pathologic features. IV. Treatment. *Brit. Vet.* 114: 105–125.
31. Leonard, E.P. (1971). *Orthopedic Surgery of the Dog and Cat*, 2e, 115–117. Philadelphia, PA: WB Saunders.
32. Ross, G.E. (1969). Surgical treatment of intervertebral disk disease. *Proc. Am. Anim. Hosp. Assoc. 36th Annu. Meet.* 409–411.
33. Northway, R.B. (1965). A ventrolateral approach to lumbar intervertebral disk fenestration. *Vet. Med. Small Anim. Clin.* 60: 884–889.
34. Hoerlein, B.F. (1968). Various surgical methods for repair of intervertebral disk protrusions. *Anim. Hosp.* 4: 12–18.

35. Flo, G.L. and Brinker, W.O. (1975). Lateral fenestration of thoracolumbar disks. *J. Am. Anim. Hosp. Assoc.* 11: 619–621.

36. Yturraspe, D.J. and Lumb, W.V. (1973). A dorsolateral muscle-separating approach for thoracolumbar intervertebral disk fenestration in the dog. *J. Am. Vet. Med. Assoc.* 162: 1037–1042.

37. Seeman, C.W. (1968). Lateral approach for thoracolumbar disk fenestration. *Mod. Vet. Pract.* 49: 73–77.

38. Braund, K.G., Taylor, T.K., Ghosh, P., and Sherwood, A.A. (1976). Lateral spinal decompression in the dog. *J. Sm. Anim. Pract.* 17: 583–592.

39. Brook, G.B. (1936). *The Spine of The Dog*, 95–96. Baltimore, MD: W. Wood Co.

40. Redding, R.W. (1951). Laminectomy in the dog. *Am. J. Vet. Res.* 12: 123–128.

41. Hoerlein, B.F. (1956). Further evaluation of the treatment of disk protrusion in the dog. *J. Am. Vet. Med. Assoc.* 129: 495–502.

42. Swaim, S.F. (1976). Bilateral hemilaminectomy: a technique for extensive spinal decompression. *Auburn Vet.* 62: 32–38.

43. Swaim, S.F. (1977). Clinical and histologic evaluation of bilateral hemilaminectomy and deep dorsal laminectomy for extensive spinal cord decompression in the dog. *J. Am. Vet. Med. Assoc.* 170: 407–413.

44. Funkquist, B. (1962). Thoraco-lumbar disk protrusion with severe cord compression in the dog. I. Clinical and patho-anatomic observations with special reference to the rate of development of symptoms of motor loss. II. Clinical observations with special reference to prognosis in conservative treatment. III. Treatment by decompressive laminectomy. *Acta Vet. Scand.* 3: 256–274.

45. Trotter, E.J. and deLahunta, A. (1975). Modified deep dorsal laminectomy in the dog. *Cornell Vet.* 65: 402–427.

46. Prata, R.G. (1981). Neurosurgical treatment of thoracolumbar disks: the rationale and value of laminectomy with concurrent disk removal. *J. Am. Anim. Hosp. Assoc.* 17: 17–26.

47. Hoerlein, B.F. (1978). Intervertebral disks. In: *Canine Neurology*, 3e (ed. B.F. Hoerlein), 549–550. Philadelphia, PA: WB Saunders.

48. Brisson, B.A. (2017). Pediculectomy/mini-hemilaminectomy. In: *Current Techniques in Canine and Feline Neurosurgery* (ed. A. Shores and B.A. Brisson), 183. Hoboken, NJ: Wiley.

49. Hoerlein, B.F. (1953). Successful correction of a vertebral fracture in a dog. *Auburn Vet.* 10: 15–17.

50. Hoerlein, B.F. (1956). Traumatic lesions of the canine spine. *Am. J. Vet. Res.* 17: 685–689.

51. Swaim, S.F. (1971). Vertebral body plating for spinal immobilization. *J. Am. Vet. Med. Assoc.* 158: 1683–1695.

52. Gage, E.D. (1969). A new method of spinal fixation in the dog. *Vet. Med. Small Anim. Clin.* 64: 295–303.

53. Gage, E.D. (1969). *Surgical Repair of Spinal Fractures in Toy Breed Dogs*, 29–36. Southwestern Veterinarian; Fall.

54. Rouse, G.P. and Miller, J.I. (1975). The use of methylmethacrylate for spinal stabilization. *J. Am. Anim. Hosp. Assoc.* 11: 418–423.

55. Blass, C.E. and Seim, H.B. (1984). Spinal fixation in dogs using Steinmann pins and methylmethacrylate. *Vet. Surg.* 13: 203–210.

56. Wong, W.T. and Emms, S.G. (1992). Use of methylmethacrylate in stabilization of spinal fractures and luxations. *J. Sm. Anim. Pract.* 33: 415–422.

57. Brasmer, T.H. and Lumb, W.V. (1972). Lumbar vertebral prosthesis in the dog. *Am. J. Vet. Res.* 33: 493–499.

58. Yturraspe, D.J., Lumb, W.V., Young, S., and Gorman, H.A. (1975). Neurological and pathological effects of second lumbar spondylectomy and spinal column shorting in the dog. *J. Neurosurg.* 42: 47–50.

59. Knecht, C.D. (1972). Results of surgical treatment for thoracolumbar disc protrusion. *J. Sm. Anim. Prac.* 13 (8): 449–453.

60. Northway, R.B. (1966). Fusion of the lumbar vertebrae in the dog. *Vet. Med. Small Anim. Clin.* 61: 1190–1196.

61. Slocum, B. and Rudy, R.L. (1975). Fractures of the seventh lumbar vertebra in the dog. *J. Am. Anim. Hosp. Assoc.* 11: 167–172.

62. Dulisch, M.L. and Nichols, J.B. (1981). A surgical technique for management of lower lumbar fractures: case report. *Vet. Surg.* 10: 90–91.

63. Ullman, S.L. and Boudrieau, R.J. (1993). Internal skeletal fixation using a Kirschner apparatus for stabilization of fracture/luxation of lumbosacral joint in six dogs. A modification of the transilial pin technique. *Vet. Surg.* 22: 11–17.

64. McAnulty, J.F., Lenehan, T.M., and Maletz, L.M. (1986). Modified segmental spinal instrumentation in repair of spinal fractures and luxations in dogs. *Vet. Surg.* 15: 143–149.

65. Shores, A., Nichols, C., Koelling, H.A., and Fox, W.R. (1988). Combined Kirschner-Ehmer apparatus and dorsal spinal plate fixation of caudal lumbar fractures in dogs: biomechanical properties. *Am. J. Vet. Res.* 49: 1979–1982.

66. Oliver, J.E., Selcer, R.R., and Simpson, S. (1978). Cauda equina compression from lumbosacral malarticulation and malformation in the dog. *J. Am. Vet. Med. Assoc.* 173: 207–214.

67. Tarvin, G. and Prata, R.G. (1980). Lumbosacral stenosis in dogs. *J. Am. Vet. Med. Assoc.* 177: 154–159.

68. Slocum, B. and Devine, T. (1986). L7-S1 fixation-fusion for treatment of cauda equina compression in the dog. *J. Am. Vet. Med. Assoc.* 188: 31–35.

69. Bietto, W.V. and Thatcher, C. (1987). A modified lateral decompression technique for treatment of canine intervertebral disk disease. *J. Am. Anim. Hosp. Assoc.* 23: 409–413.

70. McCartney, W. (1977). Partial pediculectomy for treatment of thoracolumbar disk disease. *Vet. Comp. Orthop. Traumatol.* 10: 117–121.

71. Hoerlein, B.F. (1952). The treatment of intervertebral disk protrusion in the dog. *Proc. Am. Vet. Med. Assoc.* 89: 206–208.

72. Funkquist, B. (1962). Decompressive laminectomy for cervical disk protrusion in the dog. *Acta Vet. Scand.* 3: 88–101.

73. Hoerlein, B.F. (1962). Cervical spinal surgery – ventral and dorsal approach. *Proc. Am. Vet. Med. Assoc.* 103–104.

74. Popovic, N.A., VanderArk, G., and Kempe, L. (1971). Ventral approach for surgical treatment of cervical disk disease in the dog. *Am. J. Vet. Rsch.* 32: 1155–1161.

75. Cloward, R.B. (1958). The anterior approach for removal of ruptured cervical disks. *J. Neurosurg.* 15: 602–617.

76. Swaim, S.F. (1973). Ventral decompression of the cervical spinal cord in the dog. *J. Am. Vet. Med. Assoc.* 162: 276–277.

77. Prata, R.G. and Stoll, S.G. (1973). Ventral decompression and fusion for the treatment of cervical disk disease in the dog. *J. Am. Anim. Hosp. Assoc.* 9: 462–472.

78. Gilpin, G.N. (1976). Evaluation of three techniques of ventral decompression of the cervical spinal cord in the dog. *J. Am. Vet. Med. Assoc.* 168: 325–328.

79. Goring, R.L., Beale, B.S., and Faulkner, R.F. (1991). The inverted cone decompression technique: a surgical treatment for cervical vertebral instability "Wobbler Syndrome" in Doberman Pinchers. *J. Am. Anim. Hosp. Assoc.* 27: 403–409.

80. Pettit, G.D. and Whittaker, R.P. (1963). Hemilaminectomy for cervical disk protrusion in a dog. *J. Am. Vet. Med. Assoc.* 143: 379–383.

81. Parker, A.J. (1973). Surgical approach to the cervico-thoracic junction. *J. Am. Anim. Hosp. Assoc.* 9: 374–377.

82. Felts, J.F. and Prata, R.G. (1983). Cervical disk disease in the dog: intraforaminal and lateral extrusions. *J. Am. Anim. Hosp. Assoc.* 19: 755–760.

83. Lipsitz, D. and Bailey, C.S. (1992). Lateral approach for cervical spinal cord decompression. *Prog. Vet. Neurol.* 3: 39–44.

84. Geary, J.C., Oliver, J.E., and Hoerlein, B.F. (1967). Atlanto axial subluxation in the canine. *J. Small Anim. Pract.* 8: 577–582.

85. Gage, E.D. and Smallwood, J.E. (1970). Surgical repair of atlanto-axial subluxation in a dog. *Vet. Med. Small Anim. Clin.* 65: 583–592.

86. Oliver, J.E. and Lewis, R.E. (1973). Lesions of the atlas and axis in dogs. *J. Am. Anim. Hosp. Assoc.* 9: 304–313.

87. Chambers, J.N., Betts, C.W., and Oliver, J.E. (1977). The use of nonmetallic suture material for stabilization of atlantoaxial subluxation. *J. Am. Anim. Hosp. Assoc.* 13: 602–605.

88. Renegar, W.R. and Stoll, S.G. (1979). The use of methylmethacrylate bone cement in the repair of atlantoaxial subluxation stabilization failures-case report and discussion. *J. Am. Anim. Hosp. Assoc.* 15: 313–318.

89. LeCouteur, R.A., McKeown, D., Johnson, J., and Eger, C.E. (1980). Stabilization of atlantoaxial subluxation in the dog, using the nuchal ligament. *J. Am. Vet. Med. Assoc.* 177: 1011–1017.

90. Kishigami, M. (1984). Application of an atlantoaxial retractor for atlantoaxial subluxation in the cat and dog. *J. Am. Anim. Hosp. Assoc.* 20: 413–419.

91. Jeffery, N.D. (1996). Dorsal cross pinning of the atlantoaxial joint: new surgical technique for atlantoaxial subluxation. *J. Sm. Anim. Pract.* 37: 26–29.

92. Sorjonen, D.C. and Shires, P.K. (1981). Atlantoaxial instability: a ventral surgical technique for decompression, fixation, and fusion. *Vet. Surg.* 10: 22–29.

93. Denny, H.R., Gibbs, C., and Waterman, A. (1988). Atlanto-axial subluxation in the dog: a review of thirty cases and an evaluation of treatment by lag screw fixation. *J. Small Anim. Pract.* 29: 37–47.

94. Blass, C.E., Waldron, D.R., and vanEe, R.T. (1988). Cervical stabilization in three dogs using Steinmann pins and methylmethacrylate. *J. Am. Anim. Hosp. Assoc.* 24: 61–68.

95. Stead, A.C., Anderson, A., and Coughlan, A. (1993). Bone plating to stabilize atlantoaxial subluxation in four dogs. *J. Sm. Anim. Pract.* 34: 462–465.

96. deLahunta, A. (1971). Cervical cord contusion from spondylolisthesis (A wobbler syndrome in dogs). In: *Current Veterinary Therapy*, 4e (ed. R.W. Kirk), 917–930. Philadelphia, PA: WB Saunders.

97. Gage, E.D. and Hall, C.L. (1972). Surgical repair of caudal cervical subluxation in a dog. *J. Am. Vet. Med. Assoc.* 160: 424–426.

98. Dueland, R., Furneaux, R.W., and Kaye, M.M. (1973). Spinal fusion and dorsal laminectomy for midcervical spondylolisthesis in a dog. *J. Am. Vet. Med. Assoc.* 162: 366–369.

99. Gage, E.D. and Hoerlein, B.F. (1973). Surgical repair of cervical subluxation and spondylolisthesis in the dog. *J. Am. Anim. Hosp. Assoc.* 9: 385–390.

100. Swaim, S.F. (1975). Evaluation of four techniques of cervical spinal fixation in dogs. *J. Am. Vet. Med. Assoc.* 166: 1080–1086.

101. Trotter, E.J., deLahunta, A., Geary, J.C., and Brasmer, T.H. (1976). Caudal cervical vertebral malarticulation-malformation in Great Danes and Doberman Pinchers. *J. Am. Vet. Med. Assoc.* 168: 917–930.

102. Lincoln, J.D. and Pettit, G.D. (1985). Evaluation of fenestration for treatment of degenerative disk disease in the caudal cervical region of large dogs. *Vet. Surg.* 14: 240–246.

103. Ellison, G.W., Seim, H.B., and Clemmons, R.M. (1988). Distracted cervical spinal fusion for management of caudal cervical spondylomyelopathy in large-breed dogs. *J. Am. Vet. Med. Assoc.* 193: 447–453.

104. Bruecker, K.A., Seim, H.B., and Blass, C.E. (1989). Caudal cervical spondylomyelopathy: decompression by linear traction and stabilization with Steinmann pins and polymethyl methacrylate. *J. Am. Anim. Hosp. Assoc.* 25: 677–683.

105. McKee, W.M., Lavelle, R.B., Richardson, J.L., and Mason, T.A. (1990). Vertebral distraction-fusion for cervical spondylopathy using a screw and double washer technique. *J. Small Anim. Pract.* 31: 22–27.

106. Lyman, R. (1991). Continuous dorsal laminectomy is the procedure of choice. *Prog. Vet. Neurol.* 2: 143–146.

107. Hettlich, B. (2017). Vertebral fracture and luxation repair. In: *Current Techniques in Canine and Feline Neurosurgery* (ed. A. Shores and B.A. Brisson), 211. Hoboken, NJ: Wiley.

108. Gage, E.D. (1968). Surgical repair of a fractured cervical spine in the dog. *J. Am. Vet. Med. Assoc.* 153: 1407–1411.

109. Hoerlein, B.F. (1958). Traumatic lesions of the canine spine. *Mod. Vet. Pract.* 39: 31–37.

110. Gendreau, C.L. and Cawley, A.J. (1969). Repair of fractures of the axis. *Can. Vet. J.* 10: 297–301.

111. Rouse, G.P. (1979). Cervical spine stabilization with methylmethacrylate. *Vet. Surg.* 8: 1–6.

112. Basinger, R.R., Bjorling, D.E., and Chambers, J.N. (1986). Cervical spinal luxation in two dogs with entrapment of the cranial articular process of C6 over the caudal articular process of C5. *J. Am. Vet. Med. Assoc.* 188: 865–867.

113. Boudrieau, R.J. (1997). Distraction-stabilization using the Scoville-Haverfield self-retaining laminectomy retractors for repair of 2nd cervical vertebral fractures in 3 dogs. *Vet. Comp. Orthop. Traumatol.* 10: 71–76.

114. Hawthorne, J.C., Blevins, W.E., Wallace, L.J. et al. (1999). Cervical vertebral fractures in 56 dogs: a retrospective study. *J. Am. Anim. Hosp. Assoc.* 35: 135–146.

115. Brinker, W.O. (1957). *Canine Surgery*, 4e (ed. K. Mayer, J.V. Lacroix and H.P. Hoskins), 666. Evanston, IL: American Veterinary Publications.

116. Leonard, E.P. (1960). Fractures of the skull, spine and pelvis. In: *Orthopedic Surgery of the Dog and Cat* (ed. E.P. Leonard), 247. Philadelphia, PA: WB Saunders.

117. Andersson, B. (1956). A case of nervous canine distemper treated with prefrontal lobotomy. *Nord. Vet. Med.* 8: 179–182.

118. Redding, R.W. (1972). Prefrontal lobotomy of the dog. Scientific presentations. *J. Am. Anim. Hosp. Assoc.* 374–378.

119. Allen, B.D., Cummings, J.F., and deLahunta, A. (1974). The effects of prefrontal lobotomy on aggressive behavior in dog. *Cornell Vet.* 64: 201–215.

120. Hart, B.L. (1982). Neurosurgery of behavioral problems. A curiosity or the new wave. *Vet. Clin. North Am. Small Anim. Pract.* 126: 707–714.

121. Few, A. (1966). The diagnosis and surgical treatment of canine hydrocephalus. *J. Am. Vet. Med. Assoc.* 149: 286–292.

122. Gage, E.D. and Hoerlein, B.F. (1968). Surgical treatment of canine hydrocephalus by ventriculoatrial shunting. *J. Am. Vet. Med. Assoc.* 153: 1418–1431.

123. Markowitz, J. and Archibald, J. (1956). Transbuccal hypophysectomy in the dog. *Can. J. Biochem. Physiol.* 34: 422–428.

124. Alvarez-Buylla, R., Segura, E.T., and Alvarez Buylla, E.R. (1961). Participation of the hypophysis in the conditioned reflex which reproduces the hypoglycemic effect of insulin. *Acta Physiol. Lat. Am.* 11: 113–119.

125. Henry, R.W., Hulse, D.A., Archbald, L.F., and Barta, M. (1982). Transoral hypophysectomy with mandibular symphysiotomy in the dog. *Am. J. Vet. Res.* 43: 1825–1829.

126. Niebauer, G.W. and Evans, S.M. (1988). Transsphenoidal hypophysectomy in the dog. A new technique. *Vet. Surg.* 17: 296–303.

127. Meij, B.P. (1998). Transsphenoidal hypophysectomy for treatment of pituitary-dependent hyperadrenocorticism in dogs. *Vet. Quart. Suppl.* 20: S98–S100.

128. Oliver, J.E. (1965). Surgical relief of epileptiform seizures in the dog. *Vet. Med. Small Anim. Clin.* 60: 367–368.

129. Hoerlein, B.F., Few, A.B., and Petty, M.F. (1963). Brain surgery in the dog-preliminary studies. *J. Am. Vet. Med. Assoc.* 143: 21–29.

130. Oliver, J.E. (1968). Surgical approaches to the canine brain. *Am. J. Vet. Res.* 29: 353–378.

131. Parker, A.J. (1972). Transfrontal craniotomy in the dog. *Vet. Rec.* 90: 622–624.
132. Swaim, S.F. (1973). Use of pneumatic surgical instruments in neurosurgery. *Vet. Med. Small Anim. Clin.* 68: 1404–1412.
133. de Wet, P.D. (1977). Some anatomical and functional considerations with regard to general and experimental canine brain surgery. *Zbl. Vet. Med. C Anat. Histol. Embryol.* 6: 87–88.
134. de Wet, P.D., Alt, I.I., and Peters, D.N. (1982). Surgical approach to the rostral cranial fossa by radical transfrontal craniotomy in the dog. *J. South African Vet. Assoc.* 53: 40–51.
135. Parker, A.J. and Cunningham, J.G. (1971). Successful surgical removal of an epileptogenic focus in a dog. *J. Small Anim. Pract.* 12: 513–521.
136. Bagedda, G. (1972). The EEG as an aid to the topographical diagnosis of a cerebral lesion in a puppy: neurosurgical treatment and the post-operative EEG-clinical course. *J. Small Anim. Pract.* 13: 185–192.
137. Niebauer, G.W., Dayrell-Hart, B.L., and Speciale, J. (1991). Evaluation of craniotomy in dogs and cats. *J. Am. Vet. Med. Assoc.* 198: 89–95.
138. Jeffery, N. and Brearley, M.J. (1993). Brain tumors in the dog: 10 cases and review of recent literature. *J. Small Anim. Pract.* 34: 367–372.
139. Sorjonen, D.C., Thomas, W.B., Myers, L.J., and Cox, N.R. (1993). Radical cerebral cortical resection in dogs. *Prog. Vet. Neurol.* 2: 225–236.
140. Harari, J., Moore, M.P., Leathers, C.W. et al. (1992). Computed tomographic-guided free-hand needle biopsy of brain tumors in dogs. *Prog. Vet. Neurol.* 4: 41–44.
141. Thomas, W.B., Sorjonen, D.C., Hudson, J.A., and Cox, N.R. (1993). Ultrasound-guided brain biopsy in dogs. *Am. J. Vet. Res.* 54: 1942–1947.
142. Koblik, P.D., LeCouteur, R.A., Higgins, R.J. et al. (1999). CT-guided brain biopsy using a modified Pelorus Mark III stereotactic system: experience with 50 dogs. *Vet. Radiol. Ultrasound* 40: 434–440.
143. Shores, A. (1991). Use of the ultrasound aspirator in intracranial surgery: technique and case reports. *Prog. Vet. Neurol.* 2: 89–94.
144. Feder, B.M., Fry, T.R., Kostolich, M. et al. (1993). Nd:YAG laser cytoreduction of an invasive intracranial meningioma in a dog. *Prog. Vet. Neurol.* 4: 3–9.
145. Bagley, R.S., Baszler, T.V., Harrington, M.L. et al. (1995). Clinical effects of longitudinal division of the corpus callosum in normal dogs. *Vet. Surg.* 24: 122–127.

146. Pluhar, G.E., Bagley, R.S., Keegan, R.D. et al. (1996). The effect of acute, unilateral transverse venous sinus occlusion on intracranial pressure in normal dogs. *Vet. Surg.* 25: 480–486.
147. Bagley, R.S., Harrington, M.L., Pluhar, G.E. et al. (1997). Acute, unilateral transverse sinus occlusion during craniectomy in seven dogs with space-occupying intracranial disease. *Vet. Surg.* 26: 195–201.
148. Bagley, R.S., Wheeler, S.J., Klopp, L. et al. (1998). Clinical features of trigeminal nerve-sheath tumor in 10 dogs. *J. Am. Anim. Hosp. Assoc.* 34: 19–25.
149. Glass, E.N., Kapatkin, A., Vite, C., and Steinberg, S.A. (2000). A modified bilateral transfrontal sinus approach to the canine frontal lobe and olfactory bulb: surgical technique and five cases. *J. Am. Anim. Hosp. Assoc.* 36: 43–50.
150. Kostolich, M. and Dulisch, M. (1987). A surgical approach to the canine olfactory bulb for meningioma removal. *Vet. Surg.* 16: 273–277.
151. Smith, H.A. and Jones, T.C. (1957). *Veterinary Pathology*, 208. Philadelphia, PA: Lea & Febiger.
152. McGrath, J.T. (1960). *Neurologic Examination of the Dog*, 152. Philadelphia, PA: Lea & Febiger.
153. Luginbuhl, H. (1961). Studies of meningiomas in cats. *Am. J. Vet. Res.* 22: 1030–1040.
154. Nafe, L. (1979). Meningiomas in cats: a retrospective clinical study of 36 cases. *J. Am. Vet. Med. Assoc.* 174: 1224–1227.
155. Lawson, D.C., Burk, R.L., and Prata, R.G. (1984). Cerebral meningiomas in the cat: diagnosis and surgical treatment of ten cases. *J. Am. Anim. Hosp. Assoc.* 20: 333–342.
156. Gallagher, J.G., Berg, J., Knowles, K. et al. (1993). Prognosis after surgical excision of cerebral meningiomas in cats: 17 cases (1986–1992). *J. Am. Vet. Med. Assoc.* 203: 1437–1440.
157. Gordon, L.E., Thacher, C., Matthiesen, D.T., and Joseph, R.J. (1994). Results of craniotomy for treatment of cerebral meningiomas in 42 cats. *Vet. Surg.* 23: 94–100.
158. Abrams-Ogg, A.C.G., Holmberg, D.L., Stewart, W.A., and Claffey, F.P. (1993). Acromegaly in a cat: diagnosis by magnetic resonance imaging and treatment by cryohypophysectomy. *Can. Vet. J.* 34: 682–685.
159. Simpson, D.J., Hunt, G.B., Tisdall, P.L. et al. (1999). Surgical removal of an ependymoma from the third ventricle of a cat. *Aust. Vet. J.* 77: 645–648.

2

Applications of 3D Printing in Veterinary Neurosurgery

Fred Wininger

Charlotte Animal Referral & Emergency, Charlotte, NC, USA

"Necessity is the mother of invention" is an idiom that pertains to veterinary medicine in ways unthinkable to other fields. The anatomic variation of domestic animals and relative financial limitations of treating them have emboldened veterinarians to be entrepreneurial and creative in their approach to treating animals. Makeshift instrumentation to suit the needs of the individual practitioner is commonplace. 3D printing (3DP) lends itself to this spirit of ingenuity as any structure can be created with exquisite detail and limitless customization to suit an individual animal's needs and be available to general consumers, representing >80% of the current market share. These printers are now cost affordable to the hobbyist, often less than a few hundred dollars. The technology (also known as fused filament fabrication) uses a filament (often a thermoplastic) that can be melted by a heated extruder creating successive layers that melt and then harden, binding them in 3DP.

3DP, also known as additive modeling (AM), is the practice of joining or fusing materials by an automated process in a 3D envelope. The original iterations of 3DP were created in the 1980s and slowly have become more widely available in the marketplace. The practice was initially thought of as a prototyping mechanism but in recent years has evolved into large-scale production techniques. The two commonplace 3DP technologies currently available are Fused Deposition Modeling (FDM) and Stereolithography (STL).

FDM is the most commonly available form of 3DP predesigned orientation. In this regard the extruder moves in an x and y plane and then the z plane is created as the extruder moves away from the print bed after each layer. Support structures ("rafts and bridges") can be created to permit for more complicated overhanging structures and are removed

in post print processing. The thermoplastics most often used are acrylonitrile butadiene styrene (ABS) and polylactic acid (PLA). FDM prints have a characteristic ridged appearance from the distinct layered plastic which can be minimized but not removed through sanding and acetone polishing. ABS is the plastic used for mass production injection molding industry. PLA is a biodegradable thermoplastic derived from renewable resources such as corn starch or sugarcane and is thought of as "softer." Both plastics are of similar tensile strength, elasticity, and cost. ABS is more heat resistant than PLA but is considered more difficult to print with and is more failure prone. Neither material can be steam autoclaved. More recent material options include filled nylon which shares the ideal properties of both. PEEK (polyetheretherketone) is a plastic with desirable biomechanical properties often used in medical devices. The material can be manipulated as a filament in FDM printers but requires specialized extruders and both printers and the filaments are expensive.

STL printing was the original form of 3DP. Through photopolymerization, liquid resins are hardened layer by layer through a transparent silicone basin by an ultraviolet laser onto a rising build platform. The technology has become more readily available with initial setups in the $4000 range[1]. STL prints require more extensive post-print-processing than FDM, including removal of supports, clearing of residual resin by alcohol baths, and resin curing in UV chambers. STL prints have a higher part accuracy than FDM (1 mm vs. 25 μm) with more defined and resolved details and no ridges. STL print equipment is sensitive as it relies on lasers and mirrors for accuracy which can lead to print failure.

----

1 Formlabs, Inc.; Somerville, MA, USA

Advanced Techniques in Canine and Feline Neurosurgery, First Edition. Edited by Andy Shores and Brigitte A. Brisson.
© 2023 John Wiley & Sons, Inc. Published 2023 by John Wiley & Sons, Inc.
Companion site: www.wiley.com/go/shores/advanced

The primary advantage of STL printers is the variety of resins available. Most of the polymers are predominantly based on methacrylate oligomers of multiple colors, including a clear one. The resins can be tailored to the different needs of the print, including their tensile strength, elasticity, weight, and thermal resistance. Standard and engineering resins can be interchanged on the same printer. There are also zero ash-content after burnout resins that can be used for casting/metallurgy and medical resins that have been tested for their biocompatibility with tissue contact. A disadvantage of STL 3DP is a lack of biodegradable materials, though "green resins" are under development.

Other 3DP techniques include powder bed fusion techniques that have recently entered the general consumer space. These printers are historically expensive but have the advantage of novel materials including metals such as titanium. They are also less restricted in shape options than other techniques. In a similar methodology to STL printing, selective laser sintering uses a layer to fuse powder particles into fused nylon or polyamides. Electron beam melting is the analogue for use with titanium alloys. At this time this technology is in specialized 3DP labs and parts are often consigned for rather than created on site.

Steps of the 3D Printing Process

Acquisition

3D models can be created as virtual shapes on a computer or imported as digital projections of real objects. These digital projections are made from 3D scans that create surface projections by interconnecting polygons into a manifold or wire mesh. In the medical fields, traditional tomographic modalities make digital models of anatomic regions of interest, including ultrasonography, computerized tomography (CT), or magnetic resonance imaging (MRI).

The most commonly used modality for 3DP acquisition is CT as it inherently has several advantages when creating surface renderings from acquired volumes. Contrast resolution is the ability to distinguish different tissue based on image intensity. Contrast resolution is inherent to individual modalities and with regards to CT is based on tissue density. Tissue density is defined by numerical Hounsfield units (HU). The large variety of bone HU and its high value makes it easy to identify bone from itself and other tissues and gives the ability of an imaging modality to differentiate two adjacent structures as being distinct from one another. CT has excellent spatial resolution and is improved by minimizing voxel size which it can do with limited signal-noise degradation. With advanced printers'

resolution at $10\,\mu m$, image acquisition is often the rate limiter of print accuracy and CT provides the highest quality body representation.

MRI is a lesser used modality for 3DP, because of its lesser spatial and contrast resolving properties relative to CT with tissues of interest. Since MR does not rely on density but rather on water content, it is ideal for soft tissue imaging. Conversely, the lack of water in bone makes it difficult to resolve the tissue given a poor signal to noise ration. MR slice thickness tends to be greater than $2\,mm$ and voxels of unequal dimensions when using traditional spin echo techniques. The preferable image acquisition for bone is often a post contrast gradient based T1 weighted 3D image dataset with isotropic voxels that are sub-1 mm. These acquisitions are often long and prone to motion and other artifacts. The ideal use of MRI in 3DP is often in images fused with matched CT. In this regard, the MRI can identify soft tissue regions of interest and their association with overlying bone.

Thresholding

The process of selecting the tissue range of interest is termed thresholding. In the case of CT, this will be specific to HU. A window width in the range specific to the tissue of interest (in the case of bone often 300–3000) is selected, removing extraneous anatomy. This is an area for potential unintentional data loss and adjustments may be necessary based on the mineralization of bone and quality of the scan. Too high a HU filter and essential bone may be lost. Too low a filter and other tissues and "noise" will obscure the image

Segmentation

Segmentation is the process by which tissues that are of interest are kept and the remainder removed post thresholding. Automated segmentation is linked to the "connectedness" of tissues. Seeds can be placed in areas of interest and computer algorithms expanded to other images in the data, extrapolating whether they should be included in the highlighted region of interest (ROI). Auto-segmentation can be done on 3D volume renderings as a whole or through individual 2D multiplanar reconstructions. Manual segmentation requires the individual hand selection of pixels and, while time consuming, is significantly more accurate.

After segmentation, it is common for the manifold (total integrity of the polygon mesh) to have inherent errors, essentially disconnected polygons or polygons that are oriented in impossible orientations. Most software platforms and have an inspector that identifies these errors and corrects them. This is also a source for automated error and should be manually inspected.

File Format Creation

The general processes are performed in image review software also used in clinical practice. The surface renderings can be exported to a 3D specific file format for manipulation and printing. The STL format is the most common and despite have the same name as a type of printing is used in all 3DP models. It is reliant on a system of triangles and is sometimes referred to as "Standard Triangle Language" to represent its more universal use. To achieve curved surfaces, triangles are made smaller to create smoother angles. The single polygon shape makes for an easier format, but the files are prone to becoming unwieldly and large as the curves become more intricate and resolved. The OBJ (waveform object) format is the second most common and uses a variety of polygon shapes. It also gives information about color which can be useful in non 3DP applications. The AMF (additive manufacturing file) format is the least commonly used, though it is expected to overtake the others in utility. It is superior to the geography formatting of the other files and stores other metadata, including information about material type.

Manifold Manipulation

Once "cleaned," the creative aspect of 3D application can begin. There is a variety of software programs (both freeware and subscription based) that are used for model manipulation. These programs are often thought of as falling into two main categories: computer aided design (CAD) or 3D sculpting. CAD programs have traditionally been used by engineers and maintain angles and preciseness of geometric shapes. Basic and complex shape designs include those used in traditional orthopedics. Screw heads and shaft parts (including thread number, angle, and width, as well as pitch and size) can be easily re-created. Sculpting programs have been typically utilized by the animation space for esthetic circular structures and textures than can be articulated and move. The distinctions between these program functions have become less distinct and medical 3DP utilizes both.

Anatomic Modeling

Anatomic models may be "cut" to have solid edges at their borders, similar to cropping a photograph. Plane cut functions can be used to section the model, enabling ideal visualization of canals and foramina not easily studied in the model whole form. Pegs and struts can be added to maintain the anatomic position of structures that are stabilized by soft tissues not present on the model (i.e. vertebral segments with minimal bone contact such as those in cases of articular facet hypoplasia). Models are often converted to a "solid" format and can be hollowed if the cancellous bone is not of interest to reserve materials (Figure 2.1).

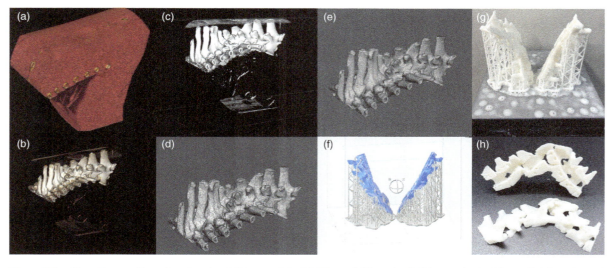

Figure 2.1 Steps for creation of anatomic additive models. (a) CT acquisition: the ROI is acquired with small (<1 mm) voxels. The imaging software creates a volume rendering. (b) Thresholding and segmentation: the prescribed Houndsfield units for bone removes the majority of soft tissue. Manual segmentations remove unneeded bone (i.e. scapula or ribs) and other artifactual pieces. In this example, segmentation is incomplete and segments of the CT bed and thoracic vascular tissues remain. (c) The model is converted to a surface rendering prior to exportation as an STL file. (d) The model is imported into 3D modeling software. Segmentation is completed. The model has several manifold errors and a roughened texture. (e) The manifold is corrected through a combination of automated and manual inspection and remeshing. The model is split for surgeon preference. (f) The model is imported into a G-Slicer print program often proprietary to the individual printer. Support struts are created for overhangs as well as a raft for model adherence to the platform. (g) The printed SLA model prior to curing. The model is removed from the bed and placed in alcohol to remove excess resin. (h) The completed model after completed photocuring.

Printing

When the modeling is complete, the file is sent to a printing program that is often proprietary to the printer being used. Printers use a slicer algorithm which converts the models to layers in a format known as a G-Code. The orientation of the print is also dictated at this point to fit inside the build platform and minimize overhanging structures. Supports are rendered and the user has the option to add or remove these struts. For the purpose of interdigitating tools, it is best to avoid strut placement with bone contact points. Printing can take hours to days depending on the number of layers, complexity of the design, type of material used, and resolution selected. Some STL printers have designated "draft" resins that can print in a fraction of the time for rapid prototyping but with poor detail and less durability.

Current Spinal Applications

Printing anatomic references was the initial purpose of 3DP in medical applications. Anatomic references are of value in the surgical theater, especially in cases of unusual anatomy particular to a specific patient. Plates can be pre-contoured to a scaled anatomic reference for ease of intra-operative placement [1]. Models are an excellent teaching tool and some materials can be drilled with tactile properties similar to bone [2]. We have also found them to be excellent client communication tools that make unfamiliar concepts more tangible. Examples of diseases (i.e. bone tumors) and pre-made surgical corridors can be created to better illustrate surgical procedures.

Another potential application for printing unaltered anatomy is for biomechanical testing. Biomechanical testing requires the harvesting of spines from cadavers, removing soft tissues, and often multiple freeze–thaw cycles which can alter the biomechanical properties of bone. Standardized printed models alleviate many of the challenges including: eliminating the need to find specimens, standardization of subject anatomy, and the absence of soft tissue which can alter the physical properties. Further, the model can be standardized across multiple studies and institutions as an open-source control. There is a precedent documenting that certain plastics, even in basic cylindrical shapes, have similar biomechanical properties to the spine [3]. However, they cannot mimic the anatomic contours that alter the tested implant–bone interface. Cadaver spines need to be "potted" in a compatible mount to connect with biomechanical testing machines. The interface between the potting material and the spine can create artifactual changes to testing [4]. 3DP spines can be designed with these interfaces to eliminate these challenges.

Customized Tools

The primary application of 3DP for spinal applications is the creation of customized jigs for implant guidance [5] (Figure 2.2). The estimated rate of canal violation approaches 33% [6] when placing thoracolumbar implants with anatomic landmarks and goniometers using standardized corridor entry points and trajectory angles. Though alternative techniques, including real time fluoroscopy and neuronavigation, have been described, they are cumbersome, increase the rate of infection, and are expensive. 3DP jigs can be applied to any pre-determined surface of bone that can be cleared of superficial tissues. The general concept of 3DP tools is that instruments can interdigitate with a novel contour of bone specific to that site enabling accurate bone resection. The surface must be novel enough that it will not fit in alternative positions and large enough for firm contact. Often, multiple vertebral motion units are included to increase accuracy. Though incorporating motion units can introduce angles different from those when imaged, making the jig fit less precisely, in most parts of the spine this difference is nominal. The accuracy of customized jigs has been reported in the veterinary literature [7–9]. In addition to increased safety and efficiency, the procedures are more rapid with less need for post-operative imaging. Unreported benefits include the confidence to place implants in more aggressive corridors that cross midline for greater bone purchase. Jigs can be used with known drill lengths to dual serve as depth gauges which may minimize the risk for ventral soft tissue damage.

There are limitations on the use of 3DP jigs in the clinical setting. The process can be time consuming making it less clinically useful in cases of external trauma or those that require immediate stabilization. In addition to imaging, the model and jigs need to be created, printed, and then sterilized. Newer "draft resins" can print five implant jigs in under one hour. Many of the sterolithographic resins can be steam or plasma sterilized. The adaptations make 3DP more rapid but still difficult to utilize in the patient that requires same-day surgery.

Another limitation is bone integrity and contact. All soft tissues must be removed for ideal jig–bone contact. Decompressive procedures may create defects that alter the bone contact, preventing seating of the jig. Though unconventional in traditional surgery, implants are often placed prior to decompressive procedures. A possible advantage of this is that the decompression can be performed while the vertebral column is in its final reduced state.

Transarticular implants are often used in atlantoaxial and lumbosacral stabilizations. The challenge of 3DP for transarticular implants in these joints is their high degree

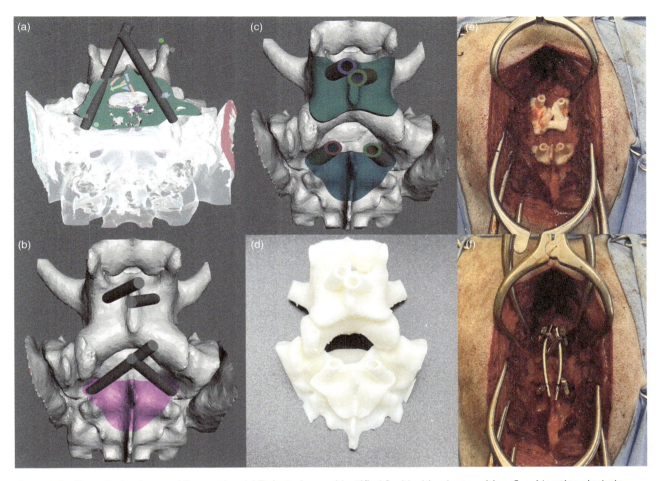

Figure 2.2 Steps for lumbosacral jig creation. (a) Trajectories are identified for ideal implant position. Considerations include described corridors, degree of bone stock, proximity to neurovascular structures, and implant size. (b) Once all trajectories are planned, areas of novel bone contours are identified for jig–bone interface. (c) The trajectories are converted to channels and integrated into the foot of the jig. (d) Final print of jig on the printed bone model for surgical practice. (e) Placement of the jig intraoperatively. Soft tissues are completely removed for maximal jig–bone contact. In this iteration of the jig, transarticular screws have been added. (f) Implant placement after jig removal.

of movement. One option for these jigs is to place the implant based on the "cis" bone and use natural landmarks with the" assumption" that the trans bone will be adequately implanted. Alternatively, the bones can be digitally aligned into the ideal anatomic position during the modeling process and then a jig created that both guides that alignment intraoperatively and places the implants. Challenges with the latter are that segmenting the bones digitally can be time consuming and the digital orientation can create a reduction which cannot be realized in the operating anatomic space. There is a paucity of literature evaluating the efficacy of 3DP transarticular implants.

Perhaps the "brass ring" of 3DP in the spine is the creation of customized implants that have biomechanical properties and biocompatibility to maintain distraction and stabilization with potential bone incorporation [10].

Human implants are generally created as a "one-size fits all" and do not accommodate the anatomy of the dog/cat spine (i.e. the ventral processes of the cervical spine). Customized 3DP implants could not only overcome these challenges but create patient specific distraction based on pre-imaging studies.

The creation of 3DP titanium for cervical body cages in dogs has been reported [11].

Current Brain Applications

Anatomic 3DP can be helpful as a surgical reference and for pre-contouring cranioplasty prosthetics for both skull and brain pathology. For this use, CT and MRI are often fused so that regions of the brain, brain lesions, and brain

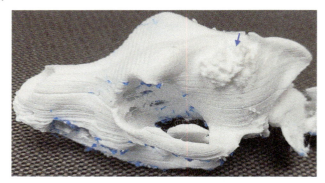

Figure 2.3 A multilobular tumor of bone (blue arrow) shown in a 3D printed skull. The patient was imaged using a CT scanner and the 3D reconstruction was converted to an STL file and printed using 1.75 mm PLA filament.

vasculature can be co-localized with normal and abnormal skull anatomy. A common skull tumor is a multilobular of tumor of bone (Figures 2.3 and 2.4). This tumor causes significant osteolysis and proliferation in conjunction with invading local vasculature. Skull prints can be vital in surgical preparedness and are often designed with cross sections removed and printed in clear resin. For tumors that are not apparent on CT but on MR (i.e. gliomas), the fusion can allow for the mass to be thresholded in such a way that it is printed on the skull surface.

The next iteration of 3DP use beyond anatomic modeling is in creating craniectomy jigs. Prior to 3DP, craniectomy defects were created by a combination of pre-surgical image measurements based on natural skull landmarks that could be co-localized in surgery. These defects were often not precise enough and localizing the mass would require enlarging the defect and intraoperative imaging assistance. Neuronavigation devices ameliorated this challenge, but systems are expensive and cumbersome and require significant planning, complete patient stabilization, and intraoperative setup time. 3DP surgical jigs based on fusion images create a simple and fast solution. The surgical jigs articulate with a novel surface on the skull and outline the ideal craniectomy for lesion access.

Similar to spinal applications, trajectory assist jigs can be used for the skull. This space has been largely used by

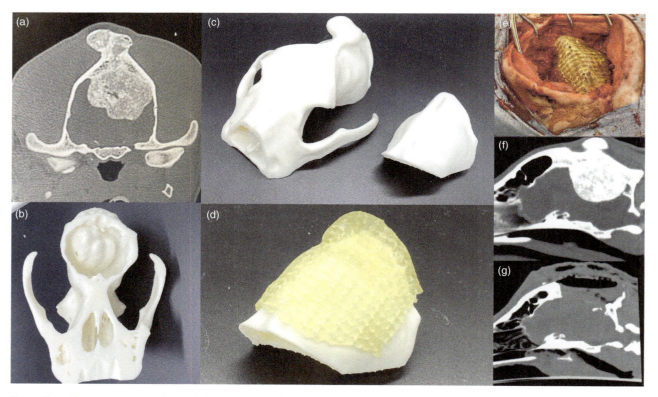

Figure 2.4 Case example of a large skull osteoma in a two-year-old dog. (a) Transverse CT image (bone window) of occipital bone osteoma. There is both intra- and extracranial extension of the mass. (b) Printed model with the calvarial floor removed, demonstrating the extent of intracranial mass extension. (c) Same model as (b) demonstrating the extent of extracranial mass extension. The calvarium is remodeled with the tumor removed. (d) A 3D-printed cranioplasty is created over the reassigned craniectomy site for complete tumor excision. (e) Placement of the cranioplasty intraoperatively post mass removal. The implant is secured with self-drilling titanium screws. (f) Pre- and postoperative CT. At the time of publication, the patient is approximately 750 days from the surgery without complications.

neuronavigation instrumentation. 3DP jigs are extremely accurate and more rapid in brain biopsies, brain injections, deep brain stimulator electrodes, and local catheter placement [12]. However, 3DP does not allow for intraoperative trajectory modification or alterative entry point manipulations like neuronavigation does.

Cranioplasties are necessary for large skull defects, and common materials used include polymethylmethacrylate and titanium meshes/matrices because they are bioinert and MR compatible. 3DP makes pre-contouring possible, increasing surgical ease and efficiency. Digital skull manipulations are sometimes required to remove external abnormalities to promote more esthetic contouring resembling the pre-diseased skull. On occasions where the defect is too large for commercially available meshes, 3DP cranioplasties have been printed in both titanium and STL resin. While the former is a metal with a precedent for implantation, the latter is off-label use. The STL dental resin is FDA approved for surface contact but not permanent implantation. However, the material once cured has excellent biocompatibility properties and its biomechanics are not a concern for this style of implant. The long-term durability of these implants is questionable but likely acceptable within the lifespan of domestic animals. The author has placed three of these cranioplasties with three years' follow-up and no clinical complaint.

Alternative skull adaptations are based on need based on individual cases. Traditional implants may require modifications for optimal use. We have created specialized anchors specific to individual skull conformation for ventricular catheter adhesion. 3DP can be created based on skin contours with a 3D scanner or CT. This application has been used to create external coapative devices temporarily worn by domestic animals. Cases of comminuted skull fractures maybe be treated with helmets to prevent floating segments from becoming depressed. 3DP can be used to optimize neuronavigation systems. Fiducial arrays and long-term channels can be adhered to specific skull topography, decreasing landmark movement and increasing accuracy.

Future Applications of 3D Printing in Veterinary Neurosurgery

The current applications of 3DP in veterinary medicine presented thus far focus on the use of "non-biological materials" such as plastics and resins to construct models and devices that can be used for a variety of medical and surgical applications. While these materials and applications have proven to be extremely useful, they present limitations for broad use in the context of therapeutic or replacement treatments; especially in vivo, due to their potentially toxic nature during degradation.

The search for acceptable "biocompatible" materials (i.e. materials able to be used externally or internally to provide desired function without detrimental effects to the overall health of the organism) that can be 3D printed into biologically active structure/tissues/organs, and improving the techniques for 3DP, or "bio-printing," are the next crucial steps for the advancement of 3DP in a clinical setting. Bio-printing can be defined as the fabrication of 3D constructs using biocompatible/biodegradable materials, such as organic polymers and viable living cells, to help repair or replace biological structures and/or systems. Generation of tissue architecture is accomplished via one of two methods: scaffold-based bio-printing, which utilizes an exogenous scaffold to provide mechanical support during tissue development, or scaffold-free bio-printing, which exploits the intrinsic ability of cells to generate adjacent tissue architecture [13].

Recent research in bio-printing has uncovered a wide variety of biocompatible materials, or "bio-inks" as well as improved 3DP techniques, such as biocompatible scaffolds (internal framework suitable for cellular in-growth and proliferation) for the engineering of bone regrowth [14]. Additionally, 3D bio-printed vascular grafts, comprised of autologous mesenchymal stem cells printed onto conventional artificial grafts, have been implanted into canine bilateral carotid and femoral arteries, resulting in increased endothelialization and decreased inflammation [15].

Limitations, such as the inability of bio-printers to print at both high resolution and viscosity and bio-inks to maintain cell viability during printing and the successful vascular integration of printed tissues, have impeded clinical translation of bio-printing; however, it is thought to be likely that 3D bio-printing will soon emerge as a powerful tool for regenerative medicine in the veterinary sciences. It could improve the treatment of several veterinary conditions such as diabetes, cancer, and musculoskeletal injuries, and 3D bio-printed organ transplantation may one day become commonplace [16].

References

1. Mathiesen, C.B., de la Puerta, B., Groth, A.M. et al. (2018). Ventral stabilization of thoracic kyphosis through bilateral intercostal thoracotomies using SOP (string of pearls) plates contoured after a 3-dimensional print of the spine. *Vet. Surg.* 47 (6): 843–851. https://doi.org/10.1111/vsu.12939. Epub 2018 Aug 9. PMID: 30094860.

2. Neves, E.C.D., Pelizzari, C., Oliveira, R.S. et al. (2020). 3D anatomical model for teaching canine lumbosacral epidural anesthesia. *Acta Cir. Bras.* 35 (6): e202000608. https://doi.org/10.1590/s0102-865020200060000008. Epub 2020 Jul 13. PMID: 32667587; PMCID: PMC7357831.

3. Hermann, A., Voumard, B., Waschk, M.A. et al. (2018). in vitro biomechanical comparison of four different ventral surgical procedures on the canine fourth-fifth cervical vertebral motion unit. *Vet. Comp. Orthop. Traumatol.* 31 (6): 413–421. https://doi.org/10.1055/s-0038-1667200. Epub 2018 Sep 20. PMID: 30235472.

4. Pfeiffer, M., Gilbertson, L.G., Goel, V.K. et al. (1996). Effect of specimen fixation method on pullout tests of pedicle screws. *Spine (Phila Pa 1976)* 21 (9): 1037–1044. https://doi.org/10.1097/00007632-199605010-00009. PMID: 8724087.

5. Zhao, Y., Ma, Y., Liang, J. et al. (2020). Comparison of the 3D-printed operation guide template technique and the free-hand technique for S2-alar-iliac screw placement. *BMC Surg.* 20 (1): 258. https://doi.org/10.1186/s12893-020-00930-5. PMID: 33121450; PMCID: PMC7596934.

6. Hettlich, B.F., Fosgate, G.T., Levine, J.M. et al. (2010). Accuracy of conventional radiography and computed tomography in predicting implant position in relation to the vertebral canal in dogs. *Vet. Surg.* 39 (6): 680–687. https://doi.org/10.1111/j.1532-950X.2010.00697.x. Epub 2010 Apr 29. PMID: 20459486.

7. Guevar, J., Bleedorn, J., Cullum, T. et al. (2021). Accuracy and safety of three-dimensionally printed animal-specific drill guides for thoracolumbar vertebral column instrumentation in dogs: bilateral and unilateral designs. *Vet. Surg.* 50 (2): 336–344. https://doi.org/10.1111/vsu.13558. Epub 2020 Dec 19. PMID: 33340136.

8. Elford, J.H., Oxley, B., and Behr, S. (2020). Accuracy of placement of pedicle screws in the thoracolumbar spine of dogs with spinal deformities with three-dimensionally printed patient-specific drill guides. *Vet. Surg.* 49 (2): 347–353. https://doi.org/10.1111/vsu.13333. Epub 2019 Oct 16. PMID: 31617955.

9. Oxley, B. and Behr, S. (2016). Stabilisation of a cranial cervical vertebral fracture using a 3D-printed patient-specific drill guide. *J. Small Anim. Pract.* 57 (5): 277. https://doi.org/10.1111/jsap.12469. Epub 2016 Mar 23. PMID: 27004483.

10. Wallace, N., Schaffer, N.E., Aleem, I.S., and Patel, R. (2020). 3D-printed patient-specific spine implants: a systematic review. *Clin Spine Surg.* 33 (10): 400–407. https://doi.org/10.1097/BSD.0000000000001026. PMID: 32554986.

11. Joffe, M.R., Parr, W.C.H., Tan, C. et al. (2019). Development of a customized interbody fusion device for treatment of canine disc-associated cervical Spondylomyelopathy. *Vet. Comp. Orthop. Traumatol.* 32 (1): 79–86. https://doi.org/10.1055/s-0038-1676075. Epub 2019 Jan 15. PMID: 30646415.

12. Chen, J., Chen, X., Lv, S. et al. (2019). Application of 3D printing in the construction of Burr hole ring for deep brain stimulation implants. *J. Vis. Exp.* 151: https://doi.org/10.3791/59560. PMID: 31545320.

13. Ovsianikov, A., Khademhosseini, A., and Mironov, V. (2018). The synergy of scaffold-based and scaffold-free tissue engineering strategies. *Trends Biotechnol.* 36 (4): 348–357. https://doi.org/10.1016/j.tibtech.2018.01.005. Epub 2018 Feb 20. PMID: 29475621.

14. Williams, J.M., Adewunmi, A., Schek, R.M. et al. (2005). Bone tissue engineering using polycaprolactone scaffolds fabricated via selective laser sintering. *Biomaterials* 26 (23): 4817–4827. https://doi.org/10.1016/j.biomaterials.2004.11.057. Epub 2005 Jan 23. PMID: 15763261.

15. Jamieson, C., Keenan, P., Kirkwood, D. et al. (2021). A review of recent advances in 3D bioprinting with an eye on future regenerative therapies in veterinary medicine. *Front Vet. Sci.* 16 (7): 584193. https://doi.org/10.3389/fvets.2020.584193. PMID: 33665213; PMCID: PMC7921312.

16. Jang, E.H., Kim, J.H., Lee, J.H. et al. (2020). Enhanced biocompatibility of multi-layered, 3D bio-printed artificial vessels composed of autologous mesenchymal stem cells. *Polymers (Basel).* 12 (3): 538. https://doi.org/10.3390/polym12030538. PMID: 32131428; PMCID: PMC7182803.

3

Postoperative Radiation Therapy of Intracranial Tumors

M. W. Nolan

North Carolina State University, Raleigh, NC, USA

Introduction

Because resection of large volumes of normal brain tissue is unsafe, the outcome of any brain tumor surgery is that either: (i) the tumor has been marginally excised (*gross total resection*), or (ii) the tumor has been debulked (*subtotal resection*). In the case of a marginal excision, all visible tumor has been removed and the only tumor remaining in the body is that microscopic disease burden which locally invaded into adjacent neuroparenchyma. By contrast, a debulked tumor is one for which surgery involved incomplete resection of the gross tumor volume (GTV); this may have been planned (e.g. emergency cytoreduction to alleviate intracranial pressure) or unplanned (e.g. inability to safely access the entire tumor). In either situation, adjunctive (postoperative) RT should be considered if there is a moderate to high likelihood that tumor recurrence will negatively impact quality or quantity of life. Risk factors may include completeness of resection, patient age and overall health status, tumor type (and associated metastatic potential), and tumor histology.

Overview of Radiation Therapy

Tumors develop when a series of gene mutations cause cell cycle perturbations that result in dysregulated cell division; the end result is an unusually high rate of cell proliferation and tumor growth. With this understanding, it should make sense that one way to stop tumor growth is to disrupt the cell cycle in a way that prevents cell division; indeed, this is the *biological basis of therapeutic radiation*. Radiation dose is measured in units of Gray (Gy). One Gray is equal to one Joule per kilogram. That is: one Joule per kilogram of mass irradiated, not one Joule per kilogram of body weight. This is an important distinction, and reflects the fact that radiotherapy (RT) is rarely used as an antimetastatic therapy; instead, it is primarily a tool for achieving local tumor control. Thus, to avoid radiation injury, therapeutic irradiations must be focused on the tumor and/or tumor bed, with minimal "spillage" into surrounding normal tissues. Methods for delivering tumoricidal doses of radiation to the intended target form the basis of *radiation physics and treatment planning*.

Radiobiology

DNA as The Target for Radiation

The most common method by which tumors of the nervous system are irradiated is external beam RT. The beams are sometimes composed of gamma rays that are produced during nuclear decay of radioactive cobalt-60 (e.g. Gamma Knife radiosurgery). As is more often the case in modern clinics, however, the beams are made of x-rays that have been generated by and then emitted from high-energy x-ray machines that are called linear accelerators. These so-called "linacs" can also emit therapeutic electrons; however, electron beam therapy is rarely utilized in veterinary neuro-oncology.

The beams, whether gamma- or x-ray, can be thought of as being made up of a stream of tiny energy packets. Those packets are called photons. And when the energy of the photon interacts with a cell, various types of physical damage can occur, including base damage, DNA single-strand breaks, DNA double-strand breaks, DNA-protein cross-links, etc. Clinically, it is the DNA double-strand breaks that are most valuable. While cells have molecular machinery that is capable of repairing DNA double-strand

---

Advanced Techniques in Canine and Feline Neurosurgery, First Edition. Edited by Andy Shores and Brigitte A. Brisson.
© 2023 John Wiley & Sons, Inc. Published 2023 by John Wiley & Sons, Inc.
Companion site: www.wiley.com/go/shores/advanced

breaks, if enough of those breaks are left unrepaired, the cell will undergo a process called mitotic cell death.

In mitotic death, the cell may remain physically present and metabolically functional, but it becomes incapable of completing the cell cycle. Without being able to undergo mitosis, the cell can no longer divide. It is through this manner of targeting and damaging nuclear DNA that ionizing radiation can reproductively sterilize a cell. That cytotoxic effect is not specific to tumor cells, but as compared with normal healthy tissues, neoplastic cells are generally more sensitive to the effects of radiation. One reason for this relative radiosensitivity is that a driver for development of many cancers are mutations that contribute to defects in the major DNA repair pathways. A classic example of this comes from human breast cancers, which often have mutant BRCA1 and BRCA2 genes. Those genes critically regulate non-homologous end joining and homologous recombination repair, which are two key DNA double-strand break repair pathways. When radiation is absorbed by a cell that has dysfunctional or abnormally low levels of BRCA1 or BRCA2 protein, DNA damage repair will be inefficient and incomplete, and the cell will be more likely to die than a neighboring normal cell that has intact repair machinery.

Normal Tissue Injury

While the cells of normal tissues do have intact and functional DNA repair pathways, it is possible to overload that repair capacity and cause injury. Radiation injuries are generally classified as being either acute (early) or late (delayed). In the brain, there is also a third category of radiation toxicity, called an "early-delayed" effect.

Acute toxicities are those which occur during a course of RT, or within a few weeks of completing therapy. Acute effects develop in tissues composed of cells that have rapid turnover. Acute injury begins as soon as the tissue is exposed to radiation; the injury is not clinically manifested until enough cells have died that the morphology or function of the affected tissue is altered; the acute effects then resolve as new cells replace those which had been lost. The classic example of acute tissue injury is moist desquamation of skin. This is something that develops two to three weeks into a course of radiation treatment, often becomes most severe a week after finishing therapy, and heals a few weeks later. These types of acute effects can be painful, and have adverse effects on quality of life. However, they are generally considered acceptable in the context of definitive-intent radiotherapy because the tradeoff for a bad but self-limiting side effect is an excellent long-term prognosis for survival. Older reports of brain tumor irradiation in dogs and cats included descriptions of acute effects that encompassed such problems as keratitis, keratoconjunctivitis sicca, otitis,

and pharyngeal mucositis, and occasional dermatitis. However, with modern conformal irradiation techniques, these types of complications are quite uncommon. Instead, acute toxicity is typically now limited to mild somnolence that may last a few weeks.

Early-delayed (or "subacute") central nervous system (CNS) effects are limited to the brain; they are not a recognized complication of spinal irradiation. While early-delayed effects can be severe, and may indeed be lethal, they tend to manifest as a mild to moderate and transient worsening of the presenting neurologic signs. They occur in the window of time that is one to five months post-irradiation, and when they do occur, they seem to last an average of one to two weeks. Historically, early-delayed effects were not commonly documented in the veterinary neuro-oncology literature. However, in recent years, they have been suspected to affect upwards of 30–40% of dogs undergoing stereotactic irradiation of intracranial meningiomas [1,2]. There are no known imaging or lab tests that aid in diagnosis; the diagnosis is clinical, and the major differential diagnosis is tumor progression. The underlying pathophysiology is unclear, but early-delayed effects may result from transient demyelination. They are usually self-limiting; as a component of supportive care, patients are often prescribed orally administered corticosteroids.

Late effects manifest months to years after treatment. They occur due to vascular injury and tissue fibrosis. The most worrisome late effect that can occur with brain irradiation is brain necrosis. This is a particularly challenging problem because the potential ramifications of brain necrosis are significant, and there is no effective treatment – any such changes that occur are permanent. For this reason, in definitive-intent RT, late effects become the dose-limiting toxicities. While in theory any tumor could be cured if it were treated with a high enough dose of radiation, clinical RT prescriptions are made with the idea that an acceptable rate of severe CNS toxicity is 1% at 2–3 years post-treatment. In line with this paradigm, perhaps the most commonly used radiation prescription in current veterinary practice is 50–54 Gy, delivered in 20 consecutive daily fractions of 2.5–2.7 Gy. There are trends toward more succinct courses of treatment, and similar risk has been associated with doses of about 40–42 Gy in 10 consecutive daily fractions [3,4].

There are two strategies for reducing risk of severe (late) radiation toxicity: biological avoidance (fractionation) and physical avoidance.

Rationale for Radiation Fractionation

Conventionally, radiation therapy has involved the delivery of large total doses of radiation, broken up, and given in many small daily dose "fractions." The benefits of fractionation have been summarized as the "4 Rs" of radiobiology [5];

1) *Repair*: As long as one does not administer too much radiation dose all at once, most of the DNA damage that happens in slowly dividing normal tissues can be repaired. In the brain and spinal cord, this repair takes place over several hours, and perhaps up to a day. Thus, to allow for optimal protection of normal CNS tissue during a course of RT, fractions are given no more often than once daily.
2) *Reoxygenation*: Tumors can outgrow their blood supply, and develop regions of necrosis and hypoxia. That hypoxia is a challenge because the availability of molecular oxygen within the tumor microenvironment is strongly predictive of a tumor's radiosensitivity. Fortunately, the very process of irradiating a tumor allows a subset of hypoxic cells to become better oxygenated. Therefore, the clinical impact of hypoxia will be minimized as long as: (i) sufficient time is allowed between dose fractions, and (ii) the process of reoxygenation is repeated many times (i.e. over multiple fractions).
3) *Redistribution*: The many cells of a tumor are always going to be distributed across the various phases of the cell cycle. For example, it will always be true that some cells are in G0 at the same time that others are in S or M-phase. At present, there is just no way to get this synchronized, *in vivo*. Interestingly, the relative radiosensitivity of a cell changes as it progresses through the various phases of the cell cycle. Therefore, if you were to deliver the entire dose of radiation all at once, some cells would be more susceptible than others would to radiation-induced cell death. This differential effect is easily overcome by administering the radiation dose over a long period of time, during which the radioresistant cells can progress to a more radiosensitive phase of the cell cycle.
4) *Repopulation*: Tumor cells that have not yet been terminally injured will continue to divide during a course of RT. In fact, radiation can cause the rate of tumor cell proliferation to increase; that is called "accelerated repopulation." Accelerated repopulation is best described in head and neck cancer; the phenomenon is generally considered to begin counteracting the efficacy of RT when a course of treatment exceeds a few weeks. Thus, while there are many benefits to fractionation, there must be a limit!

Together, the 4Rs help explain the benefits of radiation fractionation – benefits that include maximizing radiosensitivity of the tumor, and protecting normal tissues. A wide range of fractionation schemes have been described for irradiation of canine and feline brain and spinal tumors; preferences have shifted with time, and they also vary between clinicians and institutions. In today's world, most veterinary radiation oncologists would consider a standard (or conventional) course of definitive-intent RT to deliver a total dose of 40–54 Gy in 10–20 daily (Monday through Friday) fractions. That radiation is targeted to include the tumor (or the tumor bed, as is the case in postoperative RT) plus a margin of surrounding tissue. The margin is based on two expansions. The first expansion is designed to incorporate within the RT field any tissue that the prescriber believes may harbor tumor cells. The size of that expansion depends on how invasive the tumor is expected to be. For example, in the case of a meningioma, it may be that the microscopic tendrils of invasive tumor extend only a few millimeters beyond what can be seen as the GTV on cross-sectional imaging; and in the case of a high-grade glial tumor, that leading edge of subclinical disease burden may extend several centimeters. There are no standards for how large this expansion should be; the decision is at the discretion of the prescriber(s). And regardless of magnitude, all tissue included within that expansion is termed the "Clinical Target Volume" (CTV). Starting at the outer edge of the CTV begins the second expansion, and all tissue within that area is denoted as the "Planning Target Volume" (PTV). The PTV expansion is designed to account for motion that may occur during treatment delivery and/or inaccuracies in the way the patient is set up for treatment on a day-to-day basis. The size of the PTV expansion may vary, but it is most often 1 cm or less. A graphical representation of these treatment volumes is presented in Figure 3.1.

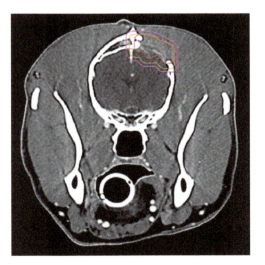

Figure 3.1 Graphical representation of radiation targets. This is a transverse plane image from the post-contrast simulation CT scan acquired for planning postoperative RT in a dog having undergone resection of a meningioma. The red line demarcates the surgically disrupted field (SDF). The orange line shows the clinical target volume (CTV) which was generated by making a 3 mm expansion from the SDF, into the calvarium and neuroparenchyma. The magenta line represents the planning target volume (PTV), which was made by isotropically expanding the CTV by 2 mm.

Stereotactic radiosurgery (SRS) represents a departure from the paradigms of conventional RT. In SRS, the entire course of radiation therapy is condensed into a single treatment session. Stereotactic radiotherapy (SRT) is similar in that it represents a succinct course of treatment, typically no more than five consecutive daily fractions. There are instances where SRT is given on non-consecutive days (e.g. every other day); however, that is uncommon in neuro-oncology.

Radiation Physics and Treatment Planning

The goal of treatment planning is to first identify what tissues need to be targeted (i.e. define a GTV, CTV, and PTV), and then create a volume of radiation dose that matches the PTV in shape and size, with rapid falloff of dose outside of the PTV. There multiple strategies for creating that conformal radiation dose "cloud," and choices include the energy, number, shape, and location of the beams. Once the plan is created, it undergoes quality assurance testing that is overseen by a therapeutic medical physicist. Next, the patient must be readied for daily treatment, including some strategy to ensure appropriate tumor localization prior to treatment delivery.

Beam Energy Selection

Once the PTV has been defined, the next step in planning RT is to decide what type of radiation to use. As mentioned earlier, the choice is between photons (gamma or x-rays) or electrons. Electrons deposit their maximum dose near the surface, and they do not penetrate very far into the patient. Photons deposit their maximum dose under the surface, and penetrate deeply. That ability to spare skin while reaching deep-seated targets provides the rationale for using photons far more often than electrons when treating tumors of the brain and spine.

Cobalt-60 machines come with no choice; the beam energy is an average of 1.25 mega electron volts (MeV), and that is entirely dependent upon the nuclear decay of cobalt, which is continual and natural. With linacs, there may be more choice. While many linacs are built with capacity to only emit one photon energy (most often 6 megavolts [MV]), others have 2–3 photon energy options. Common photon beam energy options that modern linacs can be equipped with include 4, 6, 10, and 18 MV. The higher energy beams deposit their maximum dose more deeply (e.g. 2.4 cm for a 10 MV beam, versus 1.5 cm for a 6 MV beam), and the dose falloff is slower. Those differences are rarely relevant in neuro-oncology; most brain and spinal tumors can be effectively treated with a standard 4 or 6 MV beam. In the event that electrons are chosen, the general idea is that the depth of beam penetration increases with beam energy. Most linacs are built with multiple electron beam energies, ranging from about 4 to 20 MeV. As a general rule of thumb, the "usable" dose will sit at a depth (in centimeters) that is about $1/3^{rd}$ to $1/4^{th}$ of beam energy (in MeV); so a tumor that is 3.5 cm deep might be approached with a 12 MeV beam, which has its usable dose in range of about 3–4 cm.

Dose Calculations

Radiation dose can be calculated either manually, or in an automated fashion using mathematical algorithms that are built into specialized software packages designed for radiation treatment planning. Manual dose calculations can be done quickly and with little financial expense; they are typically utilized when treatment field geometries are simple (squares and rectangles), the number of fields is small (1–2), and the goal is to create a homogeneous dose distribution across the treatment field. However, in modern practice, computerized treatment planning is far more commonly used for definitive-intent treatment of brain tumors. Almost all computerized treatment planning involves use of cross-sectional imaging. Delineation of an appropriate radiation target (i.e. PTV) is aided with the use of MRI, and CT is used by the computer algorithm in a manner that accounts the effects had by tissue composition heterogeneity on dose calculations.

There are two basic types of computerized treatment plans that can be generated: three-dimensional conformal radiotherapy (3DCRT) and intensity-modulated radiotherapy (IMRT). There are advantages and disadvantages to each. While 3DCRT and IMRT are both strategies for creating conformal radiation treatment plans, IMRT has the upper hand, and generally results in better conformity. Indeed, IMRT has been described as a "dose-painting" technique, which allows the prescriber to create radiation dose clouds that are closely matched to the PTV in both shape and size. Superficially, that sounds as if it would always be advantageous. However, there are other considerations. Perhaps the biggest concern is that improved conformity increases the risk of a marginal or geographic miss. Mitigating that risk requires accurate target delineation and accurate patient localization for each treatment session. Another consideration is that the total treatment time for an individual dose fraction is often shorter for 3DCRT than IMRT; this is useful for optimizing workflow efficiency, and for minimizing the amount of time a patient is under anesthesia. Additionally, IMRT requires more specialized treatment planning software, more complex treatment

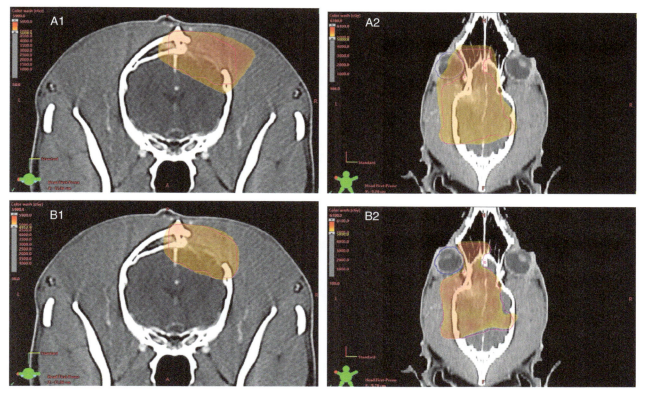

Figure 3.2 Three-dimensional conformal radiotherapy (3DCRT; A1, A2) versus intensity modulated radiotherapy (IMRT; B1,B2). In each image, the PTV is outlined in magenta. The orange/red fill shows the areas where radiation dose is at or above the prescribed dose. The top row (A1, B1) shows a representative transverse plane slice from the post-contrast simulation CT scan of a dog that underwent postoperative RT for a marginally excised meningioma. In this case, the 3DCRT plan was used for treatment; it was simpler (three beams vs. seven) and faster to deliver (86% increase in beam-on time for the IMRT plan). The IMRT plan has improved conformity in the temporalis muscle, but that tissue is relatively tolerant of radiation, and conformity in the brain was similar for 3DCRT and IMRT. The bottom row (A2, B2) is a coronal slice from plans that were generated for postoperative treatment of a dog with histiocytic sarcoma. In this case, the IMRT plan was chosen for treatment; even with simple planning (as shown on the right, this plan has five beams, static gantry angle, and sliding window technique), IMRT was able to provide far superior ocular sparing (the left eye is outlined in blue) as compared with even a complex 3DCRT plan (8 multi-leaf collimator (MLC)-fitted beams, as shown on the left).

delivery systems, and more exacting quality assurance/control; these requirements all come with physical costs that are passed along to the consumer to make IMRT a more costly option than 3DCRT. Thus, IMRT may be optimal for tumors and targets that have complex geometries and/or are close to critical organs that need to be physically shielded from high-dose radiation, and IMRT is most likely to be advantageous when the prescribed dose is close to the maximally tolerated dose of surrounding (or in-field) normal tissues. Conversely, 3DCRT may be perfectly adequate when the shape of the PTV is simple, or when the radiation prescription is relatively conservative. The comparative efficacy of 3DCRT and IMRT have not been well-studied in veterinary neuro-oncology, but based upon available literature, and on a population basis, one is not obviously inferior to the other [6]. Representative images of 3DCRT and IMRT plans that were generated for two different clinical cases are shown in Figure 3.2.

There are multiple systems for IMRT treatment delivery; chief among those are: linac-based static gantry angle (sliding window or step-and-shoot) IMRT, volumetric arc therapy (VMAT), and tomotherapy. The technical differences that distinguish these different forms of IMRT are beyond the scope of this chapter, but suffice it to say that while there are specific situations where one technique or technology may be advantageous over another, for most cases, the differences are negligible and one form can be considered clinically equivalent to another.

Target Localization Strategies

The ideal situation would be to have systems in place that both eliminate motion during treatment delivery, and enable precise repositioning of the patient for each radiation fraction. In veterinary practice, the vast majority of small animal patients are irradiated while under general anesthesia, and this helps to minimize the amount of intrafraction motion, particularly for CNS targets whose position is minimally impacted by respiratory thoracic excursions. Further minimizing intrafraction motion, and also facilitating precise day-to-day repositioning, are external devices including: (i) mattresses that conform to the shape of an individual patient's body and that rigidly attach to the treatment table; and (ii) bespoke bite blocks and face masks.

In addition to these setup devices, imaging systems are also used to verify correct positioning prior to treatment delivery. The most traditional methods for position verification is to acquire a "port film." Port films involve exposing film (or digital panels) using the megavoltage x-ray treatment beam. The resultant images show boney anatomy reasonably well but can be blurry, and do not provide good image contrast. More modern approaches involve on-board imaging systems that house kilovoltage x-ray tubes to acquire diagnostic quality planar radiographs (in lieu of megavoltage port films), and/or computed tomography systems (e.g. megavoltage CT, or kilovoltage cone beam CT [CBCT]). Setup inaccuracies that are visualized on imaging (Figure 3.3) can then be corrected prior to treatment. Those corrections include

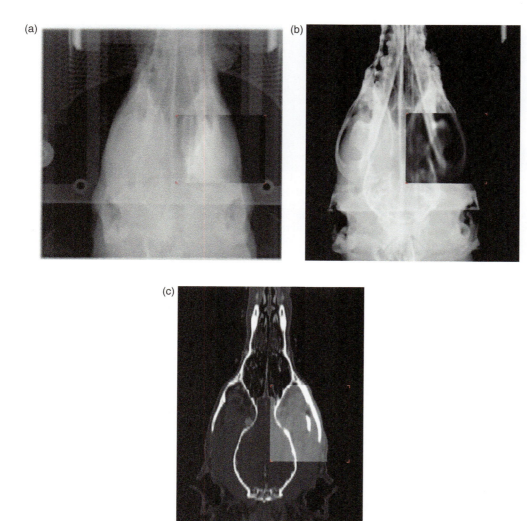

Figure 3.3 On-board imaging systems are commonly used to verify accurate positioning of the patient (and target) prior to radiation delivery. These are pretreatment images from a single dog undergoing brain irradiation. The images show the dorsal-ventral projection of a megavoltage portal radiograph (a), kilovoltage radiograph from the on-board imaging system (b), and kilovoltage cone-beam CT (CBCT); c). The image within the small green rectangle represents either the digitally reconstructed radiograph (from the simulation CT scan) in relation to the planar radiographs (left and middle) or the CBCT in relation to the simulation CT scan. This clearly demonstrates the improved visualization that is achieved by using kilovoltage radiographs rather than megavoltage portal imagining, and CBCT rather than planar imaging.

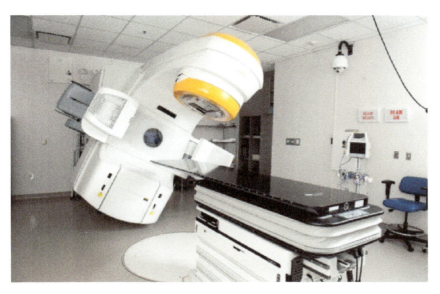

Figure 3.4 Conventional C-arm linear accelerator. The head of the linear accelerator emits the treatment beam (depicted by the red triangle), and is able to rotate around the patient (which lies on the black tabletop, called the "treatment couch.")

manual shifting/adjusting of the patient, or adjustment in position of the entire treatment table (also called the treatment "couch"). Most treatment couches move in three to four dimensions in space (X, Y, Z, and yaw). Newer systems may also allow for pitch and roll, with the ultimate allowing movement in all six dimensions.

Other systems that have been described in the literature, but are infrequently utilized in veterinary practice and thus are beyond the scope of this chapter, include implantable metallic (gold) fiducial markers and systems for rigid fixation of the skull (e.g. head frames).

Delivery Systems

With conventional teletherapy, the patient lies on their back atop a treatment couch that is parallel to the ground. The patient does not move during therapy and, instead, the linac is mounted on to a C-arm gantry that rotates around the patient (Figure 3.4). The patient is positioned such that the tumor is the axis around which the gantry rotates and is coincident with the center of the PTV, and thus as the gantry rotates, the radiation dose accumulates centrally within the tumor. The radiation beam is shaped using X and Y jaws, much as would be used to collimate square and rectangular imaging fields on a diagnostic radiograph. Additional collimation can then be achieved circular collimators, called cones, that have fixed diameters; or using multileaf collimators that can have either a static position during treatment delivery (as is the case in 3DCRT), or can move while the beam is on to create a non-uniform fluence of radiation that allows for improved beam shaping (as is the case in step-and-shoot or sliding window IMRT). Alternatives to the conventional C-arm linac include compact linear accelerators can also be mounted with a ring gantry. One example of this is TomoTherapy®, where the linac is spinning around the ring as the patient translates through the gantry. Or the compact linac can be mounted to a jointed robotic arm, as is the case in Cyberknife® treatments (Figure 3.5).

Each treatment unit has its strengths and weaknesses. Linacs are known for their versatility; they can easily be used for delivery of manual or computerized treatment

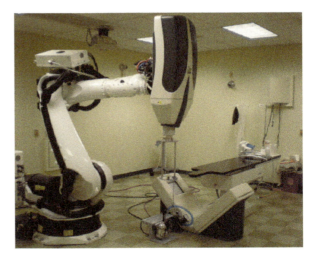

Figure 3.5 The Cyberknife® is a small 6 MV linear accelerator mounted on a KUKA® robotic arm. The head of the linear accelerator emits the treatment beam (depicted by the red triangle), and is able to move around the patient (which lies on the black tabletop, called the "treatment couch") and deliver radiation from 100 or more positions.

plans, and advanced modern linacs can delivery IMRT, VMAT, and even SRT and SRS. Tomotherapy is better suited for delivery of IMRT to long treatment fields, as might be the case in craniospinal irradiation. Cyberknife can be used for delivery of conventionally fractionated RT, but was specifically engineered for radiosurgery. Taking it a step farther, GammaKnife® (a cobalt-60 based platform) was designed for radiosurgery of intracranial targets.

Plan Evaluation

Radiation treatment planning is a complex process, and requires knowledge of tumor biology, the individual patient's disease state, therapeutic intent, the technical and technological capabilities of the treatment center, and equipment available in that center. But one constant among all of these factors are the tools and metrics that can be used to evaluate radiation treatment plan quality.

With computerized treatment planning, radiation dose can modeled directly on the simulation CT scan. The dose can visualized as a dose color wash, where different colors correspond to different doses. Dose can also be viewed as concentric isodose lines which appear much like topography lines on a map, wherein a given line encircles an area corresponding to a specific dose, and where the inner lines represent higher dose regions. In general, the prescriber will choose the isodose line which best conforms to the shape of the PTV; dose can then be "normalized" or

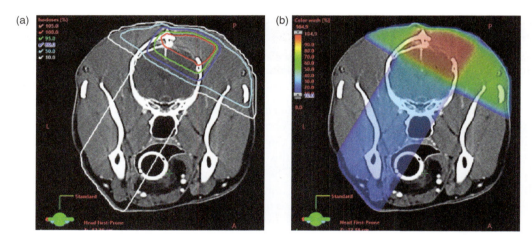

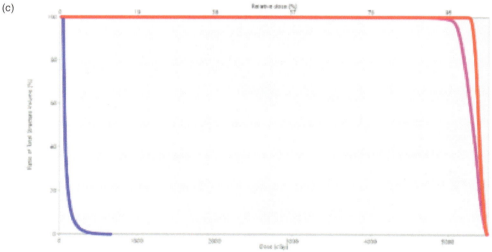

Figure 3.6 Radiation treatment plan quality is assessed visually and graphically. The image on the far left (a) shows isodose curves. These are similar to topography lines on a map; for example, everything lying inside of the green line will receive at least 95% of the prescribed dose. In the middle pane (b) the radiation dose from the same plan is depicted using a different technique. In this relative dose color wash, blue and green colors indicate low to intermediate dose, and orange and red tones represent progressively higher doses. These methods allow the prescriber to visually assess how much of the PTV is receiving the prescribed dose; it also allows for assessment of dose in organs at risk, as well as visualization of "hot spots." The far right panel is a dose–volume histogram. This allows for objective tracking of dose to both the radiation targets and the organs at risk. In this example (which corresponds to the CT images a and b), the red line shows dose to the CTV, the magenta line shows dose to the PTV, and the blue line is an organ at risk (the right eye).

prescribed to that line. However, coverage of the target with the prescription isodose is not the only consideration; there are times where an isodose line of lesser conformity will be chosen as the prescription isodose because it bends around (and thus better protects) an organ at risk (OAR) for injury.

As a complement to visual inspection of isodoses on cross-sectional images, radiation dose–volume histograms (DVH) represent another important way of expressing and evaluating radiation treatment plan quality [7]. The DVH is a graphical representation of radiation dose plotted against volume – volume of the targets (GTV, CTV, PTV) and various OAR that have been contoured (drawn) in the computer treatment planning system by the dosimetry team. There are published estimates of maximally tolerated doses for a range of OARs; thus, access to a DVH gives the prescriber an opportunity to objectively assess the toxicity profile for a given treatment plan (Figure 3.6) [8–10].

In recent years, mathematical tools have also emerged to aid in comparing the quality of different treatment plan options. Two of the most commonly utilized options are the conformity index (CI) and the gradient index (GI) or gradient measure. The CI is an expression of how well the PTV is covered by the prescription isodose. There are multiple formulas that have been described for calculating the CI, but in all cases, scores range from zero to one, with the idealized plan having a score of one [11]. The GI helps the dosimetrist understand how rapidly dose falls outside of the target, and is calculated as the volume of body receiving 50% of prescribed dose divided by the volume receiving 100%; the lower the value, the steeper the dose gradient [12].

Specific Tumor Types

Meningioma

Clinical Data
In a 2015 meta-analysis, the overall median survival time for dogs undergoing surgery as the sole treatment for intracranial meningioma was 10.4 months [13]. Meticulous surgical extirpation of intracranial meningiomas has been associated with longer survival times, but even then, local tumor control remains problematic, with nearly a quarter of cases experiencing recurrence within two years of surgery [14, 15]. It is unclear whether in dogs the risk of recurrence with surgery alone is dependent upon clinical factors, such as the surgeon's impression of resection completeness, or the histologic subtype or grade.

Radiotherapy has been used as an adjunctive therapy, with an aim of preventing or at least delaying recurrence. Indeed, in veterinary neuro-oncology, canine meningioma

is the only tumor type for which there is any direct evidence that adjunctive RT may extend survival beyond that achieved with surgery alone. Axlund and colleagues (2002) retrospectively analyzed survival in 31 dogs treated at Auburn University between 1989 and 2002 [16]. Included were 16 dogs that had undergone tumor resection (and survived at least one week postoperatively) and 15 dogs that underwent surgery followed by a course of RT. Of the dogs who underwent surgery alone, the median overall survival time was 7 months, and 3 of 16 (19%) survived at least 1 year. Of the dogs treated with surgery plus RT, the median survival time was 16.5 months, with 8 of 15 (53%) surviving 1 year or longer. In all cases, RT was planned manually, and delivered on a Monday–Wednesday–Friday schedule. Total radiation doses ranged from 40 to 49.5 Gy in all but one case, where the dog stopped treatment early (after receiving 28 Gy). Some dogs were treated with cobalt teletherapy ($N = 5$) and others ($N = 6$) were treated with 6 MV x-rays from a linear accelerator; there was no detectable difference in survival between these two approaches. During the study period, adjunctive RT was recommended for all dogs undergoing surgery for intracranial meningioma, and there is a possibility that selection bias influenced the outcomes; it may be that clinicians or pet owners opted against RT if surgery and/or postoperative recovery was problematic. Nonetheless, the difference in survival was significant ($p < 0.005$), and outcomes are generally in line with those of other studies [17].

Interestingly, while postoperative RT has been associated with improved survival as compared with surgery alone, it is unclear whether on a population basis, the provision of surgery improves outcomes over RT alone. A 2013 study by Keyerleber et al., reported the outcomes of 31 dogs having undergone RT for intracranial meningiomas; the overall median survival time was 19 months, and prior surgical excision did not confer a survival advantage [18]. Indeed, long-term survival after conventionally fractionated full-course RT is common, and in the past couple of decades, median survival times for dogs treated with RT alone have ranged from 19 to 25.2 months [3, 18–20].

Together these data suggest that for dogs undergoing definitive-intent RT for intracranial meningioma, the probability of long-term survival is not significantly improved when surgical debulking or excision is performed first. However, there are cases where surgery alone may be adequate. For example, if a 13-year-old Labrador retriever undergoes complete gross resection of a slow-growing, large, well-differentiated, and low mitotic index meningioma of the olfactory lobe that had caused no clinical signs other than seizures, the likelihood of that tumor growing back quickly enough to have negative impacts on patient prognosis are low, and adjunctive RT is unlikely to provide benefit even if the dog is otherwise quite healthy at the time of surgery. If that dog does experience locally recurrent disease that requires further tumor-directed intervention, then a second surgery could be considered, or alternatively RT as monotherapy is likely to be well tolerated and efficacious. There are also cases where surgery should be considered essential. The best example of that would be a dog presenting with severe neurologic signs for which short-term survival depends upon rapid tumor volume reduction; meningioma tumor volume does not predictably or rapidly reduce after irradiation [21].

Another important consideration is that there may be some cases where careful observation may be a rewarding approach. This may seem worrisome in light of published data showing that in dogs for which there is provision of no treatment, or palliative medical care alone, the median survival time is only two to three months [20]. However, many intracranial meningiomas in dogs are slow growing. Thus, in the case of an incidentally diagnosed tumor that is asymptomatic and small, serial imaging may be the best initial recommendation, with any treatment withheld until there is demonstrable tumor growth, an uptick in tumor growth rate, or development of clinical signs that are directly attributable to the intracranial mass.

In contrast to dogs, cats tend to develop benign, slow-growing meningiomas. They are most often supratentorial, and craniotomy with surgical removal is well documented as being a safe and effective therapy. The largest case series to-date is a multicenter study of 121 cats, wherein the median survival time with surgery alone was approximately three years [22]. Surgery alone is typically the preferred approach, and the only cats for which postoperative radiotherapy might be considered are those for whom histopathology indicates aggressive features (i.e. high grade), or cats with tumors that are locally recurrent (especially after multiple surgeries).

Radiotherapeutic Techniques

Postoperative RT is typically scheduled to begin two to three weeks after surgery. A postoperative CT scan is used to identify the surgical bed. The CTV is then expanded based on several considerations. To ensure that tissues which directly contacted the mass are included in the field, it is common to co-register the postoperative simulation CT scan with the preoperative MRI. The target volume is then adjusted based upon the neurosurgeon's description of the location of residual tumor, and a postoperative MRI may also be used in that regard. An additional margin expansion may then also be applied, based on knowledge of direction of spread and dural tails. A final expansion is applied (typically isotropically) to account for setup errors and motion; the size of that expansion depends on precision of the immobilization, imaging, and delivery systems, but often ranges from 2 to 5 mm. In total, the combined CTV and PTV expansion is generally 5–10 mm beyond the visible surgical bed, but in certain high-risk cases, may be even larger.

A typical plan will include three to four coplanar x-ray beams with either blocks or multileaf collimators used for field shaping. Other accessories (e.g. wedges) may be utilized. Bolus material is rarely needed, as recurrence in the skin is unlikely; however, it may be considered in very small animals, especially if the target is superficial. IMRT planning and delivery may be utilized, depending on equipment availability, and location of the tumor. For example, an olfactory lobe tumor is likely to benefit from the ocular sparing that can be achieved with IMRT, whereas there is often little to no benefit for brainstem lesions, unless particularly close to the cochlea.

Historically, practitioners prescribed 40–48 Gy in 4 Gy fractions that were administered on a Monday–Wednesday–Friday schedule. However, with the advent of modern gas anesthetics (e.g. isoflurane and sevoflurane), daily (Monday through Friday) fractionation is now the norm. For the past couple of decades, a typical postoperative radiotherapy dose for canine meningioma has been 50–54 Gy in 20 daily fractions; the higher end of that dose range is often reserved for cases in which resection was subtotal (i.e. gross residual disease). However, there is no firmly established standard dosing protocol, and some radiation oncologists instead to prefer to prescribe 45–48 Gy given in 3 Gy fractions. With advanced radiation technologies that allow improved conformity and application of smaller setup margins, there has been a move toward modest hypofractionation; recent data indicate comparable safety and efficacy when patients are treated with 40–42 Gy in 10 daily fractions, rather than the more protracted 20 fraction protocols [3, 4].

Glial Tumors

Clinical Data

In dogs, approximately 35% of primary brain tumors are gliomas. Despite the frequency with which they occur, relatively little is known about how to optimally manage the care of a dog with glioma. In theory, the optimal care path would begin with surgery, to debulk the lesion and firmly establish a diagnosis. Indeed, gliomatous tumors adopt a relatively indolent course wherein dogs respond favorably to treatment and survival is prolonged. Other dogs have a more aggressive, or apparently high grade, variant of glioma, which is clinically similar to glioblastoma multiforme (GBM) in human beings – where prognosis for survival is poor even with resection plus radiotherapy and chemotherapy. The National Cancer Institute (NCI) recently convened a panel of pathologists to develop consensus recommendations for diagnosis and grading of canine glial tumors;

however, to-date, no validated system is available to aid in robust prognostication.

With surgery alone, median survival times range from two to six months [23, 24]. When RT is used alone, outcomes vary considerably, with reported median survival times of 7–28 months [3, 25–28]. Postoperative chemoradiotherapy would be considered the most intensive treatment. In human GBM, temozolomide would be the drug of choice for many patients. However, the activity of available chemotherapeutic agents is unclear. In case series where dogs with primary brain tumors have been treated with lomustine, outcomes have been poor [29, 30], and in one study evaluating the addition of temozolomide to radiotherapy, there was no benefit [27]. There are no published data are available to describe outcomes with postoperative RT.

Radiotherapeutic Techniques

In humans with GBM, there are reports of widespread dissemination of glioma cells along white matter tracts, that can lead to postoperative recurrences in the contralateral hemisphere [31]. Indeed, there are cases of canine gliomatosis cerebri with clear evidence of extensive tumor extension throughout the brain [32]. This argues in favor of using wide margins. Nonetheless, whole brain irradiation is rarely performed after resection of a solitary gliomatous lesion in humans. The preference for localized irradiation is supported by the observation by Wallner and colleagues that 78% of unifocal GBM lesions will recur within 2 cm of the initial tumor volume, which is defined as the enhancing edge of the tumor on a CT scan; furthermore, 56% recurred within 1 cm, and in that series of 32 human patients, large tumor size was not associated with any increase in the risk of more distant recurrence [33]. If similar biology is assumed to be true for canine glioma, then a reasonable approach to defining the CTV may be to include a 2 cm margin around the lesion (or tumor bed) when planning with a CT scan alone, or a 1 cm margin if there is access to an MRI (especially fluid-attenuated inversion recovery (FLAIR) and T2-weighted images, so that regions of edema can be included in the volume from which the expansion is made). All other treatment planning and delivery parameters can be adopted from the paradigms established for management of meningioma. In cases where RT will be delivered after subtotal resection, consideration should be given to use of IMRT, such that a simultaneous integrated boost (e.g. 15–30%) can be targeted to gross residual tumor mass.

Choroid Plexus Tumors

Clinical Data

There are no known reports wherein clinical outcome is reported in sufficient numbers of dogs having been irradiated for known or presumed choroid plexus tumors to enable estimation of survival statistics. In this author's opinion, the only situation where RT might be considered as an adjunct to surgery is in the case of a narrowly excised choroid plexus carcinoma. In that scenario, definitive-intent craniospinal irradiation (CSI; i.e. irradiation of the entire CNS) might be useful for reducing risk of ventricular system carcinomatosis and/or drop metastases.

Radiotherapeutic Techniques

In humans, CSI is most commonly deployed as a treatment for medulloblastoma. There are several technical challenges which result from involvement of large treatment volumes. Conventionally, planning is performed on a CT scan (with or without MRI co-registration) and using 3DCRT techniques. The brain and spinal cord are typically treated separately. Often, two opposing lateral x-ray beams are used to treat the brain, and then the spine is treated with one posterior (x-ray or electron) beam, with the treatment couch "kicked" 90° to match the divergence of the brain and spine beams. Field matching must be done with extreme care to avoid errors than can lead to inadvertent under- or overdosing of tissues at the junction; this is often achieved with a feathering technique, wherein the junction is intentionally moved back and forth a few centimeters on a day-to-day basis. There are no published reports of CSI being used in veterinary patients. At North Carolina State University, treatment planning is just as has been described for humans, and our current practice is to prescribe 19 fractions, with a total dose of 47.5 Gy delivered to visible mass lesions, and 37.5 Gy to the entire CNS; treatment planning and delivery involves careful coordination between the medical physics team, the prescribing radiation oncologist(s), and the radiation therapists. Evolving IMRT and VMAT techniques and technologies are expected to make treatment planning more facile, and delivery safer [34]. When and where available, use of helical tomotherapy is likely to be advantageous [35].

Spinal Tumors

Clinical Data

There are few published data to drive evidence-based decision-making. However, the basic principles are the same as for postoperative irradiation of brain tumors. Treatment is considered in cases where the clinical impression indicates moderate-to-high risk of local recurrence. In the spine more so than in the brain, this may involve irradiation of gross residual disease. That is because surgery is often approached with a goal of tumor debulking, to decompress the spinal cord and allow clinical recovery.

As with primary brain tumors, the largest amount of data exists in support of postoperative irradiation of spinal meningiomas. Petersen and colleagues (2008) reported that in dogs having undergone cytoreductive surgery for spinal meningioma, postoperative radiotherapy is associated with prolongation of the interval between surgery neurologic deterioration (due to tumor recurrence or spinal cord injury) [36]. Radiotherapy can also be used as an effective salvage treatment in cases with locally recurrent meningioma [37]. Surgical decompression followed by RT is expected to offer similar opportunities for delaying neurological decline and prolonging survival in dogs with a wide range of spinal and vertebral malignancies [38].

Radiotherapeutic Techniques

The general approach is to position the patient in lateral recumbency on the treatment couch, and extend the radiation treatment field to include at least one vertebral body cranial and caudal to the tumor bed and/or surgical field. Radiation prescriptions are similar to those described for brain tumors (40–54 Gy total delivered in 2.5–4 Gy daily fractions). Because the spinal cord, vertebrae, and immediate surrounding tissues (muscles and blood vessels) are generally quite tolerant of these radiation doses, there is no need for extreme conformity or advanced forms of image guidance. For most cases, high-quality treatment plans can be achieved using bilaterally opposed and equally weighted x-ray beams. The fields are typically rectangular, thus obviating any need for extensive field shaping. Such plans are often generated using a CT scan to aid in delineation of the complete surgical field, and to assess for evidence of gross residual disease; and in cases where a postoperative CT is available, 3DCRT is almost always adequate, with no need for deploying IMRT. However, even in the absence of a CT scan, with close collaboration between the neurosurgeon and radiation oncologist, most spinal and vertebral tumors can be effectively targeted and treated using a simple manually calculated treatment plan. Because the radiation target is centered within the axial skeleton, accurate position verification can be achieved with basic and routine megavoltage portal imaging.

Stereotactic Radiosurgery and Stereotactic Radiation Therapy

SRS and SRT are thought to have a unique biological mechanism of action, which distinguishes them from conventionally fractionated radiotherapy. They achieve tumor ablation via delivery of large fractional doses of radiation with extreme conformity. To avoid injury, treatments must be planned to have steep dose gradients outside of the high-dose zone, and they must be delivered with extreme precision (which is achieved using the various aforementioned methods of stereotaxis). These treatment modalities are generally reserved for lesions that are small and have a high degree of conspicuity. They are also generally reserved for management of bulky (macroscopic) targets, and thus the primary role for SRS and SRT is as a surgical alternative.

In veterinary neuro-oncology, SRS, and SRT have been associated with clinical outcomes that are broadly similar to those reported for conventional full-course definitive-intent RT. Such is the case when SRS and SRT are applied as treatments for canine intracranial meningiomas; treatment is generally well-tolerated, and the median overall survival times are 18–24 months [1, 2, 39, 40]. Similarly, SRS and SRT can be used to improve the neurologic status and survival of dogs with presumed glial tumors [27, 28, 40].

Use of SRS and SRT as surgical adjuncts has not been reported in veterinary neuro-oncology. While the obvious appeal of such an approach would be that the treatment course is more concise than conventionally fractionated RT, there is hesitation with this approach, because delineation of the treatment target is challenging, and also because there are safety concerns. Similarly, postoperative SRS is infrequently used in human neuro-oncology. It has infrequently been reported as an option for postoperative irradiation of intracranial meningioma, and is perhaps best described as an adjunct to reduce risk of marginal recurrence in humans being treated for brain metastases [41]. However, the presence of edema and surgical changes make it difficult to identify an appropriate treatment target. To address this challenge, some clinicians have proposed neoadjuvant SRS and SRT as an alternative for brain metastases [42]. One distinct advantage of neoadjuvant treatment is that the radiation oncologist will be targeting a more conspicuous target. There is also thought that irradiating before surgery could reduce risk of leptomeningeal recurrences [43]. And in at least one case report, preoperative SRS was used to reduce tumor vascularity and improve safety of a subsequent resection [44]. With potential for extensive microscopic invasion into surrounding neuroparenchyma, it seems unlikely that any form of SRS or SRT would be both safe and effective for a canine glioma, whether delivered in the pre- or postoperative setting. However, a modestly fractionated course of preoperative SRT (e.g. 3–5 fractions, with a total dose of 24–30 Gy) with a 2–4 mm CTV expansion and minimal (if any) PTV expansion should be investigated as an opportunity for efficiently reducing the risk of local recurrence in patients that are to undergo resection of a brain or spinal meningioma.

 Video clips to accompany this book can be found on the companion website at:
www.wiley.com/go/shores/advanced

References

1. Kelsey, K.L., Gieger, T.L., and Nolan, M.W. (2018). Single fraction stereotactic radiation therapy (stereotactic radiosurgery) is a feasible method for treating intracranial meningiomas in dogs. *Vet. Radiol. Ultrasound* 59: 632–638.

2. Griffin, L.R., Nolan, M.W., Selmic, L.E. et al. (2016). Stereotactic radiation therapy for treatment of canine intracranial meningiomas. *Vet. Comp. Oncol.* 14: e158–e170.

3. Schwarz, P., Meier, V., Soukup, A. et al. (2018). Comparative evaluation of a novel, moderately hypofractionated radiation protocol in 56 dogs with symptomatic intracranial neoplasia. *J. Vet. Intern. Med.* 32: 2013–2020.

4. Rohrer Bley, C., Meier, V., Schwarz, P. et al. (2017). A complication probability planning study to predict the safety of a new protocol for intracranial tumour radiotherapy in dogs. *Vet. Comp. Oncol.* 15: 1295–1308.

5. Withers, H.R. (1975). The four R's of radiotherapy. In: *Advances in Radiation Biology* (ed. J.T. Lett and H. Adler). Elsevier.

6. Van Asselt, N., Christensen, N., Meier, V. et al. (2020). Definitive-intent intensity-modulated radiation therapy provides similar outcomes to those previously published for definitive-intent three-dimensional conformal radiation therapy in dogs with primary brain tumors: a multi-institutional retrospective study. *Vet. Radiol. Ultrasound* 61: 481–489.

7. Verhey, L.J., Koehler, A.M., McDonald, J.C. et al. (1979). The determination of absorbed dose in a proton beam for purposes of charged-particle radiation therapy. *Radiat. Res.* 79: 34–54.

8. Benedict, S.H., Yenice, K.M., Followill, D. et al. (2010). Stereotactic body radiation therapy: the report of AAPM Task Group 101. *Med. Phys.* 37: 4078–4101.

9. Emami, B., Lyman, J., Brown, A. et al. (1991). Tolerance of normal tissue to therapeutic irradiation. *Int. J. Radiat. Oncol. Biol. Phys.* 21: 109–122.

10. Bentzen, S.M., Constine, L.S., Deasy, J.O. et al. (2010). Quantitative Analyses of Normal Tissue Effects in the Clinic (QUANTEC): an introduction to the scientific issues. *Int. J. Radiat. Oncol. Biol. Phys.* 76: S3–S9.

11. Feuvret, L., Noël, G., Mazeron, J.J., and Bey, P. (2006). Conformity index: a review. *Int. J. Radiat. Oncol. Biol. Phys.* 64: 333–342.

12. Paddick, I. and Lippitz, B. (2006). A simple dose gradient measurement tool to complement the conformity index. *J. Neurosurg.* 105 (Suppl): 194–201.

13. Hu, H., Barker, A., Harcourt-Brown, T., and Jeffery, N. (2015). Systematic rreview of brain tumor treatment in dogs. *J. Vet. Intern. Med.* 29: 1456–1463.

14. Klopp, L.S. and Rao, S. (2009). Endoscopic-assisted intracranial tumor removal in dogs and cats: long-term outcome of 39 cases. *J. Vet. Intern. Med.* 23: 108–115.

15. Greco, J.J., Aiken, S.A., Berg, J.M. et al. (2006). Evaluation of intracranial meningioma resection with a surgical aspirator in dogs: 17 cases (1996–2004). *J. Am. Vet. Med. Assoc.* 229: 394–400.

16. Axlund, T.W., McGlasson, M.L., and Smith, A.N. (2002). Surgery alone or in combination with radiation therapy for treatment of intracranial meningiomas in dogs: 31 cases (1989–2002). *J. Am. Vet. Med. Assoc.* 221: 1597–1600.

17. Uriarte, A., Moissonnier, P., Thibaud, J.L. et al. (2011). Surgical treatment and radiation therapy of frontal lobe meningiomas in 7 dogs. *Can. Vet. J.* 52: 748–752.

18. Keyerleber, M.A., McEntee, M.C., Farrelly, J. et al. (2015). Three-dimensional conformal radiation therapy alone or in combination with surgery for treatment of canine intracranial meningiomas. *Vet. Comp. Oncol.* 13: 385–397.

19. Bley, C.R., Sumova, A., Roos, M., and Kaser-Hotz, B. (2005). Irradiation of brain tumors in dogs with neurologic disease. *J. Vet. Intern. Med.* 19: 849–854.

20. Treggiari, E., Maddox, T.W., Gonçalves, R. et al. (2017). Retrospective comparison of three-dimensional conformal radiation therapy vs. prednisolone alone in 30 cases of canine infratentorial brain tumors. *Vet. Radiol. Ultrasound* 58: 106–116.

21. Zwingenberger, A.L., Pollard, R.E., Taylor, S.L. et al. (2016). Perfusion and volume response of canine brain tumors to stereotactic radiosurgery and radiotherapy. *J. Vet. Intern. Med.* 30: 827–835.

22. Cameron, S., Rishniw, M., Miller, A.D. et al. (2015). Characteristics and survival of 121 cats undergoing excision of intracranial meningiomas (1994–2011). *Vet. Surg.* 44: 772–776.

23. MacLellan, J.D., Arnold, S.A., Dave, A.C. et al. (2017). Association of magnetic resonance imaging–based preoperative tumor volume with postsurgical survival time in dogs with primary intracranial glioma. *J. Am. Vet. Med. Assoc.* 252: 98–102.

24. Suñol, A., Mascort, J., Font, C. et al. (2017). Long-term follow-up of surgical resection alone for primary intracranial rostrotentorial tumors in dogs: 29 cases (2002–2013). *Open Vet. J.* 7: 375–383.

25. Rohrer Bley, C., Staudinger, C., Bley, T. et al. (2022). Canine presumed glial brain tumours treated with radiotherapy: is there an inferior outcome in tumours contacting the subventricular zone? *Vet. Comp. Oncol.* 20: 29–37.

26. Debreuque, M., De Fornel, P., David, I. et al. (2020). Definitive-intent uniform megavoltage fractioned

radiotherapy protocol for presumed canine intracranial gliomas: retrospective analysis of survival and prognostic factors in 38 cases (2013–2019). *BMC Vet. Res.* 16: 412.

27. Dolera, M., Malfassi, L., Bianchi, C. et al. (2018). Frameless stereotactic radiotherapy alone and combined with temozolomide for presumed canine gliomas. *Vet. Comp. Oncol.* 16: 90–101.

28. Moirano, S.J., Dewey, C.W., Haney, S., and Yang, J. (2020). Efficacy of frameless stereotactic radiotherapy for the treatment of presumptive canine intracranial gliomas: a retrospective analysis (2014–2017). *Vet. Comp. Oncol.* 18: 528–537.

29. Van Meervenne, S., Verhoeven, P.S., de Vos, J. et al. (2014). Comparison between symptomatic treatment and lomustine supplementation in 71 dogs with intracranial, space-occupying lesions. *Vet. Comp. Oncol.* 12: 67–77.

30. Moirano, S.J., Dewey, C.W., Wright, K.Z., and Cohen, P.W. (2018). Survival times in dogs with presumptive intracranial gliomas treated with oral lomustine: a comparative retrospective study (2008–2017). *Vet. Comp. Oncol.* 16: 459–466.

31. Dandy, W.E. (1928). Removal of right cerebral hemisphere for certain tumors with hemiplegia: preliminary report. *J. Am. Med. Assoc.* 90: 823–825.

32. Schweizer-Gorgas, D., Henke, D., Oevermann, A. et al. (2018). Magnetic resonance imaging features of canine gliomatosis cerebri. *Vet. Radiol. Ultrasound* 59: 180–187.

33. Wallner, K.E., Galicich, J.H., Krol, G. et al. (1989). Patterns of failure following treatment for glioblastoma multiforme and anaplastic astrocytoma. *Int. J. Radiat. Oncol. Biol. Phys.* 16: 1405–1409.

34. Studenski, M.T., Shen, X., Yu, Y. et al. (2013). Intensity-modulated radiation therapy and volumetric-modulated arc therapy for adult craniospinal irradiation – a comparison with traditional techniques. *Med. Dos.* 38: 48–54.

35. Schiopu, S.R.I., Habl, G., Häfner, M. et al. (2017). Craniospinal irradiation using helical tomotherapy for

central nervous system tumors. *J. Radiat. Res.* 58: 238–246.

36. Petersen, S.A., Sturges, B.K., Dickinson, P.J. et al. (2008). Canine intraspinal meningiomas: imaging deatures, histopathologic classification, and long-term outcome in 34 dogs. *J. Vet. Intern. Med.* 22: 946–953.

37. Lacassagne, K., Hearon, K., Berg, J. et al. (2018). Canine spinal meningiomas and nerve sheath tumours in 34 dogs (2008–2016): distribution and long-term outcome based upon histopathology and treatment modality. *Vet. Comp. Oncol.* 16: 344–351.

38. Siegel, S., Kornegay, J.N., and Thrall, D.E. (1996). Postoperative irradiation of spinal cord tumors in 9 dogs. *Vet. Radiol. Ultrasound* 37: 150–153.

39. Mariani, C.L., Schubert, T.A., House, R.A. et al. (2015). Frameless stereotactic radiosurgery for the treatment of primary intracranial tumours in dogs. *Vet. Comp. Oncol.* 13: 409–423.

40. Carter, G.L., Ogilvie, G.K., Mohammadian, L.A. et al. (2021). CyberKnife stereotactic radiotherapy for treatment of primary intracranial tumors in dogs. *J. Vet. Intern. Med.* 35: 1480–1486.

41. Brennan, C., Yang, T.J., Hilden, P. et al. (2014). A phase 2 trial of stereotactic radiosurgery boost after surgical resection for brain metastases. *Int. J. Radiat. Oncol. Biol. Phys.* 88: 130–136.

42. Asher, A.L., Burri, S.H., Wiggins, W.F. et al. (2014). A new treatment paradigm: neoadjuvant radiosurgery before surgical resection of brain metastases with analysis of local tumor recurrence. *Int. J. Radiat. Oncol. Biol. Phys.* 88: 899–906.

43. Routman, D.M., Yan, E., Vora, S. et al. (2018). Preoperative stereotactic radiosurgery for brain metastases. *Front. Neurol.* 9: 959.

44. Kamitani, H., Hirano, N., Takigawa, H. et al. (2004). Attenuation of vascularity by preoperative radiosurgery facilitates total removal of a hypervascular hemangioblastoma at the cerebello-pontine angle: case report. *Surg. Neurol.* 62: 238–243; discussion 43–4.

4

Practice and Principles of Neuroanesthesia for Imaging and Neurosurgery

Claudio C. Natalini

Mississippi State University, Mississippi State, MS, USA

Introduction

An understanding of the interactions between anesthetic agents and neuronal pathophysiology is necessary for the rational management of patients with central nervous system (CNS) disease or trauma. Patients with neurologic diseases may potentially recover in a worse condition because of the effects of anesthetic drugs on CNS blood flow and pressure [1].

The intact cranium does not yield to increasing internal volume, so intracranial pressure (ICP) can rise when the volume of any of the component contents increases. The two pathogenic sequelae of increased ICP are tissue ischemia and brainstem herniation through the foramen magnum [2].

The spinal component of the CNS, the spinal cord, spinal nerves, and meninges are susceptible to traumatic lesions and intervertebral disk herniation or extrusion that may cause ischemia and permanent neuronal and nerve fiber deficits. Anesthetizing these patients can be challenging as some are older or unstable. Also, during spinal surgeries, intracranial hemorrhage complicates further patient stabilization [2].

For spinal and supraspinal surgeries, maintaining appropriate oxygen delivery to the neuronal tissue is a paramount goal. Aggressively maintaining arterial blood pressure and monitoring SpO_2 and $ETCO_2$ are mandatory for these patients. Avoiding potentially hypotensive drugs, such as acepromazine, will likely contribute to better patient stabilization.

Increases in ICP

Clinical Signs

Clinical signs can include headache, nausea, vomiting, mental changes, disturbances of consciousness, and seizures. Prior to diagnostic imaging, for seizures in adult animals occurring for the first time without other apparent cause, association with a space-occupying mass is considered very high on the differential list [3].

Dynamics

The naturally occurring, space-occupying constituents of the cranium are:

- parenchymal tissue, including interstitial water – 80%
- blood (arterial and venous) – 10%
- cerebrospinal fluid (CSF) – 10%.

The volume occupied by each of these components can either increase or decrease. The most common causes of increased ICP are inflammatory or space-occupying cerebral lesions and head trauma.

Parenchyma/interstitial water: The growth of a space-occupying masses like neoplasms or granulomas causes an increase in the total volume of tissue components within the calvarium. Interstitial water can change with changing hydration status and can become elevated secondary to inflammation or trauma. Interstitial water can also change (increase) when extreme hyperglycemic episodes occur. Blood glucose levels above 250 mg/dl will increase plasma osmolarity increasing risks of interstitial edema [4].

Cerebral blood flow (CBF): CBF is normally autoregulated at mean arterial pressures (MAP) between 60–160 mmHg. Cerebral blood volume can change rapidly with changes in vascular resistance secondary to P_aCO_2 and/or drugs having vasodilatory activity [5]. There is a direct relationship between CBF and cerebral metabolic requirement of oxygen ($CMRO_2$). The changes are usually in the same direction. This is called $CBF/CMRO_2$ coupling and this relationship can be affected by anesthetic drugs [2].

Advanced Techniques in Canine and Feline Neurosurgery, First Edition. Edited by Andy Shores and Brigitte A. Brisson.
© 2023 John Wiley & Sons, Inc. Published 2023 by John Wiley & Sons, Inc.
Companion site: www.wiley.com/go/shores/advanced

CSF production: The production of CSF is relatively constant, but the resistance to CSF outflow can change dynamically. When resistance to CSF outflow increases, the volume of CSF increases.

The Monro–Kellie Doctrine (Figure 4.1) states that any change in one of the above components will result in an opposing change in the other components to maintain constant ICP (e.g. increases in parenchymal volume will result in reduced CSF production) [2]. The following formula applies to this principle:

$$Vi(\text{intracranial}) = Vb(\text{Brain}) + Vcsf + Vbl(\text{blood})$$

Cerebral Perfusion and Anesthesia

Cerebral perfusion pressure (CPP) is defined as the difference in MAP minus ICP or MAP − ICP in mmHg. Thus, an increase in ICP will decrease the CPP. The importance of maintaining normal blood pressures, and therefore perfusion during anesthesia, is paramount to a successful outcome. Hypotension is associated with increased neurologic morbidity because of reduced brain tissue perfusion in patients with extreme elevation of ICP.

Cranial nerve function is decreased after induction as the arterial blood containing anesthetic drugs will be flowing after induction through the basilar artery, reaching the cranial nerves. The classic responses are miosis in dogs and mydriasis in cats under opioid effect and complete mydriasis in dogs and cats when excessive anesthetic depth is achieved in plane IV stage III or stage IV general anesthesia [6]. Structures of the brain stem (medulla and pons) are also affected, decreasing activity in an afferent sequence. Heart and respiratory rates decrease as well as arterial blood pressure. The reverse is true during recovery.

The Cushing Reflex and Anesthesia

The Cushing reflex is a vasopressor/physiologic response to severely increased ICP and can be characterized by systemic hypertension and profound bradycardia. The hypertension is an attempt to maintain CBF in the face of increased ICP, while the bradycardia is a carotid sinus baroreceptor reflex response to the increased MAP. During intracranial surgeries, especially before the cranium is opened, a strong Cushing reflex can be critical as the bradycardia is often dramatic [7]. When faced with this in the anesthetized patient, reducing hypertension prior to relief of increased ICP can result in reduced cerebral perfusion, further compounding the problem. It is better to first reduce ICP, then treat the hypertension.

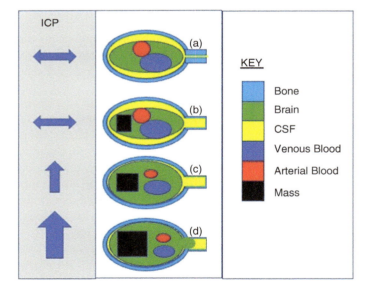

Figure 4.1 The Monro–Kellie Doctrine states that the skull is a rigid and inelastic compartment with three components: brain parenchyma, blood, and CSF. Under normal circumstances, these components exist in balanced dynamic equilibrium, where increases in volume of any will be compensated by decreases in the others. If the mechanisms become exhausted due to considerable increases in the volume of the components, or there is an additional mass (hemorrhage or hematoma can act as a mass in HT patients) with an increased volume that affects this balance, the intracranial pressure (ICP) will be elevated, and the cerebral flow (CBF) and perfusion are compromised. (a) Normal components within the calvarium with a normal amount of CSF flowing into the spinal subarachnoid space and the central canal. (b) The presence of a small mass does not increase ICP as the system compensates by shunting of additional CSF into the spinal spaces. (c) As the mass enlarges, the shunting of CSF has been maximized and there is reduced CBF and increased venous outflow. As this reaches a maximum, the ICP begins to increase and there is also an increase in the brain parenchyma because edema is developing. (d) As the mass grows much larger, the compensatory system is exhausted; consequently, brain herniation occurs.

Increases in ICP During Anesthesia

This is largely due to alterations in CBF. Normal metabolic CBF in dogs varies from 60–90 ml/min/100 g of tissue to 40–50 ml/min/100 g tissue in cats [6]. Normally, CBF is maintained and autoregulated in a range of 60–160 mm Hg mean blood pressure. For comparison, this lower than pressures for autoregulation of the kidneys (80–180 mmHg) [2]. The relationship between ICP and CBF is linear (e.g. as CBF increases, ICP also increases). An acute increase in ICP during anesthesia can be a severe setback in patients presenting with pre-existing elevated ICP. Changes in ICP during anesthesia are based on the following relationships:

a) Cerebral metabolic rate (CMR) and CBF.

- CMR refers to the rate of oxygen consumption by cerebral tissue.
- CBF varies directly with CMR.
- Most anesthetic drugs increase CBF through vasodilation while CMR is decreased.
- CBF is relatively unchanged with benzodiazepines, α-2 agonists, thiopental, propofol, etomidate, and opioids. Phenothiazines and butyrophenone tranquilizers have little effect on CBF and ICP.

Controversy exists regarding use of acepromazine in animals with history of seizures.

Of the common neuroleptic agents, only high doses of the low potency aliphatic phenothiazines, particularly chlorpromazine, are linked in humans with reduced seizure threshold and electroencephalogram (EEG) discharge patterns associated with epileptic seizure disorder; the butyrophenones rarely cause seizures [2]. As acepromazine is an aliphatic phenothiazine, similar recommendations have been applied to animals. Although abnormal EEG spiking was observed in some individuals, no seizures were reported in beagle dogs with a familial history of epilepsy when high dose chlorpromazine was administered together with intermittent light stimulation. Similarly, no seizures were reported in a retrospective study where acepromazine was administered during a seizure episode in dogs or dogs with prior history of seizures [6].

All inhaled anesthetics increase CBF and ICP (sevoflurane has the least effect at 1 MAC); however, increased CBF with isoflurane or cyclohexamines can be temporarily offset by concurrent use of IV benzodiazepines together with moderate hyperventilation. Ketamine and tiletamine increase both CMR and CBF, even at low doses.

b) CBF and $PaCO_2$.

- CBF varies directly and linearly with $PaCO_2$, because cerebral vascular resistance varies inversely with $PaCO_2$.

- Purposeful, moderate hyperventilation is a technique commonly utilized to transiently decrease CBF during anesthesia for patients suspected of having increased ICP.

The $PaCO_2$ or end-tidal CO_2 (ETCO2) is assessed using capnometry or blood gas analysis with a target $PaCO_2$ of 30–35 mmHg ($ETCO_2$ 25–30 mmHg). Excessive hyperventilation may cause cerebral ischemia secondary to inadequate perfusion of normal tissue. And although respiratory depression following opioid administration can cause hypoventilation (and increase ICP), this is usually not a significant problem in clinical patients at commonly used dosages. Nonetheless, it is judicious to withhold opioids in severely obtunded/comatose patients. More concerning is vomiting from mu agonist opioids in dogs with elevated ICP, and so hydromorphone is rarely used since emesis is a common side effect. Vomiting causes an abrupt spike in ICP. In patients with pre-existing high ICPs, vomiting can cause acute brainstem herniation [8].

c) Resistance to CSF outflow.

- Normally, increased ICP secondary to increased CBF is prevented by displacement of CSF from the cranium.
- In patients with space-occupying intracranial tumors, this compensatory mechanism is compromised and may fail, causing ICP to rapidly increase.
- The same drugs useful for maintaining balance of CMR and CBF are also best for CSF dynamics.
- Holding off the jugular veins for vena-puncture is not recommended in patients with elevated ICP. Occluding the jugular veins resist CSF outflow causing an abrupt elevation if ICP pressures.

d) Interstitial fluid volume.

- Interstitial edema forms depending on the relative balance of Starling's forces (hydrostatic, oncotic, tissue pressure).
- The hyperosmotic diuretic mannitol (0.25–1.0 g/kg) given IV over 15 minutes may be useful in decreasing interstitial fluid volume and tissue swelling, but may aggravate fluid accumulation if the blood–brain barrier is disrupted.
- Hypertonic saline (3–4 ml/kg IV; 3%) may be better choice. Clinical trials in humans have shown that hypertonic saline 3% is advantageous when compared to mannitol, producing better outcomes [9].
- Loop diuretics (furosemide, 1 mg/kg IV) can be useful, especially if pulmonary edema accompanies increased ICP.
- Corticosteroids (dexamethasone, methylprednisolone) are effective in lowering increased ICP caused by localized cerebral edema around brain tumors.

ICP and Contrast Myelography

Formerly, contrast myelography was used commonly in the diagnosis of spinal cord compression. Today, with other advanced imaging techniques, it is used less commonly but still has a placed in diagnostic imaging, combined with conventional radiographic techniques or CT, and involves injecting a volume of an iodinated contrast media into the subarachnoid or epidural space. Cervical, thoracic, or lumbar intervertebral disk protrusions are unlikely to directly affect the space-occupying constituents of the cranium, and thus are unlikely to raise ICP; however, removal of CSF prior to the injection of contrast material can precipitate herniation of the brain when ICP is high. Seizures are sometimes a side-effect following contrast myelography. In one study, 21% of dogs had at least one seizure, with a significantly greater seizure risk associated with cerebellomedullary injection compared with lumbar injection [10]. The volume of contrast agent administered to dogs having seizures was greater than to those not having seizures, and dogs >20 kg were more likely to have seizures than dogs <20 kg. Neither anesthetic regimen nor duration of anesthesia affected the frequency of complications following myelography [11].

Hydrocephalus

Hydrocephalus is often seen in miniature breed dogs, but also larger breeds as well at times. In neurologically normal neonates with open cranial sutures or older animals with an open fontanel, ICP changes associated with general anesthesia are blunted or minimized due to the compliance of the open sutures or open fontanel. With the cranium not fully intact, the Monro–Kellie Doctrine is not completely applicable here. In humans, decreased noninvasive ICP measurements may are seen in neurologically normal neonatal patients with open fontanels. This is often observed with many drugs, including ketamine, fentanyl, and isoflurane [12].

Neurologic Monitoring: Monitoring Brain State During Anesthesia

There are four key points to neurologic monitoring in anesthetized patients. First, the pathway at risk during surgery and interventions must be controllable. Second, the monitoring system should provide reliable and repeatable data. Next, when changes are detected, those should be of prognostic value. And finally, even when monitoring is possible, early detection of changes will have no advantage to the patient if no treatment or intervention is possible.

Few studies in humans have proven the efficacy of neurologic monitoring. Maintaining physiologic homeostasis and stable levels of anesthesia, and communication between neurologists and anesthesiologists, is mandatory when critical procedures and high neurologic risks are involved.

Modalities of Neurologic Monitoring

Several advanced systems for neurologic monitoring of the CNS function during surgery are available. Many of the more advanced ones are, however, not well validated in animals. Examples are global blood flow monitoring with xenon, transcranial doppler ultrasound, mixed venous blood oxygen saturation (jugular bulb, reflectance oximetry), and cerebral oximetry.

Electroencephalogram EEG

This methodology is somewhat validated in animals but with some inconsistencies. Potentially, EEG could be useful with additional investigations [13]. With induction of general anesthesia with inhalation or injectable GABAergic drugs (propofol, alfaxalone) there is a decrease in frequency and an increase in amplitude. This continues until burst suppression occurs [14]. A frequency of 10 Hz seems to be associated with unconsciousness. At this level, a loss of integration among central centers in the brain is observed.

Sensory-Evoked Responses (SERs) and Somatosensory-Evoked Potentials (SSEPs)

These are highly advanced monitoring systems that have been used experimentally in animals but are not (today) in common use clinically with small animal anesthesia. Future advances in these modalities may make them more commonplace.

Glycemic Control

Blood glucose levels of 180–250 mg/dl are associated with poor outcomes in brain injuries [15]. Blood glucose levels should be monitored during brain surgeries for traumatic injuries or neoplasia, as low values (<60 mg/dl) are also dangerous and could lead to neuronal damage and coma. If blood glucose levels are dangerously low, dextrose supplementation should be initiated [4].

Monitoring Nociception

Monitoring nociception (pain stimulation perception) and antinociception during neuroanesthesia is done presently with heart rate, blood pressure monitoring, and, in some cases, respiratory rate when the patient is not on a mechanical ventilator. These parameters should be analyzed based on patients' surgical and clinical conditions and are not reliable measurements. They are indirect markers and do not directly provide information of noxious processing in the CNS. Studies have shown that heart rate, heart rate variability (0.15–0.4 Hz), plethysmography wave amplitude, and skin conductance fluctuations, are able to predict nociceptive input, but response output is not predictable.

Other Modalities

There are other modalities available for CNS monitoring used in human patients, such as auditory and visual evoked potentials. Most anesthetic drugs such as inhalation anesthetics, sedatives (dexmedetomidine and opoids), and induction agents (propofol, etomidate, and ketamine) will interfere with neurologic monitors including electroencephalograms. There is a need for further validation and investigation on these modalities in dogs and cats. Dexmedetomidine alone has a very minimal effect on EEGs [16]. There is a need for further validation and investigation on these modalities in dogs and cats.

Sedation versus General Anesthesia for Imaging

Often, a light plane of anesthesia is recommended for imaging. Some procedures can be done under sedation or "heavy" sedation, but one should always remember that sedation by definition is a state from which an animal can be aroused with sufficient nociceptive stimulation. If noxious stimulation is expected, full general anesthesia is required including proper analgesics. Magnetic resonance imaging (MRI)-safe anesthesia machines and monitors should be considered. When these are not available, one should always consider passing the anesthesia machine and monitoring tubing through a waveguide that will filter radiofrequency and allow for plastic hoses and monitoring cables to pass to the patient [6].

Regional Anesthesia for Laminectomy, Hemilaminectomy, and Vertebral Fractures

The erector spinae plane block (ESPB) has been described in humans and dogs for surgical management as well as pain management of the thoracolumbar region. The technique involves the local anesthetic infiltration of a local anesthetic in the interfascial plane between the erector spinal muscle group and the transverse processes of the thoracic or lumbar vertebrae. In this region, the lateral and medial ramifications of the dorsal branch of the spinal nerves are located. When the block is effective, ipsilateral extensive blockade over the dorsal and dorsolateral thoracic and lumbar regions is obtained. This is a new technique that still needs additional studies before clinical application can be recommended, but there is recent evidence that supports its use [17, 18].

Anesthesia Protocol for Intracranial Surgery

A suggested protocol for intracranial surgery is summarized in Table 4.1.

Table 4.1 Suggested craniotomy anesthesia drug protocol.

Pre-Anesthetic Medications
1. **Famotidine** (10 mg/ml)
   1 mg/kg IV q 24 h for 4 d
2. **Maropitant** (10 mg/ml)
   1 mg/kg IV before induction or SC with premedication
3. **Opioid or Sedative for Pre-Medication**

Induction
1. **Propofol** (10 mg/ml)
   →4–6 mg/kg IV for induction
   →0.2–0.6 mg/kg/min IV for maintenance
   Assisted Ventilation: Maintain ETCO$_2$ between 25 and 30
   Place arterial catheter and monitor blood pressures
2. **Dexamethasone SP** (4 mg/ml)
   0.25–0.5 mg/kg IV once – Post induction, Presurgical

Maintenance
1. **Propofol**
   →0.2–0.6 mg/kg/min IV for maintenance
2. **Remifentanil** (50 mcg/ml, 1 mg powder reconstituted in 20 ml 0.9% NaCl)
   12–24 mcg/kg/h IV
3. **Atracurium** (2 mg/ml)
   0.1–0.2 mg/kg IV

Additional Intraoperative Drugs
1. **Mannitol** (0.25 g/ml) 0.5 g/kg IV once or **3% NaCl** 4 ml/kg IV once
2. **Furosemide** (50 mg/ml)
   1 mg/kg IV for three doses q 8 h

Postoperative Analgesia (tailored to the patient's need and recovery status)
1. **Methadone** (10 mg/ml)
   0.2 mg/kg IV q 4–6 h for 2 d
2. **Remifentanil** (50 mcg/ml, 1 mg powder reconstituted in 20 ml 0.9% NaCl)
   0.05–0.1 mcg/kg/min IV for 2 d
3. **Dexmedetomidine** (0.1 mg/ml)
   1.0 –2.0 mcg/kg IV q 4–8 h for 2 d or CRI 1–2 mcg/kg/h

 Video clips to accompany this book can be found on the companion website at:
www.wiley.com/go/shores/advanced

References

1. Walters, F. (1990). Neuro anaesthesia-a review of the basic principles and current practices. *Cent. Afr. J. Med.* 36: 44–51.
2. Pasternak, J.J. and Lanier, W.L. (2012). Diseases affecting the brain. In: *Stoelting's Anesthesia and Co-Existing Disease* (ed. R.L. Hines and K.E. Marschall), 218–254. Saunders.
3. Goma, H.M. and Ali, M.Z. (2009). Control of emergence hypertension after craniotomy for brain tumor surgery. *Neurosciences (Riyadh)* 14: 167–171.
4. Syring, R.S., Otto, C.M., and Drobatz, K.J. (2001). Hyperglycemia in dogs and cats with head trauma: 122 cases (1997–1999). *J. Am. Vet. Med. Assoc.* 218: 1124–1129.
5. Kaisti, K.K., Metsahonkala, L., Teras, M. et al. (2002). Effects of surgical levels of propofol and sevoflurane anesthesia on cerebral blood flow in healthy subjects studied with positron emission tomography. *Anesthesiology* 96: 1358–1370.
6. Harvey, R., Greene, S., and Thomas, W. (2007). Neurological disease. *Lumb & Jones' Vet. Anesth. Analg.* 4: 903–913.
7. Dinallo, S. and Waseem, M. (2020). Cushing reflex. *StatPearls [Internet]*.
8. Gelb, A.W., Craen, R.A., Rao, G.S.U. et al. (2008). Does hyperventilation improve operating condition during supratentorial craniotomy? A multicenter randomized crossover trial. *Anesth. Analg.* 106: 585–594.
9. Kamel, H., Navi, B.B., Nakagawa, K. et al. (2011). Hypertonic saline versus mannitol for the treatment of elevated intracranial pressure: a meta-analysis of randomized clinical trials. *Crit. Care Med.* 39: 554–559.
10. Barone, G., Ziemer, L.S., Shofer, F.S., and Steinberg, S.A. (2002). Risk factors associated with development of seizures after use of iohexol for myelography in dogs: 182 cases (1998). *J. Am. Vet. Med. Assoc.* 220 (10): 1499–1502.
11. Lewis, D. and Hosgood, G. (1992). Complications associated with the use of iohexol for myelography of the cervical vertebral column in dogs: 66 cases (1988–1990). *J. Am. Vet. Med. Assoc.* 200: 1381–1384.
12. Barash, P., Cullen, B.F., Stoelting, R.K. et al. (2013). *Handbook of Clinical Anesthesia*. Lippincott Williams & Wilkins.
13. Otto, K.A. (2007). Effects of averaging data series on the electroencephalographic response to noxious visceral stimulation in isoflurane-anaesthetized dogs. *Res. Vet. Sci.* 83: 385–393.
14. Ambrisko, T.D., Coppens, P., and Moens, Y. (2011). Continuous versus intermittent thermodilution for cardiac output measurement during alveolar recruitment manoeuvres in sheep. *Vet. Anaesth. Analg.* 38: 423–430.
15. Prisco, L., Iscra, F., Ganau, M. et al. (2012). Early predictive factors on mortality in head injured patients: a retrospective analysis of 112 traumatic brain injured patients. *J. Neurosurg. Sci.* 56: 131–136.
16. Tepper, L.C. and Shores, A. (2014). Electroencephalographic recordings in the canine: effects of low dose medetomidine or dexmedetomidine followed by atipamezole. *Open J. Vet. Med.* 4 (2): 7–13.
17. Otero, P.E., Fuensalida, S.E., Russo, P.C. et al. (2020). Mechanism of action of the erector spinae plane block: distribution of dye in a porcine model. *Reg. Anesth. Pain Med.* 45: 198–203.
18. Ferreira, T.H., St James, M., Schroeder, C.A. et al. (2019). Description of an ultrasound-guided erector spinae plane block and the spread of dye in dog cadavers. *Vet. Anaesth. Analg.* 46: 516–522.

Part I

Spinal Procedures

5

Cervical Ventral Slot Decompression

Andy Shores[1] and Allison Mooney[2]

[1] Mississippi State University, Mississippi State, MS, USA
[2] Boise, ID, USA

Cervical IVD Syndrome

History

Patients with cervical IVD protrusions often present with a history of sudden crying out in pain, neck guarding, and muscle fasciculations about the head and neck. The signs may occur spontaneously or in response to exercise or may be apparent when the animal is petted about the head. The history may include a decrease in activity, since any sudden movement elicits excruciating pain, or it may indicate intermittent episodes with varying degrees of pain. Others are presented with variable signs of severe tetraparesis, either ambulatory or non-ambulatory, from an acute disk extrusion [1].

Cervical IVD protrusion is most common in the chondrodystrophic breeds. Non-chondrodystrophic breeds can also be affected with the cervical vertebral instability ("wobbler") syndrome appear to have a higher incidence of cervical IVD protrusions than other non-chondrodystrophic breeds (Figure 5.1).

Clinical Signs

The clinical signs of cervical IVD protrusion are related to the dynamic force of compression and the mechanical displacement of the spinal cord and cervical nerve roots by the extruded disk material. The signs can include hyperesthesia of the neck and forelimbs, painful spasms of the neck muscles, ataxia, or tetraparesis. Most cervical

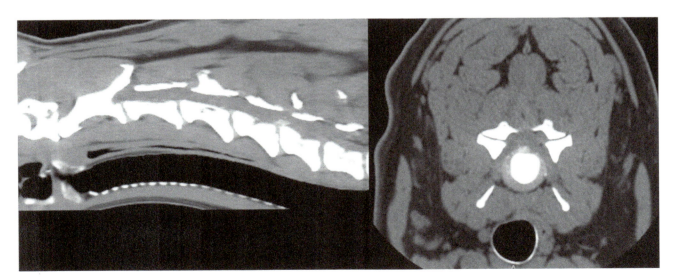

Figure 5.1 Sagittal and transverse CT images of an IVD extrusion that produced acute, severe tetraparesis in a 6-year-old male Doberman Pinscher.

Advanced Techniques in Canine and Feline Neurosurgery, First Edition. Edited by Andy Shores and Brigitte A. Brisson.
© 2023 John Wiley & Sons, Inc. Published 2023 by John Wiley & Sons, Inc.
Companion site: www.wiley.com/go/shores/advanced

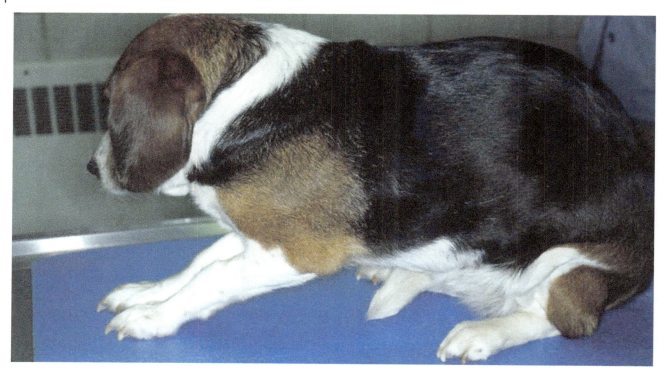

Figure 5.2 A Beagle presented for severe, persistent neck pain that was exhibited at any time the dog tried to move. Diagnostics revealed a C3–C4 IVD extrusion in this chondrodystrophic dog.

IVD protrusions, even when massive, are manifested by pain only (Figure 5.2). Pain is the hallmark of cervical IVD protrusion and may be constant or intermittent. Most of the pain is of radicular (nerve root) origin; some may be associated with meningeal initiation or "diskogenic" pain [1, 2].

Neurologic deficits are usually mild when present in cervical IVD disease (e.g., reflex alterations, proprioceptive deficits) and are often associated with progression of the disease. The acute type I protrusion can produce sudden and severe neurologic deficits (e.g., ambulatory or non-ambulatory tetraparesis), can appear clinically indistinguishable from meningitis, or can be manifested by pain only. The type II protrusion has a much slower onset but may have very similar clinical signs with progression of the protrusion [3, 4].

Radiographic Signs

The radiographic signs of cervical IVD protrusion are narrowing of the IVD space, narrowing of the intervertebral foramen, increased density ("cloudiness") in the intervertebral foramen, and the presence of a mineralized mass within the spinal canal above the IVD space (Figure 5.3). One or more of these signs may be present. Clinically, the C2–C3 and C3–C4 intervertebral disks have the highest incidence of protrusion.

Figure 5.3 A lateral radiograph demonstrating narrowing of the IVD space at C4–C5, narrowing of the intervertebral foramen, increased density ("cloudiness") in the intervertebral foramen.

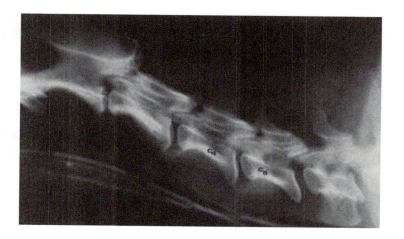

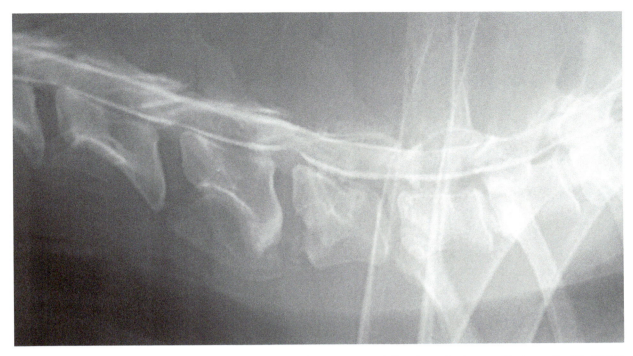

Figure 5.4 A lateral view of a myelogram study demonstrating an extramedullary/extradural mass effect over the C6–C7 IVD space, later confirmed at surgery to be an IVD extrusion.

Advanced Imaging

Myelography is also helpful in delineating the lesion (Figure 5.4). Often, for suspected cervical IVD disease, a non-ionic contrast material approved for intrathecal use is injected into the sub-arachnoid space of the anesthetized patient and is used to outline deviation in the spinal cord that would indicate an extramedullary/extradural mass (compression). Myelography is easy to perform and generally carries a minimal risk; however, it is not as detailed as cross-sectional imaging techniques (magnetic resonance imaging – MRI; computed tomography – CT).

CT is often performed in sedated patients and in chondrodystrophic dogs often provides a diagnosis without the use of contrast as these disks often contain a high mineral content (Figure 5.5). At other times, especially in non-chondrodystrophic patients, CT is combined with myelography in the anesthetized patient to provide a very definitive diagnosis of spinal cord compression (Figure 5.6).

MRI is very useful in the diagnosis of IVD disease (Figure 5.6). Its high level of tissue contrast often gives the

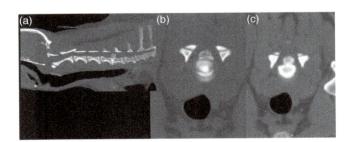

Figure 5.5 CT images of an IVD extrusion at C5–C6 in a chondrodystrophic dog. (a) Reconstructed sagittal view; (b) transverse bone window; (c) transverse soft-tissue window. The patient only required sedation for these images and did not require contrast administration for this diagnosis.

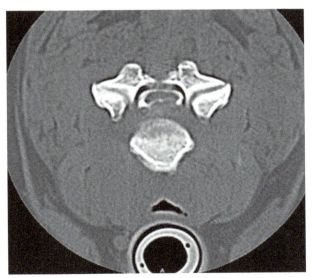

Figure 5.6 A CT-myelogram transverse view demonstrating an IVD extrusion causing severe compression of the cervical spinal cord.

neurosurgeon a very definitive view of the herniated material in the spinal canal; however, because of its sensitivity, some subtle or non-clinical lesions may also be identified – hence the need for a very through clinical examination and localization of the offending lesion.

Indications for Surgery

Surgical management of cervical IVD syndrome is often warranted. Mild pain and muscle spasms can be amenable to conservative therapy. The merits of medical versus surgical therapy and the incidence of recurrence should be discussed with the owner; however, advanced imaging early in the course of the disease may dictate earlier surgical intervention with CT or MRI findings of an especially large extrusion that is unlikely to respond to medical management long term (Figure 5.3). Proper medical management may be of particular importance when there are financial considerations. Surgical candidates should be carefully evaluated through examination procedures and presurgical laboratory profiles and thoracic radiographs in patients over 5 years of age or with cardiac disease. Thorough knowledge of the anatomy and surgical approaches to the cervical vertebrae is essential in performing the described procedures (Figure 5.7).

The indications for surgical management of cervical IVD syndrome are persistent pain, muscle spasms, or paresis, and certainly after prolonged failed conservative therapy and marked neurologic deficits (proprioceptive deficits, ataxia, tetraparesis); and pain with imaging showing evidence of extruded disk material in the cervical spinal canal. Surgical management consists of decompression of the cervical spinal cord. Fenestration of other cervical disks (C2–C3 through C5–C6) is often performed as a prophylactic procedure in chondrodystrophic dogs. Decompression is performed to remove IVD material from the spinal canal and to relieve pressure on the spinal cord [1].

Ventral Approach to the Cervical Spine

The patient is anesthetized and positioned in perfect dorsal recumbency with the neck hyperextended over a sandbag or rolled towel (Figure 5.8). The area prepared for surgery extends from the middle of the ventral surface of the mandible to a point at least 2 cm caudal to the manubrium and laterally on each side to an imaginary line drawn from the wings of the atlas to the point of the shoulder [5]. The head is secured to the table with 1-inch adhesive tape, and the forelimbs are pulled caudally to facilitate exposure of the cervical disks. Poor positioning of the patient often results in dissection off the ventral midline and considerable hemorrhage. When approaching a more caudal IVD space (C6–C7), the authors have found that having the patient's neck flat against the table surface with the head extended and the thoracic limbs pulled caudally with maximal extension improves surgical access/visualization of that site. In many instances, when the neck is flexed over a sandbag or towel, this moves the C6–C7 space caudally and under the manubrium, making exposure very difficult.

The surgical approach is always made from the patient's left side. A ventral midline incision is made from the base of the larynx to the sternum (Figure 5.9). The underlying connective tissue can be divided with Metzenbaum scissors to expose the paired sternohyoideus muscles. After the sternohyoideus muscles are exposed, they can be separated on the midline (median raphe) using Metzenbaum scissors (Figure 5.10). During the muscle separation, the caudal thyroid vein is encountered (note that this vein is not present in the cat). Branches of the vein are cauterized using

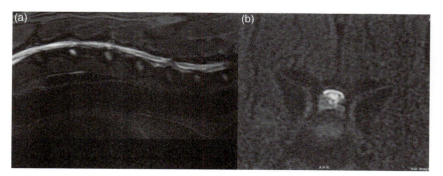

Figure 5.7 Sagittal and transverse T2-weighted MRI sequences of a C6–C7 IVD compression of the cervical spinal cord at that site.

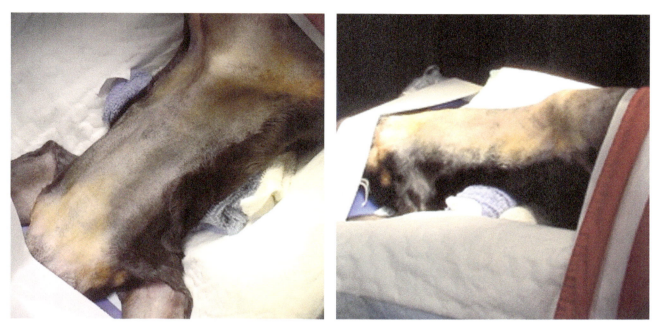

Figure 5.8 Two views of a patient positioned for a mid-cervical ventral slot. Note the rolled towel under the neck and the extension of the head and neck.

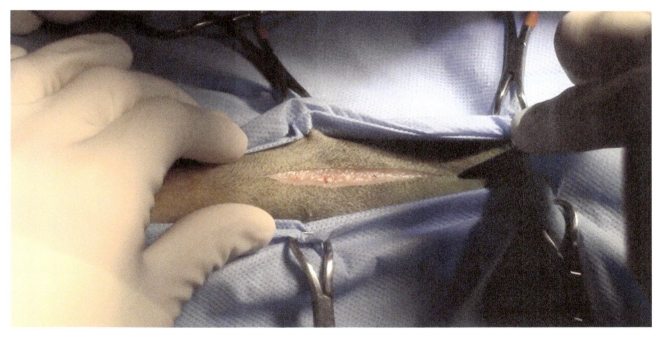

Figure 5.9 A ventral midline incision is made from the base of the larynx to the sternum.

bipolar cautery and the main vein is retracted with one of the sternohyoideus muscle bellies. Separation of these muscles exposes the trachea and its closely associated recurrent laryngeal nerve (Figure 5.11). To the surgeon's left is the right vasosympathetic trunk and the carotid sheath. To the surgeon's right are the trachea, recurrent laryngeal nerve, and esophagus. These structures are digitally separated to expose the underlying paired longus coli muscles which lie on the ventral surface of the cervical vertebrae. These muscles attach diagonally to the caudal

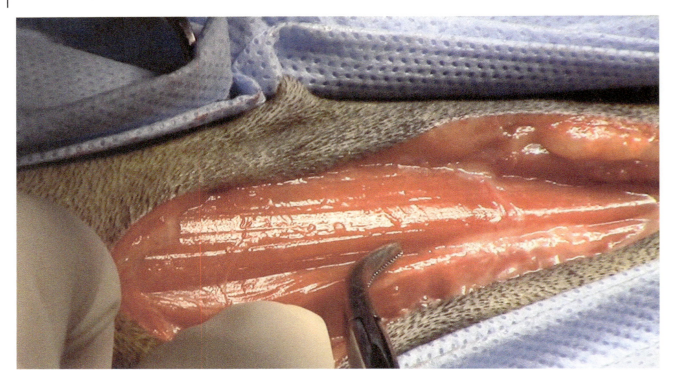

Figure 5.10   Exposure of the paired sternohyoideus muscles on the ventral midline.

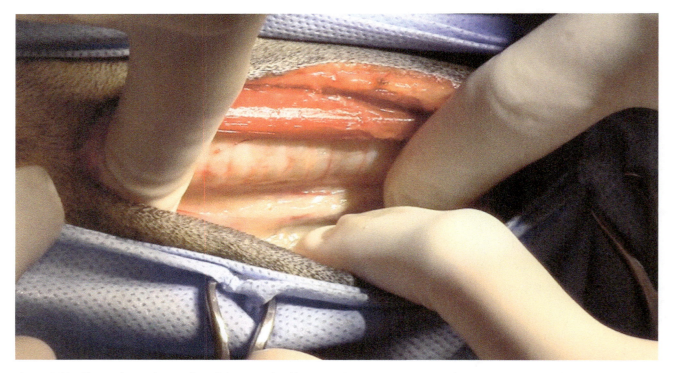

Figure 5.11   Separation and retraction of the sternohyoideus muscles reveals the underlying trachea and the adjacent recurrent laryngeal nerve.

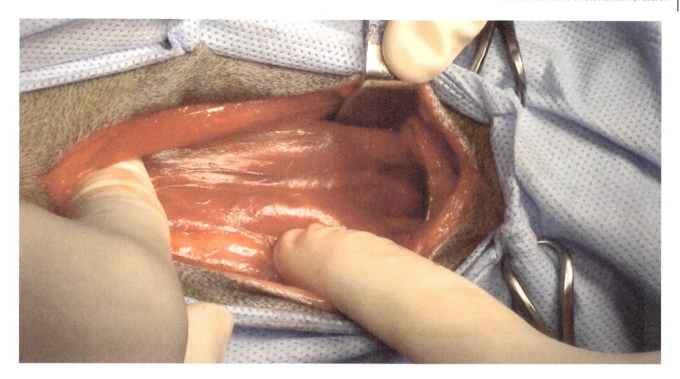

Figure 5.12 After retraction of the trachea to the surgeon's right and the right carotid sheath and vasosympathetic truck to the surgeon's left, the paired longus coli muscles are exposed. These muscles lie on the ventral surface of the cervical vertebrae. These muscles attach diagonally to the caudal ventral processes of the cervical vertebrae.

ventral processes of the cervical vertebrae (Figure 5.12). If available, an assistant uses Army-Navy retractors to retract the trachea, esophagus, and recurrent laryngeal nerve to the surgeon's right. Alternatively, self-retaining Frazier laminectomy retractors are positioned to retract the nearest carotid sheath toward the surgeon and the trachea, esophagus, and the opposite carotid sheath away from the surgeon.

Two landmarks for identification of the cervical IVD spaces are located (Figure 5.13). The cranial landmark is found by palpating the caudal borders of the wings of the

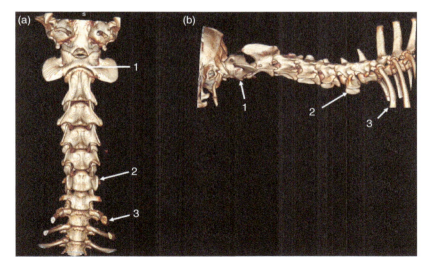

Figure 5.13 (a) Ventral and (b) lateral anatomic representations of the landmarks for identifying/locating the cervical vertebrae. 1: A sharp ventral prominence is palpated, which represents the C1–C2 interspace. 2: The large transverse processes of the C6 vertebra. 3: The first rib that attaches to the cranial aspect of the T1 vertebra.

atlas and following them to the ventral midline. At this point, a sharp ventral prominence is palpated, which represents the C1–C2 interspace. The first cervical IVD (C2–C3) is located by palpating caudally along the ventral midline until the next ventral prominence is encountered. The caudal landmark is the large transverse processes of the sixth cervical vertebra. These processes extend in a ventrolateral direction from the vertebral body and are lateral to the ventral midline. The surgeon should not mistake these transverse processes for the midline processes, an error that can lead to excessive hemorrhage. For additional identification, the surgeon can often continue careful digital palpation caudally and feel the first rib as it attaches to the cranial and lateral aspect of the T1 vertebrae.

Decompression of the Cervical Spinal Cord

The techniques described for decompression of the cervical spinal cord are the dorsal laminectomy, hemilaminectomy, and the ventral slot. Indications for decompression are the presence of motor deficits in one or more limbs or severe pain unresponsive to proper medical management and associated with extruded disk material within the spinal canal [1].

Ventral Slot Method

The involved disk is located by palpating the aforementioned landmarks and small curved hemostats are used to separate the longus coli muscle overlying the ventral annulus (Figure 5.14). The longus coli muscles are elevated periosteally and retracted laterally from the most caudal aspect of the targeted intervertebral disk through the entire length of one the cranial vertebra. The ventral annuli of the cervical disks are located just caudal to the caudal ventral-cervical processes. After elevation of the longus coli, a No. 15 or No. 11 scalpel blade is used to cut a window in the ventral annulus (Figure 5.14). The excised annulus is removed to expose the nucleus pulposus. A small tartar scraper or a 3–0 to 4–0 bone curette can be positioned in the disk space to remove the nucleus pulposus.

Gelpi retractors are positioned to retract the dissected musculature (Figure 5.15). All hemorrhage from the musculature is controlled before continuing the procedure.

Drilling is begun using a surgical drill equipped with an oblong bur (Figure 5.16). The elongated cutting surface of the oblong (oval or pineapple shaped) bur allows

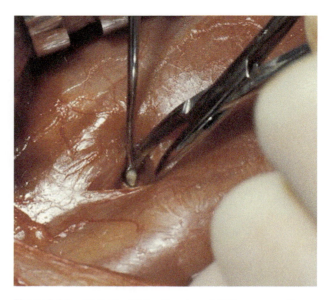

Figure 5.14 After identifying the correct IVD space, small, curved hemostats are used to separate the longus coli muscle overlying the ventral annulus. The ventral annulus is incised with a No. 15 or number 11 scalpel blade and then removed with hemostats. A small curette can be used to remove the nucleus pulposus from the disk space in chondrodystrophic dogs (fenestration technique).

for more even cutting on all sides and for the full depth of the slot. This improves the ability to maintain the entire slot perpendicular to the spinal canal. The slot should be parallel with the long axis of the vertebrae and extend from the most caudal aspect of the ventral anulus of the offending disk to approximately one-half to one-third of the cranial vertebra. Its width should not exceed one-half of the vertebral body width [1, 6, 7]. There is considerable debate about postoperative stability when considering the width of the slot and the type of slot [8, 9, 10]; however, when performing the ventral slot over one IVD space, the authors have not encountered issues with clinically relevant instability when limiting the width to one-half the width of the vertebra (Figure 5.17) if postoperative confinement is maintained for a period of at least two weeks. Limiting the width to one-third the width of the vertebral body greatly limits the visualization of the canal and the ability to remove extruded nucleus pulposus that is more lateral to the midline. Some authors have advocated the use of an inverted cone technique [9] as a means to reduce the chances of postoperative vertebral luxation, although this complication is considered a rare occurrence (8% in one study) [7]. Others recommend a slanted ventral slot technique [10] that seeks to limit the

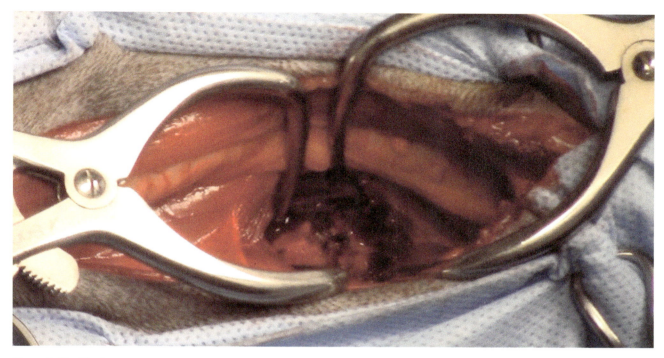

Figure 5.15 The longus coli muscle has been elevated over the ventral aspect of the vertebrae, and Gelpi retractors are positioned to retract the dissected musculature.

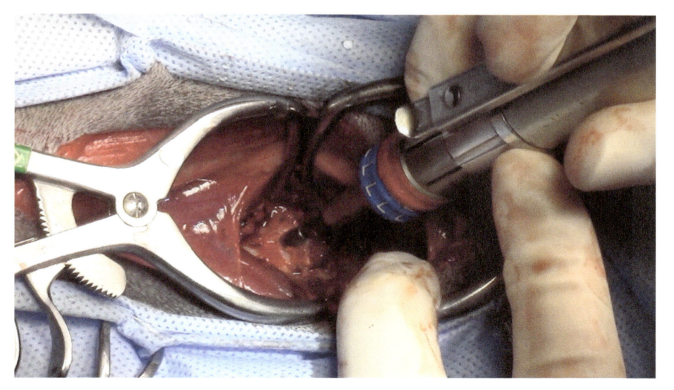

Figure 5.16 A pneumatic bur drill is positioned to begin the ventral slot. Note that an oblong/oval/pineapple shaped bur is used because it will cut evenly on all sides to produce a slot that is perpendicular on all sides.

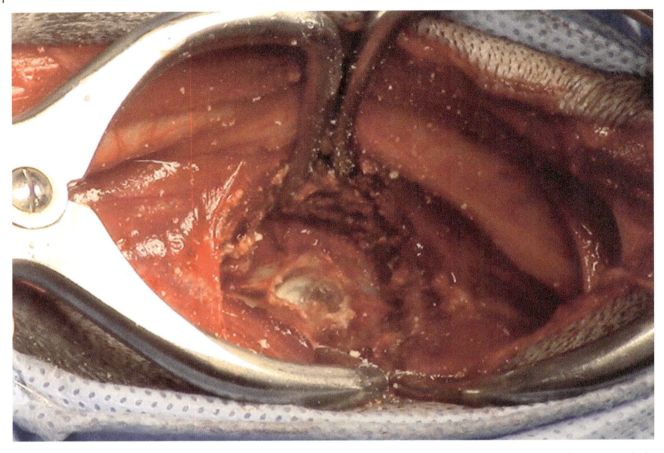

Figure 5.17 A partially completed slot. Notice that the slot is directly on midline and cranially you can see the white outer cortical bone and caudally the reddish-brown cancellous bone layer.

amount of anulus removed, but also limits visualization and perhaps excessive hemorrhage if the slanted slot extends too far cranially [5].

The surgeon begins drilling the white outer cortical bone, encounters cancellous bone next (Figure 5.18), and finally encounters the white inner cortical bone. The drilling is frequently interrupted throughout the procedure to allow irrigation of the surgical site and evaluation of the slot's depth [5, 8]. Hemorrhage from the cancellous bone is controlled by packing the area with bone wax [1, 5, 8].

The inner cortical bone is very thin and is drilled with caution to avoid damage to the spinal cord [5, 8]. With a thin shelf of cortical bone, the endosteum and the dorsal anulus are elevated and removed with small (1 mm) Love-Kerrison micro-rongeurs (Figure 5.19), a tartar scraper, curette, or similar instrument. This opens the spinal canal, exposing the dorsal longitudinal ligament, the spinal cord, and the extruded disk material. If intact, a small ear curette is used to explore the dorsal longitudinal ligament to find a rent that has allowed the extruded material to enter the canal. Rarely, the surgeon must carefully incise the dorsal longitudinal ligament with a No. 11 blade [5].

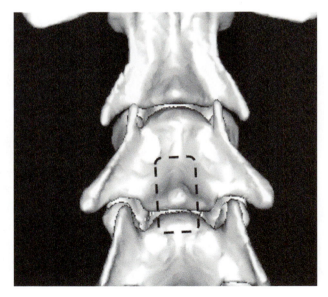

Figure 5.18 An anatomical illustration of a ventral view of the cervical vertebrae at the C3–C4 IVD space. The dotted lines represent an outline of the dimensions of the ventral slot. Adhering to this locale, the dorsal anulus will be in the middle of the slot.

5 Cervical Ventral Slot Decompression | 57

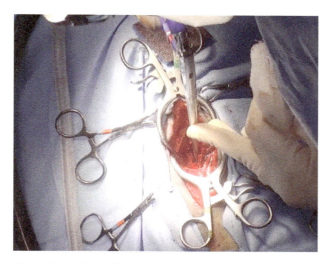

Figure 5.19 Micro-Kerrison 1 mm rongeurs are being placed into the canal and used to remove the dorsal annulus and the remaining thin layer of the inner cortical layer of bone.

The extruded disk material is removed from the spinal canal with a small, blunt neurosurgical probe or ear curette. Care is taken not to lacerate the large venous sinuses located just lateral to the slotted area. The extruded disk material may adhere to the sinuses, and removal of the material may result in hemorrhage. If hemorrhage occurs, an absorbable gelatin sponge is gently packed into the slot for a short time and the area lavaged with cold saline to aid in hemostasis. If the hemorrhage continues, the patient's head is elevated to relieve any pressure on the jugular veins that might contribute to the hemorrhage. When the canal has been cleared of the extruded disk and hemostasis is achieved, optimally the dura is visualized and the underlying spinal cord is not displaced dorsally or laterally (Figure 5.20). The surgical site is lavaged copiously and an absorbable gelatin sponge is placed ventrally over, but not into, the slot [5, 8].

The Gelpi retractors are removed and the longus coli muscle is apposed over the vertebrae, usually with a single cruciate mattress suture using 2-0 or 3-0 synthetic, resorbable, monofilament material. Prophylactic fenestration of other cervical disks concludes the procedure. Other cervical disks are often fenestrated for prophylaxis in chondrodystrophic dogs [1]. Routinely, cervical disks C2–C3 through C5–C6 are fenestrated during the operation. The incidence of C6–C7 IVD protrusions is low, and exposure of this space is sometimes difficult. Therefore, prophylactic fenestration of the C6–C7 IVD is unwarranted in most cases.

Closure of the sternohyoideus muscle is completed using a simple continuous pattern. The subcutaneous tissue and skin are closed in routine manner [1, 5].

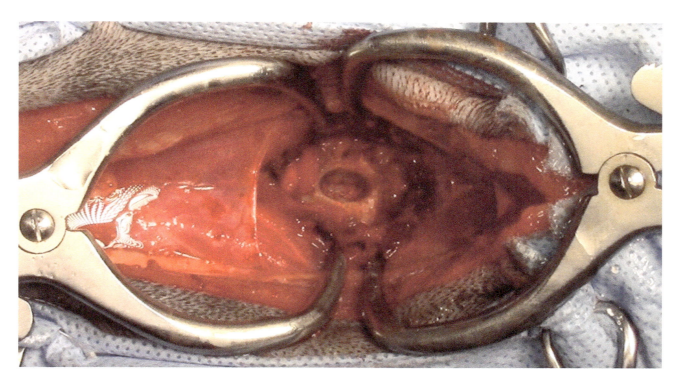

Figure 5.20 The completed slot. The inner cortical layer of the bone, the dorsal annulus, and the extruded IVD material have been removed. At the bottom of the slot, the dura is visualized.

Perioperative and Postoperative Care

Cefazolin is administered at a dose 20 mg/kg IV at the start and every 90 minutes during the surgery. If the patient does not have a history of NSAID use within the last 48 hours, methylprednisolone sodium succinate is administered at a dose of 20 mg/kg IV during the surgery. Corticosteroid usage will remain controversial and not all neurosurgeons will agree with this practice.

Pain management in our practice generally consists of an immediate initiation of midazolam at 0.3 mg/kg IV and either a low dose fentanyl CRI or every six-hour dosages of methadone at 0.1 mg/kg. When combining a benzodiazepam and an opioid, we tend to lower the opioid dose to mitigate any alterations in the swallowing reflex. The morning after surgery, the patient is transitioned to oral diazepam, acetaminophen, and gabapentin. Postoperative care includes two to three days hospitalization if ambulatory and cage rest for 14 days at home followed by a gradual return to function. For non-ambulatory patients, physical therapy is instituted soon after surgery and continues until the patient can be cared for in the home environment.

Video clips to accompany this book can be found on the companion website at: www.wiley.com/go/shores/advanced

References

1. Shores, A. (1985). Intervertebral disk disease. In: *Textbook of Small Animal Orthopaedics* (ed. C.D. Newton and D.M. Nunamaker), 739–764. Philadelphia: JD Lippincott Company.
2. Prata, R.G. and Stroll, S.G. (1973). Ventral decompression and fusion for the treatment of cervical disc disease in the dog. *J. Am. Anim. Hosp. Assoc.* 1: 462.
3. Hoerlein, B.F. (1978). Intervertebral disks. In: *Canine Neurology*, 3e (ed. B.F. Hoerlein), 470–560. Philadelphia: WB Saunders.
4. Shores, A. (1981). The intervertebral disk syndrome in the dog: Part 1. Pathophysiology and management. *Compend. Cont. Edu. Pract. Veterinarian* 3: 639.
5. Dewey, C.W. (2013). Surgery of the cervical spine. In: *Small Animal Surgery*, 4e (ed. T.W. Fossum), 1467–1507. Philadelphia: Mosby, Inc.
6. Swaim, S.F. (1973). Ventral decompression of the cervical spinal cord in the dog. *J. Am. Vet. Med. Assoc.* 162: 276.
7. Gilpin, G.N. (1976). Evaluation of three techniques of ventral decompression of the cervical spinal cord in the dog. *J. Am. Vet. Med. Assoc.* 168 (4): 325–328. PMID: 943386.
8. da Costa, R.C. (2017). Ventral cervical decompression. In: *Current Techniques in Canine and Feline Neurosurgery* (ed. A. Shores and B.A. Brisson), 157–162. Hoboken, NJ: Wiley.
9. Goring, R.L., Beale, B.S., and Faulkner, R.F. (1991). The inverted cone technique: a surgical treatment for cervical vertebral instability "wobbler syndrome" in Doberman pinchers. *J. Am. Anim. Hosp. Assoc.* 27: 403–409.
10. McCartney, W. (2007). Comparison of recovery times and complication rates between a modified slanted slot and the standard ventral slot for treatment of cervical disc disease in dogs. *J. Small. Anim. Pract.* 48: 498–501.

6

Thoracolumbar Decompression: Hemilaminectomy and Mini-Hemilaminectomy (Pediculectomy)

Brigitte A. Brisson

University of Guelph, Guelph, Ontario, Canada

Indications

Hemilaminectomy and mini-hemilaminectomy are considered the standard of care for removal of extruded disk material in the thoracolumbar region [1]. Additional indications for mini-hemilaminectomy and hemilaminectomy include decompression of inflammatory lesions (e.g. discospondylitis/osteomyelitis), decompression following spinal trauma (e.g. fracture, hematoma, protrusion of bony fragments), removal of laterally or ventrally located tumors to address appropriately located subarachnoid diverticula, and for removal of foreign material.

Procedures

Hemilaminectomy removes the articular processes of two adjacent vertebrae as well as a portion of the associated pedicles (Figure 6.1a). Mini-hemilaminectomy, also termed pediculectomy, consists of removing a portion of the pedicle bone of two adjacent vertebrae to enlarge the existing intervertebral foramen while preserving the articular processes [2–7] (Figure 6.1b). Although the partial pediculectomy technique described by McCartney [8] spares the accessory process (Figure 6.1c), the pediculectomy procedure removes the accessory process to form the dorsal margin of the laminectomy [4–6]. Removal of the accessory process has been shown to result in mild to moderate invasion of the ventral aspect of the articular processes in most dogs [9, 10].

The window provided by the mini-hemilaminectomy is adequate to visualize the ventrolateral aspect of the vertebral canal and provides excellent access to retrieve ventrally or laterally extruded disk material while limiting intraoperative spinal cord manipulation [2, 4, 9, 10]. Although direct access to the dorsal aspect of the canal may be limited compared to hemilaminectomy [9], this was not shown to have an impact on the ability to retrieve disk material in a series of clinical patients [10]. Mini-hemilaminectomy offers good visualization of the dorsal nerve root and ganglia and of the venous plexus located on the floor of the spinal canal [4, 9]. Preservation of the majority of the articular processes reduces postoperative vertebral instability compared to hemilaminectomy [11]. Effective spinal cord decompression can be achieved from T10 to L6 using this procedure [4]. The dorsolateral and lateral approaches used for mini-hemilaminectomy and hemilaminectomy also allow direct access to the IVD for fenestration [2, 4, 8]. As with hemilaminectomy, the mini-hemilaminectomy window is created close to the vertebral venous plexus (sinus) and foraminal structures, requiring care to prevent hemorrhage and nerve root damage [4, 10].

A mini-hemilaminectomy can easily be converted into a hemilaminectomy or be extended over several adjacent vertebrae if required [4]. This author has performed continuous mini-hemilaminectomies over as many as five contiguous vertebrae without complication. The latter is also reportedly possible with hemilaminectomy [5, 12]. Because mini-hemilaminectomy does not significantly invade the articular processes, it can also be performed bilaterally without causing vertebral instability. This is, however, dependent on a portion of the pedicle being left intact (cranial and/or caudal to the pediculectomy window) to prevent disconnecting the dorsal lamina from the vertebral body [13]. Similarly, mini-hemilaminectomy can easily be extended into a corpectomy if desired.

Advanced Techniques in Canine and Feline Neurosurgery, First Edition. Edited by Andy Shores and Brigitte A. Brisson.
© 2023 John Wiley & Sons, Inc. Published 2023 by John Wiley & Sons, Inc.
Companion site: www.wiley.com/go/shores/advanced

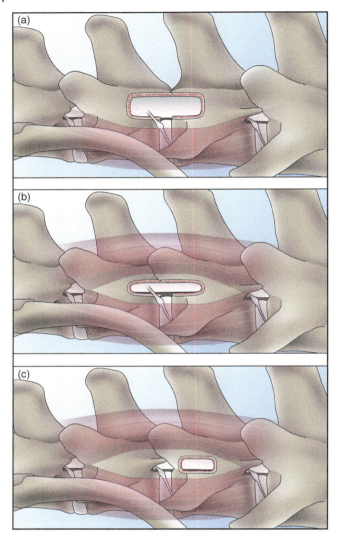

Figure 6.1 Illustrations depicting the approach and bony defect of (a) hemilaminectomy, (b) mini-hemilaminectomy or pediculectomy or foraminotomy, and (c) partial pediculectomy.

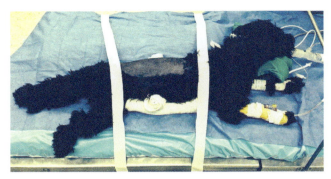

Figure 6.2 Oblique patient positioning (midway between sternal and lateral) with the spine rotated away from the surgeon and with the affected side facing up. A sandbag is placed behind the patient and under the table cover to maintain the oblique position. A rolled towel of appropriate size is placed under the patient's spine at the level of the lesion to open the disk space and facilitate fenestration of the affected disk. In some patients, as shown here, a small sandbag or towel can be tucked under the abdomen in order to straighten the spine and further stabilize the patient.

Technique: Surgical Approach for Mini-Hemilaminectomy (Video 6.1)

Mini-hemilaminectomy can be performed through a lateral or dorsolateral approach. An area caudal to the scapula and cranial to the wing of the ilium is clipped bilaterally but more so on the side of the lesion and is prepared for aseptic surgery. The patient is positioned in lateral (limbs toward the surgeon) [4, 8, 14, 15] or oblique (midway between sternal and lateral recumbency with the spine rotated away from the surgeon and with the affected side facing up) recumbency for a lateral approach [16] and in sternal [14, 15] or oblique [9, 10, 17] recumbency for a dorsolateral approach [16]. This author positions the patient obliquely for mini-hemilaminectomy and uses a dorsolateral approach as it appears to provide the best surgical field and access under the facet joints (Figure 6.2).

With the lateral and oblique position, the front limbs are tied cranially and the hind limbs are tied caudally with tape or ties. A small, rolled towel is placed under the patient, perpendicular to the spine at the level of the lesion to elevate the spine toward the surgeon, open the disk space and facilitate fenestration of the affected disk space. A small sand bag or towel is tucked under the abdomen in order to straighten the spine cranio-caudally and to further stabilize the patient. When performing surgery in a sternal position, the hind limbs are flexed cranially to maintain the normal curvature of the spine.

Review of the diagnostic images prior to surgery is essential to ensure there are no missing ribs or unusually shaped transverse processes that could confuse lesion localization.

Dorsolateral Approach [14–17] (Video 6.2)

The thoracolumbar area is palpated to identify the last rib and grossly localize the site of herniation. With the dorsolateral approach, a skin incision is made toward the affected side, approximately 1–2 cm lateral to dorsal midline over the area of interest and extending over 1–2 vertebrae cranial and caudal to the lesion as required. The incision is carried through the subcutaneous fat and fascia to identify the thick lumbo-dorsal fascia. Although some descriptions recommend undermining the fat on either side of the proposed incision through the lumbo-dorsal fascia to facilitate closure [15, 17], this is not necessary; it creates dead space and increases the risk of postoperative seroma formation. An incision through the

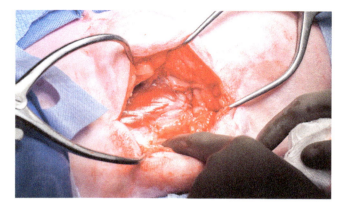

Figure 6.3 Focal finger palpation between the fascicles of the iliocostalis musculature in a large breed dog undergoing mini-hemilaminectomy allows the surgeon to palpate and count the ribs and transverse processes for orientation.

thoracolumbar fascia exposes a second layer of fat of variable thickness. In the caudal thoracic region, the caudal border of the spinalis and semispinalis thoracis muscles must also be incised. Focal finger palpation between the fascicles of the iliocostalis musculature allows the surgeon to palpate and count the ribs and transverse processes for orientation (Figure 6.3). The last rib and transverse process of L1 are landmarks used to localize the lesion site. Once the desired space is identified, the intermuscular plane between the multifidus and longissimus lumborum musculature is identified and bluntly dissected leaving the attachments of the multifidus muscle along the articular processes intact. Once the bone of the pedicle is identified, the longissimus muscle is elevated with a periosteal elevator to expose the pedicle and the attachment of the tendon of the longissimus muscle to the accessory process. This tendon is transected using a blade or Mayo scissors; the author typically uses bipolar cautery to cauterize and separate this attachment. Gelpi retractors are used to provide retraction of the multifidus muscle dorso-medially and the longissimus muscle ventrolaterally.

Variation

Bitetto and Thacher [2] described a modified lateral decompression technique that used a dorsal midline approach like that described for hemilaminectomy (see hemilminectomy approach below). This approach has since been used and reported on by others [5–7]. While the dorsal approach would allow easy conversion to a hemilaminectomy or dorsal laminectomy if this was required, it lengthens the procedure time and increases tissue dissection and trauma and is not considered the approach of choice for mini-hemilaminectomy by this author.

Recommended Variation

This author uses a modified dorsolateral approach that incises through the longissimus muscle fibers, directly over the area of the intervertebral foramen of interest. This previously described approach [13] was also described in a case series [9, 18]. As per the other approaches, focal finger palpation between the fascicles of the iliocostalis musculature allows the surgeon to palpate and count the ribs and transverse processes for orientation (Figure 6.3). After exposing the epaxial musculature through a dorsolateral approach made 1–2 cm lateral to the dorsal midline on the side of the lesion, a #15 blade is used to create a focal incision and dissection plane along and through the fibers of the m. longissimus thoracis and lumborum. The incision is made midway between the articular processes and the rib heads or transverse processes (Figure 6.4 and Video 6.2). Through this small incision, pedicle bone is identified and the incision is extended as required cranially and caudally using a combination of sharp dissection, periosteal elevation and muscle retraction (Gelpi) (Figure 6.5). In small dogs, the

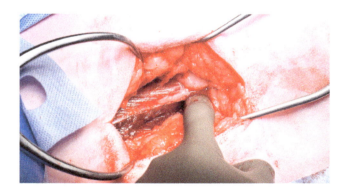

Figure 6.4 The incision is made midway between the articular processes and the rib heads or transverse processes in a large breed dog undergoing mini-hemilaminectomy. Palpation is repeated to confirm accurate surgical site.

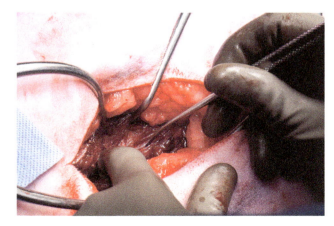

Figure 6.5 The pedicle bone is identified and the incision is extended as required cranially and caudally using a combination of sharp dissection, periosteal elevation, and muscle retraction (Gelpi).

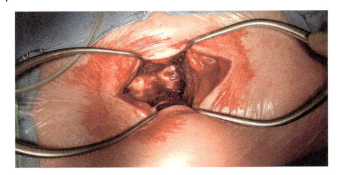

Figure 6.6 Short jawed (1-in.), right-angled Gelpi rectractors are preferred for mini-hemilaminectomies in small dogs.

author uses two 1-in. right-angled Gelpi (Figure 6.6) for their low profile. The attachment of the tendon of the longissimus muscle to the accessory process is cauterized and transected using a blade, scissors, the sharp edge of the periosteal elevator, or preferably bipolar cautery. Gelpi retractors are used at either end of the incision to provide retraction of the dorsal portion of the longissimus muscle dorsally and of the remainder of the longissimus and iliocostalis muscles ventrally. Sometimes, a third Gelpi or a weitlaner retractor is added midway through the incision to improve visualization. With this approach, only the desired adjacent pedicle bones and a small portion of the rib head/base of transverse process are exposed (Figure 6.7; Video 6.3). Although this approach traumatizes the fibers of the longissimus muscle focally, it reduces the overall amount of muscle dissection required for exposure (faster) and leads to a smaller mass of muscle that must be elevated and retracted either ventrally or dorsally compared to the other approaches. This results in an overall smaller incision and is especially helpful in the lumbar area of larger dogs where dorsal retraction of the bulky

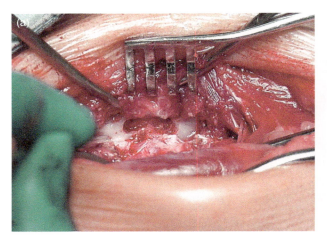
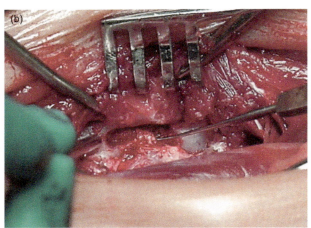
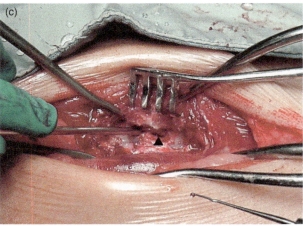

Figure 6.7 Mini-hemilaminectomy performed to remove extruded disk material in a 5.5 kg dog using a modified dorsolateral approach that separates the longissimus lomborum muscle fibers. (a) Before, (b) during, and (c) after removal of extruded disk material. Note that the spinal cord (arrow head) has returned to its normal position within the spinal canal and is clearly visible after removal of the extruded disk material (c).

iliocostalis muscle can be challenging [3]. By providing direct access to the site of surgery, this modified dorsolateral approach also facilitates ventral drilling for mini-hemilaminectomy or corpectomy and provides a direct access to the intervertebral disk for fenestration.

Technique: Mini-Hemilaminectomy Procedure

Once the lateral pedicles of the two vertebrae of interest are identified, they are cleared of soft tissues using a periosteal elevator until the tendinous attachment of the longissimus muscle is visualized on the accessory process of the cranial most vertebra. The tendon is cauterized using diathermy and then sharply transected at the level of its insertion on the accessory process which exposes the desired intervertebral foramen (Figure 6.8). The self-retaining retractors are adjusted to provide further exposure of the bony structures. When exposure seems limited, muscle retraction and visualization can be facilitated by "blindly" transecting the tendon of the longissimus muscle attachment to the vertebra cranial and/or caudal to the decompression site. Any remaining soft tissue attachments along the pedicles of the two vertebrae of interest are cleared off using a periosteal elevator and retraction continues to be maintained with self-retaining retractors; typically two Gelpi retractors. The surgical exposure spans a space dorsal to the level of the rib head/transverse process, and ventral to the base of the articular processes, without exposing the articular processes. Cranially and caudally, the dissection extends to, but does not expose the adjacent intervertebral foraminae unless an extended decompression is sought (Figure 6.7).

Mini-hemilaminectomy is performed using a drill. The accessory process that overlies the dorsal aspect of the foramen is first removed using rongeurs or preferably a drill and this forms the dorsal-most extent of the mini-hemilaminectomy, thus leaving the zygapophyseal joint intact [4, 5, 9]. The small artery located just medial to the accessory process is coagulated with bipolar diathermy [5]. Ventral to this, the pedicle is thinned cranially and caudally to essentially enlarge the intervertebral foramen over approximately 1/2 to 2/3 of the length of each vertebra; or longer if the extruded disk extends beyond [4, 9, 10]. The ventral extent of the mini-hemilaminectomy is as much as possible the ventral aspect of the intervertebral foramen/spinal canal [4]. The cranial and caudal aspects of the laminectomy are based on advanced imaging and can be extended as required until normal epidural fat is identified or until the surgeon believes all extruded disk material has been removed [4, 9, 10].

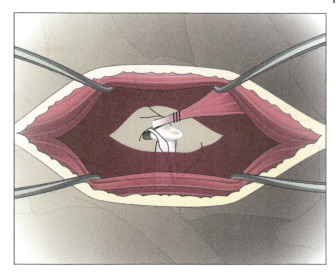

Figure 6.8 Illustration demonstrating that the lateral pedicles of interest are identified, cleared of soft tissues using a periosteal elevator, and the tendinous attachment of the longissimus musculature is cauterized and then sharply transected at the level of its insertion on the accessory process, exposing the desired intervertebral foramen.

The pedicle bone is drilled using a high-speed air or electric drill taking notice of the change from cortical (white) to more spongy (red) cancellous bone (Figure 6.9 and Video 6.4). As much as possible, the bone should be thinned evenly, preventing early focal penetration in any one area of the canal (Figure 6.10). Sterile saline lavage and suction is performed regularly to remove bony debris and cool the bone. Cancellous bone hemorrhage can be controlled as needed using small amounts of bone wax. Note that cancellous bone will not be present at the edge of the foramen and that the bony edge will also be thinner in this area. The surgeon should assess bony thickness visually and by palpating with a small blunt probe (e.g. Iris spatula, small curette, static drill bit) as often as needed. Once the cancellous bone is removed and the inner cortical bone is thinned out to a moveable, thin layer of periosteum, it can be penetrated using a 22 gauge needle with the tip bent at 90° and a #11 scalpel blade (Figure 6.11; Video 6.5), or with a dural hook or tartar scraper exposing the spinal canal over the entire length of the laminectomy. Some surgeons prefer to use a house curette or Kerrison rongeur to remove the inner periosteal edges. Should the laminectomy site need to be extended ventrally or cranio-caudally, it is best done before removing the extruded disk material because this will allow the displaced spinal cord to return to a more normal position within the laminectomy site exposing it to potential iatrogenic trauma.

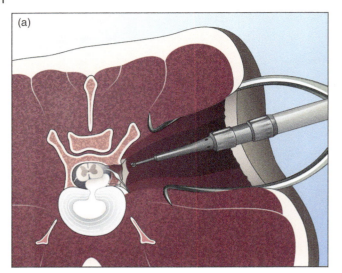
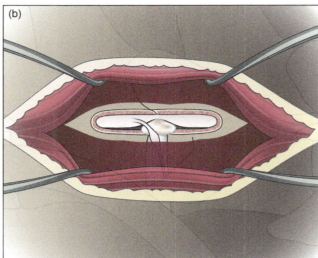

Figure 6.9 Illustration of cross-section and sagittal view of the vertebral spine depicting the bone window provided by the pediculectomy approach. This procedure provides direct access to the lateral and ventral spinal canal for removal of extruded disk material while leaving the articular facets intact.

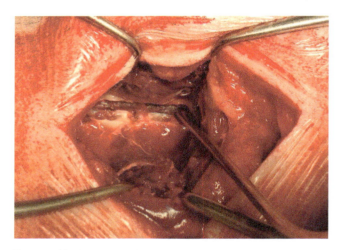

Figure 6.10 Intraoperative image showing a long pediculectomy with the bone thinned evenly across the length of the pediculectomy. Dark hemorrhage/disk can be seen through the thin remaining inner cortical bone layer.

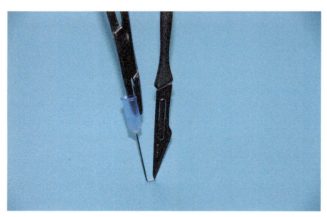

Figure 6.11 Bent needle (90°) and #11 blade used to enter the spinal canal after drilling the pedicle bone to a paper thin layer of cortical bone/periosteum.

Technique: Surgical Approach for Hemilaminectomy

A dorsolateral [19–22] or a lateral [4] approach to the thoracolumbar spine is used for the hemilaminectomy procedure. The dorsolateral approach provides the best exposure [20, 23] and is the more commonly used approach [22].

The patient is placed in sternal recumbency. A sandbag or rolled towel can be placed under the abdomen to slightly arch the spine. An area 7–10 cm on either side of the dorsal midline and from T7 to approximately L5 is clipped and prepared for surgery. Depending on the desired exposure, the midline skin incision should extend one to three vertebrae cranial and caudal to the lesion. The cutaneous trunci muscle is usually incised with the skin followed by the subcutaneous tissue and fat. If desired, a section of fat (~ 3 cm long × 2 cm wide) is excised, wrapped in a saline moistened gauze and stored sterilely for use at the end of the procedure (Figure 6.12) [23].

With the thick, thoracolumbar fascia exposed, the midline is identified by palpating the spinous processes of the thoracolumbar vertebrae. The fascia is incised beginning at the dorsal midline between the first two spinous processes

Technique: Hemilaminectomy Procedure

Palpation through or between the fibers of the longissimus muscle allow the surgeon to identify the most caudal rib and transverse process of L1 to confirm correct location. Hemilaminectomy begins by removing the articular processes directly over the involved IVD with a bone rongeur or surgical drill (Figures 6.14–6.16) [19–21]. As described for mini-hemilaminectomy, a surgical drill is typically used to create the hemilaminectomy [20, 25]. Alternatively, rongeurs can be used in smaller (<10 kg) dogs [20]. A typical hemilaminectomy extends one vertebral body length cranial and caudal to the affected IVD (Figures 6.14 and 6.17). The final length of the hemilaminectomy defect is governed by the appearance of the spinal cord and adjacent tissue within the canal. The length is extended until normal appearing tissue is encountered (presence of epidural fat; absence of IVD material or cord swelling). Lempert rongeurs, Kerrison rongeurs, or the surgical drill can be used to lengthen the hemilaminectomy when necessary [26]. Of critical importance is assuring the opening extends ventrally to the floor of the spinal canal. Failure to do this often results in failure to visualize and remove portions of the

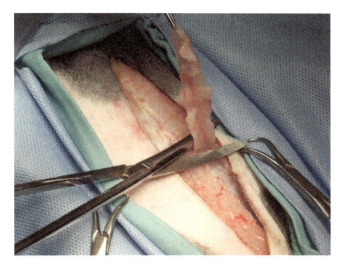

Figure 6.12 A approximately 3 cm long × 2 cm wide × 0.3 cm thick portion of the thoracolumbar subcutaneous adipose tissue is excised at the *beginning* of surgery, then wrapped in a moistened gauze sponge and stored for use at the end of the procedure.

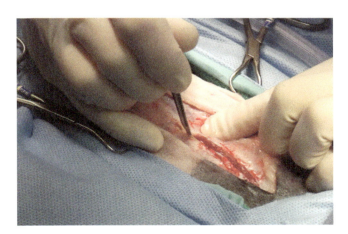

Figure 6.13 The thoracolumbar fascia is incised in a scalloped fashion, beginning at the dorsal midline between the first two spinous processes, hugging the near lateral aspect of the spinous process, returning to midline between each vertebra.

and undulating around the spinal processes and returning to midline between each vertebra (Figure 6.13) exposing the underlying multifidus muscle. Starting at the caudal aspect of the incision, the multifidus muscle is then elevated (using a periosteal elevator, the blunt end of a scalpel, or osteotomes) from the lateral aspect of the spinal processes and the articular facets and the tendinous attachments severed at each vertebra as the dissection is carried cranially [21]. Retraction is maintained using Gelpi retractors. A dry gauze sponge can be used to remove any remaining muscular attachments over the exposed vertebrae [21].

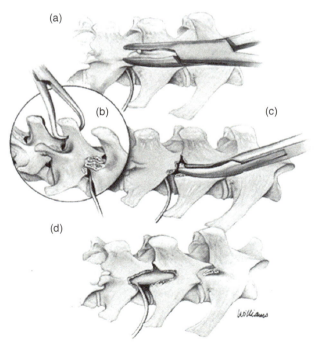

Figure 6.14 The hemilaminectomy. (a) Removal of the articular processes with rongeurs. (b) Elevation of the vertebra with a towel clamp to widen the articular space. (c) Performing the hemilaminectomy with Lempert rongeurs. (d) The completed hemilaminectomy [24].

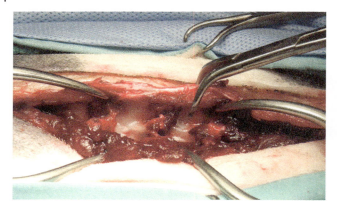

Figure 6.15 Placement of Backhaus towel forceps through the spinous process of the vertebra just cranial to the extruded disk. An assistant gently elevates the forceps to open the vertebral articulation, expanding the surgeon's access for placement of the Lempert rongeurs used to perform the hemilaminectomy.

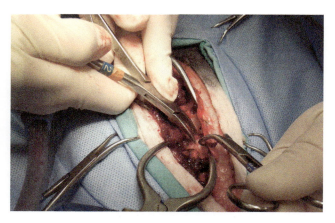

Figure 6.16 Placement of the Lempert rongeur tips in the small separation between the articular facets to begin the hemilaminectomy. Note the surgeon places the index finger from the opposite hand against the shaft of the rongeur to prevent inadvertent slipping of the instrument toward the canal as the cut is made.

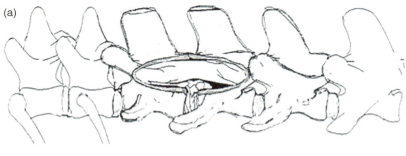

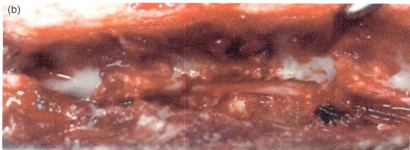

Figure 6.17 (a) Illustration and (b) intraoperative photograph of the completed hemilaminectomy. Note the ventral extent of the opening to the floor of the spinal canal. Failure expose to this level may prevent visualization and removal of portions of the extruded disk material or undue trauma when sweeping underneath the spinal cord to remove disk material.

extruded disk material or undue trauma when sweeping underneath the spinal cord to remove disk material.

Removal of Disk Material: Mini-Hemilaminectomy and Hemilaminectomy

Necrotic fat, hemorrhage, as well as soft and hard disk material are retrieved using a blunt probe (Iris spatula or ophthalmic strabismus hook), small curette or suction (the suction tip should never be allowed to contact the dura) while avoiding manipulation of the spinal cord and trauma to the dorsal nerve root. After removal of the disk material located lateral to the spinal cord (visible upon entry), sweeping extends ventrally and then dorsally to ensure as much extruded disk material as possible is removed. When sweeping the canal, care should be taken to retrieve disk material rather than push it toward the opposite side or beyond the laminectomy window. The author prefers to use a bent Iris spatula that moves from cranio-dorsal and from dorso-caudal toward the mid-section of the bony window ventrally (Video 6.6). Hard or adherent disk material may also be removed with a #11 scalpel blade [3, 17, 27]. Chronically extruded disk material may form adhesions to the venous sinus, the nerve root, and vascular bundle or the dura mater and could result in laceration of the venous sinus and hemorrhage during removal. Venous sinus hemorrhage can be controlled by applying direct pressure using an Iris spatula or placing a small block of gelatin sponge directly at the site of hemorrhage [27]. Although the gelatin sponge can be left in place if required [27], it should be removed, if possible, prior to closing the surgical defect. A preferred alternative is to fill the entire laminectomy defect with a pre-cut piece of gelatin sponge and to fill the surgical site with cool or room temperature saline to increase pressure at the laminectomy site and promote clotting without direct contact between the gelatin sponge and the vascular defect. After three to five minutes, the saline can be suctioned and the gelatin sponge gently removed without peeling away a blood clot at the level of the vascular defect, usually ventral to the spinal cord. Hemorrhage caused by a laceration of the spinal artery or vein should be controlled using diathermy.

Once the extruded disk material is removed, the spinal cord should return to a normal position within the spinal canal. In instances where the spinal cord remains displaced, the surgeon should consider that additional disk material might be present either cranially, caudally, or on the contralateral side (rare with preoperative advanced imaging) requiring extension of the laminectomy in either direction or that a contralateral procedure should be performed. Indentation of the spinal cord at the site of extrusion is possible and most common in chronic cases and does not require treatment as long as the compressive mass is removed.

If sufficient disk material is not retrieved, the surgeon should verify that the correct site and side was approached surgically. If the correct site/side was approached, the surgeon might consider extending the mini-hemilaminectomy cranially (most common), or caudally to find disk material extruded further away within the spinal canal. When significant amounts of disk material are not recovered, high impact, low volume disk extrusion or an incorrect diagnosis should also be considered. In such cases, imaging should be reviewed and possibly repeated.

Durotomy may be of interest in patients with severe neurological signs as it may improve the outcome and lessen the risk of development of myelomalacia in dogs with loss of deep pain perception [1, 28]. Durotomy can be initiated and extended using a #12 blade (cutting tip facing up) or with a bent hypodermic needle and a #11 scalpel blade.

In situations where a more chronic disk protrusion is identified, the laminectomy window can be extended to include a corpectomy. Chronically adhered disk material may not peel off the dura as easily as acute disk material and some material can be left in situ as long as the main compressive lesion is removed.

If desired, fenestration of the affected and adjacent disk spaces can be performed through these approaches (See Chapter 7).

A lumbar fat graft or gelatin sponge are used to cover the surgical site after hemilaminectomy [20, 29], but are not usually placed over the mini-hemilaminectomy site [3, 10].

Closure

Hemostasis is ascertained prior to closure. Lavage of the surgical site with warm sterile saline is performed to suction residual bony debris and any blood clots. Standard closure of the deep and superficial thoracolumbar fascia is performed using a simple continuous pattern of absorbable monofilament (3-0 or 2-0 PDS) suture. The subcutaneous tissues (3-0 Monocryl) and skin are closed routinely (Video 6.7).

Complications

The presence of residual disk material is noted in as many as 100% of patients that recover satisfactorily after hemilaminectomy and is rarely found to be clinically significant [30]. In contrast, residual disk material (7.7%, range 0–27.3%) was found in 44% of 9 patients undergoing mini-hemilaminectomy when pre- and postoperative MRI were compared [10]. Delayed recovery or lack of postoperative improvement has been associated with the presence of large amounts of residual disk material related to the wrong approach, shifting of disk material during surgery, and to the herniation of additional disk material within the spinal canal, sometimes requiring further imaging and surgery [31–33]. Failure to retrieve disk material, requiring extension to a different disk space or a bilateral procedure, is considered a major complication [3]. A disadvantage of the mini-hemilaminectomy vs hemilaminectomy is that the lateral or oblique positioning of the dog requires that the surgical site be closed and the patient be repositioned if the wrong side was initially approached surgically [3]. Nowadays, this is less likely to occur with the routine use of preoperative advanced imaging [31]. When lateralization is not evident (ventral lesion), most surgeons choose the side based on preference; most right-handed surgeons prefer approaching the left side [34]. An advantage of the mini-hemilaminectomy over the hemilaminectomy is that it can be performed bilaterally without compromise to the bony support or soft tissues [13].

Hemorrhage is typically minor and in most instances is easily controlled; but in cases where severe hemorrhage is encountered, it can hinder visualization and prevent adequate spinal decompression or lead to marked blood loss [35].

Postoperative Care

Following mini-hemilaminectomy or hemilaminectomy, dogs are hospitalized on intravenous fluids and injectable analgesics until comfortable enough to receive oral medications (typically 24 hours). Discharge is most commonly within 48 hours of surgery in patients that retain motor function. Dogs with loss of motor function are typically discharged once voluntary urinary control is confirmed or when the owners are comfortable expressing the bladder at home. Postoperative rehabilitation is recommended in most cases.

As for hemilaminectomy, overall recovery rates of greater than 90% have been reported following mini-hemilaminectomy with or without prophylactic fenestration [2, 3, 5–7, 35, 36].

 Video clips to accompany this book can be found on the companion website at: www.wiley.com/go/shores/advanced

References

1. ACVIM (2022). Consensus statement on diagnosis and management of acute canine thoracolumbar intervertebral disc extrusion. *J. Vet. Intern. Med.*, Forthcoming.
2. Bitetto, W.V. and Thacher, C. (1986). A modified lateral decompression technique for treatment of canine intervertebral disk disease. *J. Am. Anim. Hosp. Assoc.* 23: 409–413.
3. Black, A.P. (1988). Lateral spinal decompression in the dog: a review of 39 cases. *J. Small Anim. Pract.* 29: 581–588.
4. Braund, K.G., Taylor, T.K., Ghosh, P. et al. (1976). Lateral spinal decompression in the dog. *J. Small Anim. Pract.* 17: 583–592.
5. Jeffery, N.D. (1988). Treatment of acute and chronic thoracolumbar disc disease by "mini hemilaminectomy". *J. Small Anim. Pract.* 29: 611–616.
6. Lubbe, A.M., Kirberger, R.M., and Verstraete, F.J.M. (1994). Pediculectomy for thoracolumbar spinal decompression in the dachshund. *J. Am. Anim. Hosp. Assoc.* 30: 233–238.
7. Yovich, J.C., Read, R., and Eger, C. (1994). Modified lateral spinal decompression in 61 dogs with thoracolumbar disc protrusion. *J. Small Anim. Pract.* 35: 351–356.
8. McCartney, W. (1997). Partial pediculectomy for the treatment of thoracolumbar disc disease. *Vet. Comp. Orthop. Traumatol.* 10: 117–121.
9. Huska, J.L., Gaitero, L., Brisson, B.A. et al. (2014). Comparison of the access window created by hemilaminectomy and mini-hemilaminectomy in the thoracolumbar vertebral canal using computed tomography. *Can. Vet. J.* 55 (5): 449–455.
10. Huska, J.L., Gaitero, L., Brisson, B.A. et al. (2014). Presence of residual material following mini-hemilaminectomy in dogs with thoracolumbar intervertebral disc extrusion. *Can. Vet. J.* 55 (10): 975–980.
11. Hill, T.P., Lubbe, A.M., and Guthrie, A.J. (2000). Lumbar spine stability following hemilaminectomy, pediculectomy, and fenestration. *Vet. Comp. Orthop. Traumatol.* 13: 165–171.
12. Corse, M.R., Renberg, W.C., and Friis, E.A. (2003). in vitro evaluation of biomechanical effects of multiple hemilaminectomies on the canine lumbar vertebral column. *Am. J. Vet. Res.* 64 (9): 1139–1145. https://doi.org/10.2460/ajvr.2003.64.1139. PMID: 13677392.
13. Slocum, B. and Slocum, T.D. (1998). Thoracolumbar spine: pediculotomy in the thoracolumbar vertebra. In: *Current Techniques in Small Animal Surgery*, 4e (ed. M.J. Bojrab, G.W. Ellison and B. Slocum), 835–858. Baltimore: Williams & Wilkins.
14. Kerwin, S.C., Levine, J.M., and Hicks, D.G. (2012). Thoracolumbar spine. In: *Veterinary Surgery Small Animal* (ed. K.M. Tobias and S.A. Johnston), 449–475. St-Louis: Elsevier.

15. Piermattei, D.L. and Johnson, K.A. (2004). The vertebral column. In: *An Atlas of Surgical Approaches to the Bones and Joints of the Dog and Cat*, 4e, 47–105. Philadelphia: Saunders.

16. Dewey, C. (2013). Surgery of the thoracolumbar spine. In: *Small Animal Surgery*, 4e (ed. T.W. Fossum), 1508–1528. St-Louis: Elsevier.

17. Sharp, N. and Wheeler, S. (2005). Thoracolumbar disc disease. In: *Small Animal Spinal Disorders: Diagnosis and Surgery* (ed. N. Sharp and S. Wheeler), 121–159. Philadelphia: Elsevier Mosby.

18. Tanaka, N., Kitagawa, M., Ito, D., and Watari, T. (2013). A modified lateral muscle-separation approach for mini-hemilaminectomy. *Vet. Rec.* 173 (12): 296.

19. Gage, E.D. (1975). Modifications in dorsolateral hemilaminectomy and disc fenestration in the dog. *J. Am. Anim. Hosp. Assoc.* 11: 407.

20. Hoerlein, B.F. (1978). The status of the various intervertebral disc surgeries for the dog in 1978. *J. Am. Anim. Hosp. Assoc.* 14: 563–570.

21. Shores, A. (1985). Intervertebral disk disease. In: *Textbook of Small Animal Orthopaedics* (ed. C.D. Newton and D.M. Nunamaker), 739–764. Philadelphia: JB Lippincott.

22. Toombs, J.P. and Waters, D.J. (2003). Intervertebral disc disease. In: *Textbook of Small Animal Surgery*, 3e (ed. D. Slatter), 1193–1209. Philadelphia: WB Saunders.

23. Shores, A. (1982). The intervertebral disk syndrome in the dog: part III. Thoracolumbar disk surgery. *Compend. Contin. Educ. Pract. Vet.* 4: 24.

24. Shores, A. (1982). Intervertebral disk surgery in the dog: Part III. Thoracolumbar disk surgery. *Compend. Contin. Educ. Pract. Vet.* 4: 24–34.

25. Swaim, S.F. (1973). Use of pneumatic surgical instruments in neurosurgery: part I. spinal surgery. *Vet. Med. Small Anim. Clin.* 68: 1404.

26. Gage, E.D. (1980). Practical management of thoracolumbar disc disease. *Proc. Am. Anim. Hosp. Assoc.* 47: 283.

27. Bitetto, W.V. and Kapatkin, A.S. (1989). Intraoperative problems associated with intervertebral disc disease. *Probl. Vet. Med.* 1: 434–444.

28. Jeffery, N.D., Mankin, J.M., Ito, D. et al. (2020). Extended durotomy to treat severe spinal cord injury after acute thoracolumbar disc herniation in dogs. *Vet. Surg.* 49: 884–893.

29. Prata, R.G. (1981). Neurosurgical treatment of thoracolumbar disks: the rationale and value of laminectomy with concomitant disk removal. *J. Am. Anim. Hosp. Assoc.* 17: 17.

30. Roach, W.J., Thomas, M., Weh, J.M. et al. (2012). Residual herniated disc material following hemilaminectomy in chondrodystrophic dogs with thoracolumbar intervertebral disc disease. *Vet. Comp. Orthop. Traumatol.* 25: 109–115.

31. Forterre, F., Gorgas, D., Dickomeit, M. et al. (2010). Incidence of spinal compressive lesions in chondrodystrophic dogs with abnormal recovery after hemilaminectomy for treatment of thoracolumbar disc disease: a prospective magnetic resonance imaging study. *Vet. Surg.* 39: 165–172.

32. Hettlich, B.F., Kerwin, S.C., and Levine, J.M. (2012). Early reherniation of disk material in eleven dogs with surgically treated thoracolumbar intervertebral disk extrusion. *Vet. Surg.* 41: 215–219.

33. Stigen, O. (2010). Early recurrence of thoracolumbar intervertebral disc extrusion after surgical decompression: a report of three cases. *Acta Vet. Scand.* 52: 10.

34. Simpson, S.T. (1998). Thoracolumbar spine: hemilaminectomy of the caudal thoracic and lumbar spine. In: *Current Techniques in Small Animal Surgery*, 4e (ed. M.J. Bojrab, G.W. Ellison and B. Slocum), 844–849. Baltimore, MD: Williams and Wilkins.

35. Brisson, B.A., Holmberg, D.L., Parent, J. et al. (2011). Comparison of the effect of single-site and multiple-site disk fenestration on the rate of recurrence of thoracolumbar intervertebral disk herniation in dogs. *J. Am. Vet. Med. Assoc.* 238: 1593–1600.

36. Brisson, B.A., Moffatt, S.L., Swayne, S.L. et al. (2004). Recurrence of thoracolumbar intervertebral disk extrusion in chondrodystrophic dogs after surgical decompression with or without prophylactic fenestration: 265 cases (1995–1999). *J. Am. Vet. Med. Assoc.* 224: 1808–1814.

7

Thoracolumbar Disk Fenestration

Brigitte A. Brisson

University of Guelph, Guelph, Ontario, Canada

Indications

Fenestration of the herniated disk space at the time of decompressive surgery is recommended to prevent further extrusion of disk material through the ruptured annulus fibrosus (AF) in the early postoperative period [1–13]. Reports documenting early recurrent disk extrusion at a decompressed site [5, 10, 14] do not support the previous claims that recurrent herniated disk material would likely move spontaneously outside of the canal through the laminectomy site and be of no clinical consequence. It is, however, possible that the previously made laminectomy offers some relief from spinal cord or nerve root compression soon after surgery which could explain why some dogs documented as having recurrent herniated material do not develop neurological deficits [5].

Prophylactic fenestration of unaffected, adjacent thoracolumbar (TL) disks has been shown to significantly reduce confirmed late recurrence in dogs undergoing prophylactic disk fenestration in the TL region [9, 11, 12]. Prophylactic fenestration should be considered in dogs with mineralized disks [10, 11, 15, 16] and dogs of breeds predisposed to recurrence (Dachshunds and French Bulldogs) even when disks are not mineralized [7, 9, 13, 15, 17].

Intervertebral disk (IVD) fenestration can be performed using a drill and burr, known as power-assisted fenestration, or with a scalpel blade, known as blade fenestration (Figure 7.1) [8, 18]. The simple creation of a window within the lateral AF does not result in a path for any remaining disk material to herniate, nor do postoperative chiropractic bending maneuvers result in disk material being expelled through the fenestration site [8, 10, 18, 19].

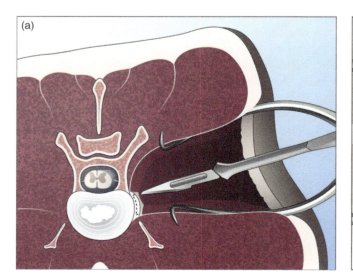 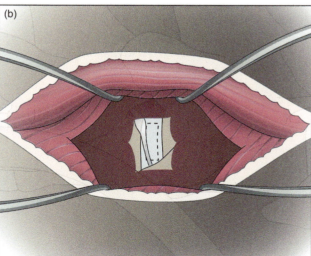

Figure 7.1 Illustration of a transverse section through a canine lumbar intervertebral disk (a) and sagittal view (b) depicting blade fenestration performed through a lateral approach.

Advanced Techniques in Canine and Feline Neurosurgery, First Edition. Edited by Andy Shores and Brigitte A. Brisson.
© 2023 John Wiley & Sons, Inc. Published 2023 by John Wiley & Sons, Inc.
Companion site: www.wiley.com/go/shores/advanced

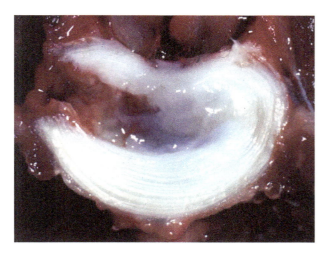

Figure 7.2 Transverse section through an intervertebral disk after fenestration was performed showing that some nucleus remains within the annulus, mostly on the side contralateral side to the fenestration.

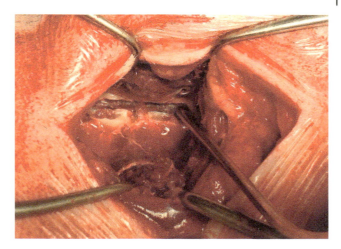

Figure 7.3 Intraoperative image of incomplete mini-hemilaminectomy (thin inner cortical bone layer still remains) showing that the exposure gained for decompression is sufficient for fenestration at the surgical site.

Furthermore, studies assessing the fate of the NP following surgical disk fenestration have failed to document a significant inflammatory reaction that would support the remaining disk material being subsequently dissolved preventing recurrence, nor has it confirmed that the window remains open to offer an alternate path for future disk extrusion, since fibrocartilage fills the void created by fenestration soon after surgery [19, 20]. Rather, the effectiveness of fenestration is thought to be governed by the amount of NP removed at the time of surgery [19] and directly related to the skill and experience of the operator [21]. Despite skill, complete removal of the remaining NP is not expected when performing fenestration [5, 8] and is likely to result in removal of more NP from the ipsilateral side and less from the contralateral side of the IVD being fenestrated [22] (Figure 7.2). This author believes that either fenestration technique can effectively remove large amounts of disk material as long as the surgeon is knowledgeable of local anatomy and is comfortable with the technique used.

Though the lateral approach may increase the effective removal of disk material compared with the dorsal or dorsolateral surgical approaches by providing a better angle and working depth for fenestration [23], the approach used for decompression will dictate the approach used for concurrent fenestration [13].

Technique – Surgical Approach

Right-handed surgeons typically find that TL fenestration is more easily performed on the left side of the spine [24], but since fenestration is most commonly performed with concurrent decompression, the approach will depend on the side of the lesion and the preferred surgical approach for decompression. When positioning the patient for decompressive surgery, a towel roll is inserted under the site of herniation to open the disk spaces on the side of surgery and to facilitate fenestration. The surgeon should review the diagnostic images for anatomical anomalies including missing or unusually shaped ribs or transverse processes in the area of interest.

The IVD is located ventral to the intervertebral foramen, immediately cranial to the rib head or the base of the transverse process. Fenestration of the affected disk space does not require much additional exposure beyond that performed for mini-hemilaminectomy or hemilaminectomy (Figure 7.3). The loose connective tissues containing the spinal nerves and vessels that overlie the disk space are retracted cranially to expose the glistening annulus for fenestration. If prophylactic fenestration of additional disks is to be performed, the skin and lumbar fascia incisions may need to be extended cranially and/or caudally accordingly. Using deep digital palpation between the fascicles of the iliocostalis musculature, the desired disk spaces are individually located and exposed by identifying the rib head or the tip of the transverse process caudal to the disk of interest. A Metzembaum scissor or Kelly forceps is used to split the iliocostalis thoracis and lumborum muscles in an oblique direction along the muscle fibers (dorsal to the tip of the transverse process or just cranial to the rib head) allowing the area of the disk space to be digitally palpated (Figure 7.4). In the lumbar region, a periosteal elevator is then used to elevate the loose layer of fascia that covers the lateral annulus from the edge of the transverse process. Dissection should proceed from the base of the transverse

72 | *Advanced Techniques in Canine and Feline Neurosurgery*

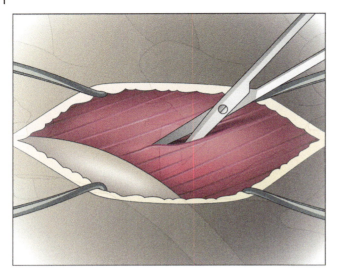

Figure 7.4 A Illustration of a Metzembaum scissor being used to split the iliocostalis lumborum muscle in the direction of its muscle fibers (dorsal to the tip of the transverse process of L1) to expose the annulus fibrosus.

process in a cranial direction exposing the fibers of the AF. Retraction of the deep muscle is most easily maintained using small tipped, right-angled Gelpi retractors (Figure 7.5). Additional retraction can be obtained using a Frasier suction tip, which has the added advantage of keeping the small field clear of blood. The exposure obtained is small but allows excellent visualization of the lateral annulus for fenestration.

Fenestration of thoracic disks is slightly more difficult and offers less visualization. After separating the fibers of the iliocostalis muscle, which attach to the 13th, 12th, 11th, and 10th ribs, an index finger is used to follow the rib

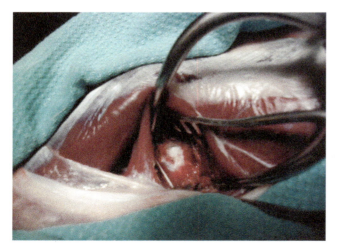

Figure 7.5 Approach for disk fenestration in a cadaver. Note that Gelpi retractors, and in this case a Weitlaner retractors, are used to maintain muscle retraction.

to the level where it articulates with the vertebral body. Alternatively, the iliocostalis muscles can be transected close to their insertion on the associated ribs [25]. The levator costae muscles originate on the transverse process of thoracic vertebrae 1–12 and insert on the anterior surface of the rib caudal to each process. This muscle is separated using a blade or periosteal elevator and is retracted ventrally. Retraction of the epaxial muscles dorsally and of the levator costae muscle ventrally is best achieved using a Gelpi retractor or handheld retractors. Care is taken to prevent pleural puncture while separating the levator costae muscle and while inserting retractors. With experience, one can "tunnel" down [26] or create a keyhole access [27] to each disk space by palpating the transverse process or rib head to avoid excessive tissue dissection and trauma.

Variations

Morelius et al. described an approach for lateral fenestration that dissects along the plane between the longissimus and iliocostalis muscles rather than through the fibers of the iliocostalis muscle [23].

Technique – Fenestration Procedure (Video 7.1)

The lateral annulus is covered by a loose fascia that contains the spinal nerve and associated vessels. A #11 blade is used to transect the soft tissue attachments along the cranial border of the rib head or transverse process and a periosteal elevator is then used to elevate these soft tissue structures in a cranial direction. Care must be taken not to injure the spinal nerve; this is especially important if fenestrating at L4–5 and L5–6. The ventral branches of the spinal nerves run along the ventrolateral aspect of the disk and can be damaged by dissecting too low along the lateral annulus [26]. Pressure or diathermy are typically effective to control hemorrhage encountered during dissection. The lateral annulus is visualized as a white, glistening, fibrous sheath. A straight hypodermic needle (22 gauge) can be used to carefully probe and confirm the exact location of the disk space and of the vertebral end plates on either side [28] (Figure 7.6), but should not be routinely necessary. Ensure that the needle is inserted as perpendicular as possible to the annulus (the required angle varies depending on patient position and surgical approach) and that it does not inadvertently penetrate the intervertebral foramen and spinal canal. Fenestration can be performed using a blade or a drill.

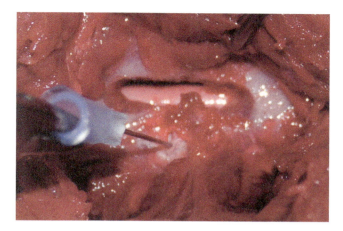

Figure 7.6 A hypodermic needle is used to palpate each of the vertebral endplates and to penetrate the annulus fibrosus, identifying the disk space for fenestration in a cadaver. Note that the exposure gained for mini-hemilaminectomy was sufficient for fenestration at this site.

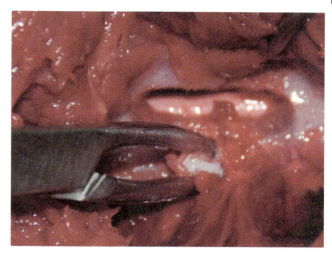

Figure 7.8 A rongeur is used to remove the fenestrated section of lateral annulus in a cadaver.

Blade Fenestration

Once the surgeon has identified the annulus, a #11 scalpel blade is used to create a rectangular window within it (Figure 7.7). The blade is oriented such that its cutting edge is directed away from the spinal cord (located dorsally) and away from the neurovascular structures (located cranially). Cranial retraction of the nerve and vessel is maintained using a periosteal elevator or suction tip during fenestration. Four adjoining cuts are made within the annulus and the rectangular piece of annulus (approximately 2 × 4–5 mm in a small dog) [8, 23] is removed using small curved hemostatic forceps or a rongeur to expose the nucleus pulposus for curettage (Figure 7.8). As large a window as possible (slightly larger than the instrument used to retrieve disk material) is created to facilitate removal of nucleus pulposus.

Power Fenestration

Power fenestration is performed through the same approach but the window is created using a high-speed pneumatic or electric drill and a 4 mm burr [8].

After creating the annular fenestration, curettes of various sizes are used to remove as much of the nucleus as possible from the disk space (Figure 7.9). Avoid directing instruments toward the spinal cord; rather, make a circular pattern that begins with entering the fenestration at the top of the window and moving in a downward "in and out" motion. Surgeons should avoid rotating curettes along their long axis within the disk space as this may result in fracture at the neck of the curette. The largest curette possible should be used for effective removal of the disk material (Figure 7.10). Smaller curettes are ineffective and are more likely to break within the disk space, making it difficult to retrieve the metal foreign body. Once fenestrated, the disk space should look and/or feel empty and might feel collapsed (more difficult to enter with a curette) (Figure 7.11).

After fenestrating the site of decompression, the spinal canal should be sweeped once again to verify that disk material was not pushed through the ruptured annulus and within the spinal canal during fenestration [5].

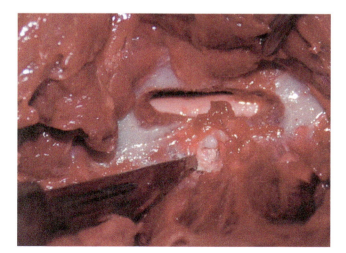

Figure 7.7 A #11 scalpel blade is used to remove a rectangular section of the lateral annulus in a cadaver. Alternatively, a drill and 4 mm burr could be used to create the fenestration.

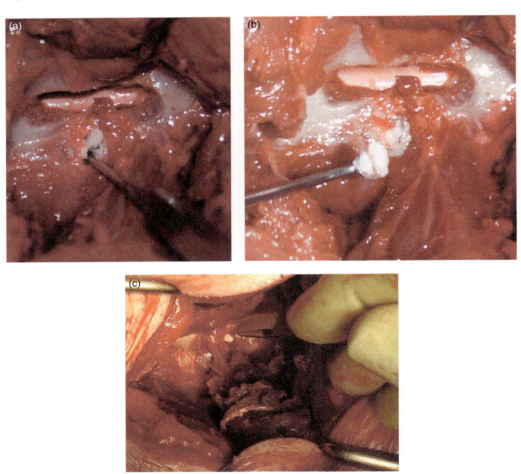

Figure 7.9 (a–c) A curette is used to retrieve the nucleus pulposus from the disk space in a cadaver (a, b) and in a patient (c). The curette with the largest diameter that will fit the disk space should be used. The curette is inserted and moved in a craniocaudal and in-and-out motion without turning within the disk space. Alternatively, a curved spatula or dental scraper can be used to retrieve the nucleus pulposus.

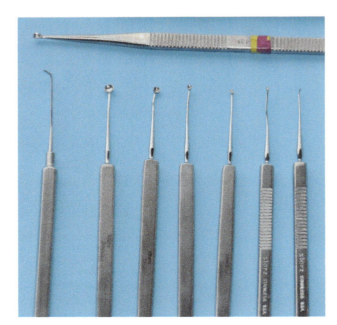

Figure 7.10 A variety of neurological curettes are shown. The largest curette possible should be used to allow effective removal of the disk material during fenestration. Smaller curettes are ineffective and are more likely to fracture within the disk space making it difficult to retrieve the metal foreign body.

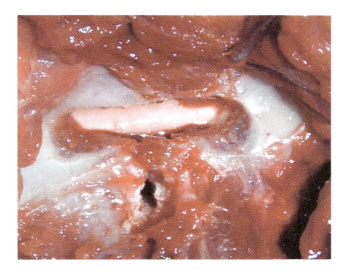

Figure 7.11 The disk space of a cadaver appears empty after fenestration has been completed. Fenestration in a live patient typically results in collapse of the disk space.

Other Requirements

Positive pressure ventilation is ideal during fenestration in the thoracic region to prevent pneumothorax should the parietal pleura be punctured during fenestration. If puncture of the pleura is suspected, one can confirm it by filling the surgical site with sterile saline and observing for the presence of air bubbles during positive pressure ventilation.

Closure

The muscle separation planes do not require closure. Closure is standard for a laminectomy.

Complications

Reported complications associated with fenestration include increased anesthetic and surgical times [1], displacement of disk material into the vertebral canal and/or spinal cord trauma causing worsening of neurologic

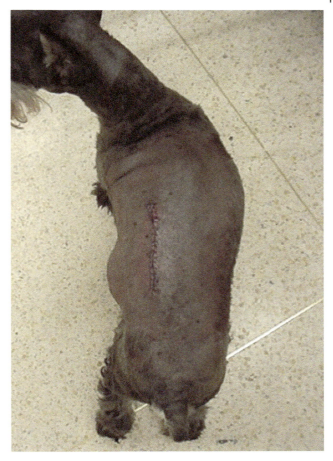

Figure 7.12 Postoperative view of a Miniature Schnauzer with abdominal wall weakness following decompression for IVD herniation and fenestration of all disks between T11–12 and L3–4.

grade [12, 27, 29–32], hemorrhage [9, 11], pleural puncture or pneumothorax when fenestrating thoracic disks [9, 27, 29], soft-tissue and nerve-root trauma leading to postoperative pain, scoliosis, and abdominal wall weakness [11, 21, 27] (Figure 7.12), bone damage (Figure 7.13), lysis and diskospondylitis, especially related to power fenestration [29, 33], difficulty identifying one or more disk spaces for fenestration [9, 11, 12],

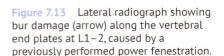

Figure 7.13 Lateral radiograph showing bur damage (arrow) along the vertebral end plates at L1–2, caused by a previously performed power fenestration.

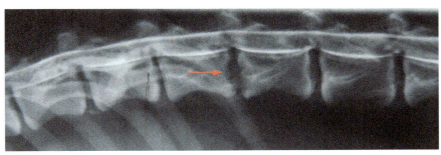

and vertebral subluxation [12]. Despite the lengthy list of potential complications, the rate of complications associated with fenestration is overall quite low. Moore et al. [34] calculated an overall 0.01% complication rate on more >1100 published cases, with most complications being minor and having no long-term negative effects [9, 11, 12, 21, 27]. Increased cost associated with longer surgical and anesthetic times, increased surgical incision length, and possibly postoperative morbidity related to additional tissue dissection and surgical trauma should however be considered on an individual basis. Recurrent disk herniation at a previously fenestrated disk space is possible and has been reported, but is rare [9–12].

Postoperative Care

There are no additional postoperative considerations following fenestration other than those required for other surgeries of the spine. Dogs that undergo multiple fenestrations may have a longer incision, which may be more painful in the initial postoperative period. Application of a soft padded bandage and cold compresses for the initial 24–36 hours can reduce swelling and appears to increase patient comfort.

Video clips to accompany this book can be found on the companion website at:
www.wiley.com/go/shores/advanced

References

1. Scott, H.W. (1997). Hemilaminectomy for the treatment of thoracolumbar disc disease in the dog: a follow-up study of 40 cases. *J. Small Anim. Pract.* 38: 488–494.
2. Funkquist, B. (1970). Decompressive laminectomy in thoraco-lumbar disc protrusion with paraplegia in the dog. *J. Small Anim. Pract.* 11: 445–451.
3. Colter, S.B. (1978). Fenestration, decompression, or both? Symposium on controversial problems in clinical practice. *Vet. Clin. North Am.* 8: 379–383.
4. Levine, S.H. and Caywood, D.D. (1984). Recurrence of neurological deficits in dogs treated for thoracolumbar disk disease. *J. Am. Anim. Hosp. Assoc.* 20 (6): 889–894.
5. Forterre, F., Konar, M., Spreng, D. et al. (2008). Influence of intervertebral disc fenestration at the herniation site in association with hemilaminectomy on recurrence in chondrodystrophic dogs with thoracolumbar disc disease: a prospective MRI study. *Vet. Surg.* 37: 399–405.
6. Fingeroth, J.M. (1989). Fenestration. Pros and cons. *Prob. Vet. Med.* 1: 445–466.
7. Dhupa, S., Glickman, N., and Waters, D.J. (1999). Reoperative neurosurgery in dogs with thoracolumbar disc disease. *Vet. Surg.* 28: 421–428.
8. Holmberg, D.L., Palmer, N.C., Van Pelt, D. et al. (1990). A comparison of manual and power assisted thoracolumbar disc fenestration in dogs. *Vet. Surg.* 19: 323–327.
9. Brisson, B.A., Moffatt, S.L., Swayne, S.L. et al. (2004). Recurrence of thoracolumbar intervertebral disk extrusion in chondrodystrophic dogs after surgical decompression with or without prophylactic fenestration: 265 cases (1995–1999). *J. Am. Vet. Med. Assoc.* 224: 1808–1814.
10. Stigen, O., Ottesen, N., and Jaderlund, K.H. (2010). Early recurrence of thoracolumbar intervertebral disc extrusion after surgical decompression: a report of three cases. *Acta Vet. Scand.* 52: 10.
11. Brisson, B.A., Holmberg, D.L., Parent, J. et al. (2011). Comparison of the effect of single-site and multiple-site disk fenestration on the rate of recurrence of thoracolumbar intervertebral disk herniation in dogs. *J. Am. Vet. Med. Assoc.* 238: 1593–1600.
12. Aikawa, T., Fujita, H., Mitsuhiro, S. et al. (2012). Recurrent thoracolumbar intervertebral disc extrusion after hemilaminectomy and concomitant prophylactic fenestration in 662 chondrodystrophic dogs. *Vet. Surg.* 41: 381–390.
13. ACVIM (2022). Consensus statement on diagnosis and management of acute canine thoracolumbar intervertebral disc extrusion. *J. Vet. Intern. Med.*, Forthcoming.
14. Hettlich, B.F., Kerwin, S.C., and Levine, J.M. (2012). Early reherniation of disk material in eleven dogs with surgically treated thoracolumbar intervertebral disk extrusion. *Vet. Surg.* 41: 215–219.
15. Mayhew, P.D., McLear, R.C., Ziemer, L.S. et al. (2004). Risk factors for recurrence of clinical signs associated with thoracolumbar intervertebral disk herniation in dogs: 229 cases (1994–2000). *J. Am. Vet. Med. Assoc.* 225 (8): 1231–1236.
16. Longo, S., Gomes, S.A., Briola, C. et al. (2021). Association of magnetic resonance assessed disc degeneration and late clinical recurrence in dogs treated surgically for thoracolumbar intervertebral disc extrusions. *J. Vet. Intern. Med.* 35 (1): 378–387.
17. Kerr, S., Crawford, A.H., and De Decker, S. (2021). Late onset recurrence of clinical signs after surgery for intervertebral disc extrusion in French bulldogs. *J. Small Anim. Pract.* 62 (8): 683–689.

18. Flo, G.L. and Brinker, W.O. (1975). Lateral fenestration of thoracolumbar discs. *J. Am. Anim. Hosp. Assoc.* 11: 619–626.

19. Shores, A., Cechner, P.E., Cantwell, H.D. et al. (1985). Structural changes in thoracolumbar disks following lateral fenestration. A study of radiographic, histologic and histochemical changes in the chondrodystrophic dog. *Vet. Surg.* 14: 117–123.

20. Wagner, S.D., Ferguson, H.R., Leipold, H. et al. (1987). Radiographic and histologic changes after thoracolumbar disc curettage. *Vet. Surg.* 16: 65–69.

21. Black, A.P. (1988). Lateral spinal decompression in the dog: a review of 39 cases. *J. Small Anim. Pract.* 29: 581–588.

22. Forterre, F., Dickomeit, M., Senn, D. et al. (2011). Microfenestration using the CUSA excel ultrasonic aspiration system in chondrodystrophic dogs with thoracolumbar disk extrusion: a descriptive cadaveric and clinical study. *Vet. Surg.* 40: 34–39.

23. Morelius, M., Bergadano, D., Schawalder, P. et al. (2007). Influence of surgical approach on the efficacy of the intervertebral disk fenestration: a cadaveric study. *J. Small Anim. Pract.* 48: 87–92.

24. Simpson, S.T. (1998). Thoracolumbar spine: hemilaminectomy of the caudal thoracic and lumbar spine. In: *Current Techniques in Small Animal Surgery*, 4e (ed. M.J. Bojrab, G.W. Ellison and B. Slocum), 844. Baltimore: Williams & Wilkins.

25. Denny, H.R. (1978). The surgical management of cervical disc protrusions in the dog: a review of 40 cases. *J. Small Anim. Pract.* 19: 251–257.

26. Creed, J.E. and Yturraspe, D.J. (1998). Thoracolumbar spine: intervertebral disc fenestration. In: *Current Techniques in Small Animal Surgery*, 4e (ed. M.J. Bojrab, G.W. Ellison and B. Slocum), 835–839. Baltimore: Williams & Wilkins.

27. Bartels, K.E., Creed, J.E., and Yturraspe, D.J. (1983). Complications associated with the dorsolateral muscle-separating approach for thoracolumbar disk fenestration in the dog. *J. Am. Vet. Med. Assoc.* 183: 1081–1083.

28. Hoerlein, B.F. (1956). Further evaluation of the treatment of disk protrusion paraplegia in the dog. *J. Am. Vet. Med. Assoc.* 129: 495–502.

29. Funkquist, B. (1978). Investigations of the therapeutic and prophylactic effects of disc evacuation in cases of thoraco-lumbar herniated discs in dogs. *Acta Vet. Scand.* 19: 441–457.

30. Tomlinson, J. (1985). Tetraparesis following cervical disc fenestration in two dogs. *J. Am. Vet. Med. Assoc.* 14: 240–246.

31. Dickey, D.T., Bartels, K.E., Henry, G.A. et al. (1996). Use of the holmium yttrium aluminum garnet laser for percutaneous thoracolumbar intervertebral disc ablation in dogs. *J. Am. Vet. Med. Assoc.* 208: 1263–1267.

32. Sterna, J. and Burzykowski, T. (2008). Assessment of the usefulness of the fenestration method in cases of disc extrusion in the cervical and thoraco-lumbar spine in chondrodystrophic dogs. *Pol. J. Vet. Sci.* 11: 55–62.

33. Hoerlein, B.F. (1952). The treatment of intervertebral disc protrusion in the dog. *Proc. Am. Vet. Med. Assoc.* 89: 206–212.

34. Moore, S.A., Andrea, T., Olby, N.J. et al. (2020). Current approaches to the management of acute thoracolumbar disc extrusion in dogs. *Front. Vet. Sci.* 7: 610.

8

Percutaneous Laser Disk Ablation

Danielle Dugat

Oklahoma State University, Stillwater, OK, USA

Introduction

Dogs experiencing an episode of intervertebral disk herniation (IVDH) have a 2.6–41.7% risk of recurrence [1–4]. Percutaneous laser disk ablation (PLDA) is a minimally invasive procedure performed on the thoracolumbar spine to reduce recurrence of IVDH. The effect of PLDA on recurrence of thoracolumbar IVDH in dogs has been described in two retrospective reports including 277 and 303 dogs [5, 6]. Prior to these publications, a pilot study was performed in 33 dogs to determine the efficacy of PLDA in dogs referred for surgical fenestration [7]. These studies documented successful outcomes with minimal, short-term complications associated with the procedure. A prospective study has since evaluated the changes that occur with PLDA to the intervertebral disk, vertebral body, and spinal cord [8].

Laser Ablation

PLDA uses laser energy transmitted through a thin optical fiber into the intervertebral disk to vaporize the nucleus pulposus [9]. The ablation of the nucleus pulposus results in a reduction of intradiskal pressure, thus inducing a reduction in recurrent disk herniation. Percutaneous disk decompression using laser ablation was first reported in 1984 as a minimally invasive therapy for lumbar disk herniation in humans [10]. With a variety of mechanical and chemical techniques available, PLDA using laser therapy was created to reduce the volume and pressure of an affected disk without damaging surrounding spinal structures. Ablation of a relatively small nucleus pulposus has been shown to result in a significant reduction in intradiskal pressure that was noted to result in persistent or recurrent back pain in humans [11–15]. Subsequently, the nucleus pulposus is gradually replaced by cartilaginous fibrous tissue [16].

Fiber-delivered, high-power lasers, including the neodymium-yttrium-aluminum-garnet (Nd:YAG, 1.064 μm), diode (0.980 μm), and holmium-yttrium-aluminum-garnet (Ho:YAG, 2.1 μm) lasers, have been used for tissue ablation, photocoagulation, and endoscopic stereotactic neurosurgical applications [17]. Reported advantages include decreased invasiveness, reduced morbidity rates, shorter intervention times, and lower recurrence rates of IVDH [10, 13, 18]. The Ho:YAG laser has been shown to provide optimum laser ablation of the nucleus pulposus in humans [10]. A particular advantage of the Ho:YAG laser is that it emits a wavelength that is strongly absorbed by water, allowing depth of penetration to be limited and zones of necrosis and collateral thermal effects to be minimized [7]. Despite this benefit in humans, one consideration is that chondrodystrophic dogs contain many disks that have undergone varying degrees of chondroid metaplasia and thus a loss of water content. This could potentially reduce the effectiveness of laser ablation of the nucleus pulposus in veterinary patients. Another reported benefit of the Ho:YAG is that it is a pulsed laser, allowing a cooling effect to occur between rapid pulses, potentially limiting tissue damage through a thermorelaxation phenomenon [19, 20].

Controversy over the efficacy of laser diskectomy in human medicine has arisen due to the lack of alteration in disk morphology using magnetic resonance imaging (MRI) after the procedure has been performed [21]. Additionally, surgical outcomes in humans may reflect a natural progression of healing [22]. Alternatively, studies have shown the procedure to be safe and effective, with reported success rates ranging from 76% to 94.5% [15, 22–24]. Proponents of the procedure in human medicine suggest that the positive effects of laser ablation are the result of decreased

---

Advanced Techniques in Canine and Feline Neurosurgery, First Edition. Edited by Andy Shores and Brigitte A. Brisson.
© 2023 John Wiley & Sons, Inc. Published 2023 by John Wiley & Sons, Inc.
Companion site: www.wiley.com/go/shores/advanced

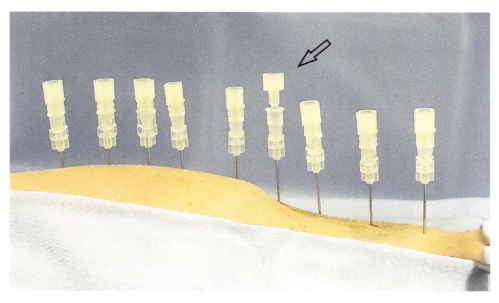

Figure 8.1 Post-needle placement into each disk space. Note the increased intradiskal pressure present, identified by the needle stylet ejection (black arrow) after placement of the needle into the nucleus pulposus.

intradiskal pressure caused by a reduction of the volume of nucleus pulposus subsequent to ablation. This effect appears to also be a benefit in dogs. One study reported that 56.3% (161/286) of owners believed their dog was improved immediately after PLDA, with many owners reporting that their dog wanted to jump and run immediately and that confinement after PLDA was difficult [5]. This was often reported as a drastic difference in the dog's demeanor after PLDA and owners were excited to report that their dog's attitude changed indefinitely after the procedure [5]. Although this may represent bias by the owners expecting improvement in their dogs after PLDA, this phenomenon can be supported by a common intraoperative finding of increased intradiskal pressure in veterinary patients, with ejection of the needle stylet after the spinal needle is placed into the nucleus pulposus (Figure 8.1).

Candidate Selection

PLDA can be performed as a true prophylactic procedure in dogs who have never experienced an episode of IVDH or can be performed as a prophylactic procedure to reduce the risk of recurrence of IVDH in dogs that have previously experienced an episode of IVDH. The author has performed PLDA in five dogs as a true prophylactic procedure. Each of these dogs have experienced successful outcomes in which owners confirmed a lack of any neurologic episodes after PLDA for at least 10 years (at time of last follow-up).

For those dogs that have previously experienced an episode of IVDH, complete resolution of active disease must be confirmed prior to PLDA. This is imperative to minimize the risk of direct ablation of the spinal cord through a weakened/disrupted annulus fibrosus. Bartels et al. documented neurologic deficits after PLDA; however, these dogs underwent PLDA while active disease was still present [6]. As a result, strict criteria have been developed to reduce the risk of an acute disk herniation secondary to ablation (Table 8.1).

IVDH most commonly affects chondrodystrophic breeds and consequently PLDA is performed most commonly in these breeds. The procedure can be, and has been, performed on multiple breeds and sizes, including a Staffordshire Terrier, as long as a spinal needle is long enough to be placed into the nucleus pulposus. In a retrospective study by Dugat et al., 61.7% (187/303) of dogs were Dachshunds [5]. In a prospective study of 30 dogs undergoing PLDA to evaluate MRI changes associated with the procedure, 73.3% (22/30) of the dogs were Dachshunds [8].

Table 8.1 Criteria required for PLDA.

1	Dogs must be recovered from an episode of confirmed or suspected IVDH
2	Dogs must receive an examination by a veterinarian a minimum of 2 weeks prior to PLDA, documenting the lack of paraspinal pain and lack of active improvement in neurologic function from a previous episode of IVDH
3	Dogs cannot receive any pain or anti-inflammatory medications for a minimum of two weeks prior to PLDA
4	Dogs must receive a second examination a minimum of two weeks after the first examination, again documenting a lack of paraspinal pain

Procedure Description

PLDA is performed on eight consecutive intervertebral disks in the thoracolumbar spine, from T10-11 to L4–5, as these disk spaces have been documented to have the highest incidence of herniation [25]. PLDA was attempted in the cervical spine of 10 dogs at the C2–3 through C4–5 intervertebral disks. Unfortunately, four of these dogs experienced significant radicular pain after PLDA and, thus, the procedure has been abandoned in the cervical spine until further studies can be performed.

The dog is placed under general anesthesia and the hair clipped and aseptically prepared on the lateral thoracolumbar spine, from dorsal midline to one-third of the distance of the flank ventrally (Figure 8.2). The dog is positioned in lateral recumbency and the surgically prepped area draped. Using fluoroscopic guidance, a 20-gauge, 2.5, or 3.5-in. spinal needle is inserted into the center of each disk space, from T10-11 to L4-5 (Figures 8.3 and 8.4). Dachshund breeds or smaller dogs generally require a 2.5-in. spinal needle, whereas French Bulldogs, Basset Hounds, or barrel-chested dogs often require a 3.5-in. spinal needle. Any

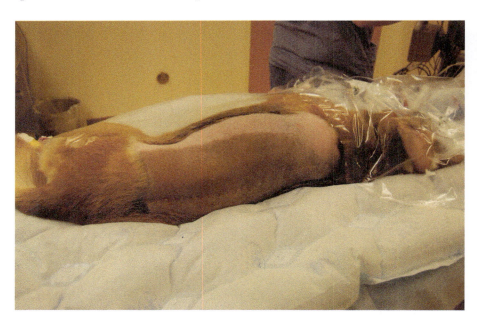

Figure 8.2 Positioning of the dog in right lateral recumbency once placed under anesthesia. The hair is clipped and aseptically prepared on the lateral thoracolumbar spine, from dorsal midline to one-third of the distance of the flank ventrally.

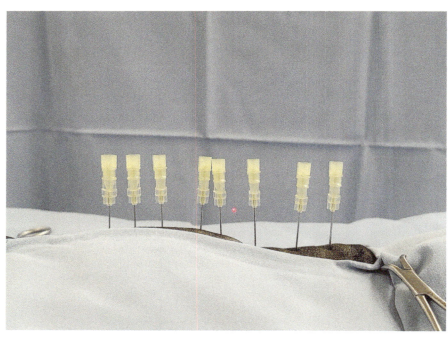

Figure 8.3 The dog is positioned in lateral recumbency and the surgically prepped area draped. 20-gauge, 2.5, or 3.5-in. spinal needles are placed percutaneously into each disk space, from T10–11 through L4–5, using fluoroscopic guidance.

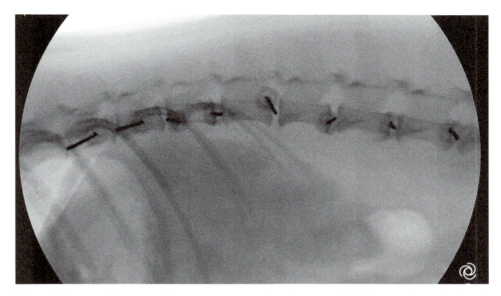

Figure 8.4 Lateral fluoroscopic image demonstrating placement of a 20-gauge, 2.5, or 3.5-in. spinal needle into the center of each disk space, from T10–11 to L4–5.

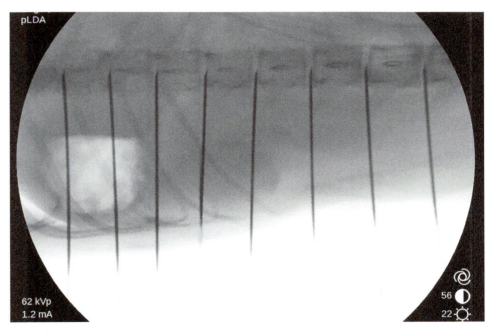

Figure 8.5 Ventrodorsal fluoroscopic image depicting accurate placement of each spinal needle. Note that the tip of each needle is centered in the disk space.

larger breed dog may require up to a 6.5-in. spinal needle. All needles are confirmed to be centered in the disk space using a ventrodorsal fluoroscopic projection of the spine (Figure 8.5). A μ-opioid is recommended at this stage for acute pain that can occur with the heat associated with laser ablation. The needle stylet is removed and a sterile, cleaved 320 μm low-quartz laser optical fiber is inserted through each spinal needle so that the tip of the fiber protrudes just at the end of the needle (Figure 8.6). A Ho:YAG laser is activated at each disk space for 40 seconds at 2 W of power with a 10-Hz pulse repetition rate. Energy per pulse delivered should be 0.2 J. Total energy over 40 seconds delivered at each disk should be 80 J. As each disk is ablated, the needle and laser fiber are removed. With

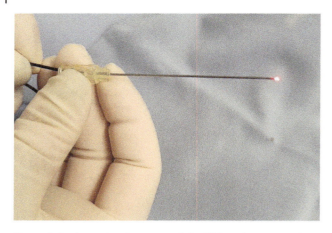

Figure 8.6 Accurate placement of the 320 μm low-quartz laser optical fiber is confirmed with a test needle by removing the needle stylet and placing the laser fiber through the spinal needle so that the tip of the fiber protrudes just past the end of the needle.

experience, mean procedure time is approximately 25 minutes. An injectable dose of a non-steroidal anti-inflammatory is administered and the dog is recovered from anesthesia. Postoperative management recommendations include strict crate rest for two weeks, including leash walks for elimination purposes only, with no jumping, running, or playing.

Procedure Complications and Recurrence

Peracute complications have been reported to occur during the procedure in up to 10% of cases, with the most common being inability to insert a needle into a disk space because of rib superimposition (3/303 dogs) or disk space narrowing (19/303 dogs) [5]. Other reported complications include mild hematoma formation at the needle insertion site [5] and pneumothorax [6]. Although pneumothorax has been reported historically, this complication is due to iatrogenic error in needle placement, by positioning the spinal needle too ventral into the thoracic cavity.

Postoperative complications have been documented in 8.6% (26/303) of dogs undergoing PLDA [5]. The most common complication reported was ataxia after the procedure for up to seven days ($N = 6$), soreness along the back ($N = 4$), mild ataxia immediately after the procedure and resolving in less than 24 hours ($N = 3$), greater pain than expected postoperatively requiring administration of pain medication for three days longer than the standard protocol ($N = 2$), and reluctance to move for eight days after PLDA ($N = 2$) [5]. The most recent prospective study of 30 dogs undergoing PLDA reports no postoperative complications (up to three months) after PLDA [8].

A recurrence rate of 19.8% (60/303 dogs) was reported in one retrospective study, including suspected or confirmed IVDH; however, this recurrence rate included dogs that developed suspected pain perceived by owners that lasted less than three days duration (19/60 dogs) [5]. Many of these dogs were not confined at all or confined to a crate for 24 hours and were subjected to owner interpretation regarding the presence of clinical signs and improvement of those signs. This questions whether some of the perceived episodes of recurrence were indeed recurrence and suggests that the overall rate of 19.8% should be interpreted cautiously. Eleven of the 303 dogs (3.6%) in this study had a recurrence of IVDH confirmed with CT or MRI and hemilaminectomy [5]. Twenty-eight of 30 dogs in another study were followed for a minimum of three years [8]. Two dogs were euthanized prior to the 3 year follow-up (13 months, 27 months) due to conditions unrelated to IVDH. Two dogs developed one episode of recurrence each, one at seven months (confirmed with MRI) and one at five months (suspected) after PLDA. Both dogs were examined by the surgeon that performed the PLDA. One dog presented with non-ambulatory paraparesis on neurologic exam and underwent a hemilaminectomy for a confirmed disk herniation at T11–12. This dog had mature mineralization documented at the T10–11 and T11–12 disk spaces at the time of PLDA. The second dog presented with paraspinal hyperesthesia only and was successfully managed medically with crate rest for four weeks and pain medications. This dog had documentation of maturely mineralized disks at T10–11 and T11–12 at the time of PLDA. The overall recurrence rate in the prospective study of 30 dogs was 6.7% (suspected and confirmed cases). The overall recurrence rate for confirmed IVDH in which surgery was recommended (modified Frankel score [4] – grade 3 or worse), was 3.3%.

In people, identification of disk mineralization at the time of decompressive surgery has been associated with a higher likelihood of recurrence [14]. Although the effects of disk mineralization were not specifically evaluated in previous studies on PLDA, it is possible that mineralization can play a role in recurrence of clinical signs after PLDA. Energy density (fluency) and power values used to perform PLDA were initially derived from in vitro research in which clear gelatin mixed with a pulverized calcium carbonate powder and contained in a culture plate was used to mimic a calcified disk. A spectrum of settings was then tested on cadaver disks to determine optimum laser settings without resulting in collateral thermal damage outside the targeted nucleus pulposus [26]. The current laser settings recommended for PLDA (2 W power, 10-Hz pulse repetition rate, 80 J /disk) are recommended to provide adequate photothermal and photoablative effects to the nucleus pulposus while minimizing damage to the annulus or vertebral endplates. There is possibility that this procedure can have less recurrence risk after being performed if done truly prophylactically, at approximately one year of age. Perhaps this can maximize the benefit of using a Ho:YAG laser, prior to the disk becoming as dehydrated and mineralized with the chondroid metaplasia that occurs.

Diagnostic Evaluation of PLDA

The effects of PLDA on the intervertebral disk, vertebral endplates, and spinal cord using MRI have been prospectively evaluated [8]. Dogs underwent a pre-PLDA MRI, immediate post-PLDA MRI, and 12 weeks post-PLDA MRI. Evaluation of the intervertebral disk revealed that PLDA did not result in a significantly identifiable change to the morphology of the disk that could be identified on MRI. Likewise, in humans, it has been documented that the disk morphology on MRI does not change with laser ablation [27–29]. This has led to historic controversy in humans as to the effectiveness of the procedure, knowing that the procedure is performed on a specific population of humans that may also naturally recover from their active disease [27–29]. Additionally, less identifiable change in disk morphology on MRI may be due to a lack of complete penetration of the volume of nucleus pulposus in a disk that is dehydrated. Despite this controversy, a previous study documented histopathologic evidence of thermal and coagulative necrosis within the disk, with tissue carbonization extending into adjacent vertebral body endplates [7].

Evaluation for diskitis revealed mild inflammation, measuring between 0% and 15% at the 12 weeks post-PLDA MRI [8]. Diskitis has been correlated with subchondral bone marrow changes in the adjacent vertebral bodies in humans [27]. Unfortunately, the definitive diagnosis of diskitis requires aspiration and culturing of the disk, which is not feasible to perform in humans or dogs. In clinical practice, MRI has been used to identify diskitis, based on the presence of contrast enhancement of the disk and the subchondral bone marrow, disk space narrowing, and endplate erosion [30].

Cvitanic et al. evaluated subchondral bone marrow changes after laser diskectomy in the lumbar spine in humans using MRI and found that 37% of dogs who underwent laser diskectomy had identifiable bone changes

present [27]. Pulsed lasers such as the Ho:YAG are designed to vaporize instantaneously; however, heating of non-target tissue due to thermal superimposition can occur as a consequence [31]. Most of the PLDA procedures are performed on chondrodystrophic breeds of dog, and the volume of disk space available is relatively small when compared to humans. Therefore, it can be justified that thermal damage can occur to structures adjacent to the laser fiber, such as vertebral endplates. Pre- and post-contrast T1 TRANS sequences evaluated for vertebral endplate lesions revealed a contrast-enhancing, hyperintense lesion with evidence of increased blood flow (Figures 8.7 and 8.8) [8]. The T2 TRANS sequences revealed a hypointense lesion suggestive of edema (Figure 8.9) [8]. Additionally, the lesion was often not as clearly seen on the

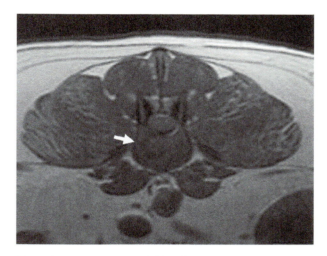

Figure 8.7 Pre-contrast T1 TRANS sequence evaluated for vertebral endplate lesions (white arrow).

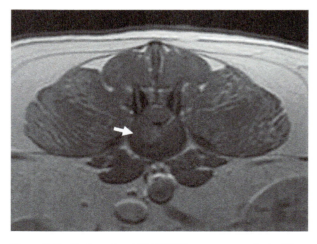

Figure 8.8 Post-contrast T1 TRANS sequence evaluated for vertebral endplate lesions revealing a contrast-enhancing, hyperintense lesion with evidence of increased blood flow (white arrow).

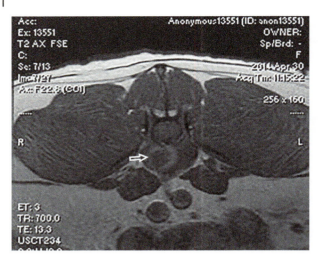

Figure 8.9 T2 TRANS sequence revealing a hypointense lesion suggestive of edema (white arrow).

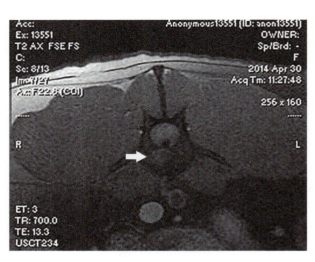

Figure 8.10 T2+FS TRANS sequence revealing a hypointense lesion suggestive of edema that was more easily identified than on the T2 TRANS due to the removal of fat (white arrow).

T2 TRANS sequence as it was on the T2+FS TRANS sequence, presumably due to the removal of fat (Figure 8.10) [8]. The mean diameter of lesions reported by Irizarry et al. were less than 1 mm at the cranial endplate and less than 2 mm at the caudal endplate, and only significant on the 12 weeks post-PLDA MRI [8]. In one study, vertebral endplate changes identified within one year of laser diskectomy were resolved when MRI was repeated after five years and each of the cases revealed lack of correlation between MRI findings and surgical outcomes [27].

Conclusion

The use of lasers in neurosurgery is well documented. PLDA is an effective, minimally invasive procedure that can be performed to reduce the recurrence of thoracolumbar IVDH. Understanding the laser–tissue interaction based on Ho:YAG laser properties is imperative to success. Future controlled studies are necessary to evaluate true success on recurrence rates on a population of dogs subjected to the risk of IVDH. Additionally, the concept of true prophylactic treatment of disks remains to be evaluated in a controlled study. Long-term success will need to be evaluated to ensure the dog does not undergo increased morbidity with the procedure.

 Video clips to accompany this book can be found on the companion website at: www.wiley.com/go/shores/advanced

References

1. Brisson, B.A., Holmberg, D.L., Parent, J. et al. (2011). Comparison of the effect of single-site and multiple-site disk fenestration on the rate of recurrence of thoracolumbar intervertebral disk herniation in dogs. *J. Am. Vet. Med. Assoc.* 238: 1593–1600.
2. Brisson, B.A., Moffatt, S.L., Swayne, S.L. et al. (2004). Recurrence of thoracolumbar intervertebral disk extrusion in chondrodystrophic dogs after surgical decompression with or without prophylactic fenestration: 265 cases (1995–1999). *J. Am. Vet. Med. Assoc.* 224: 1808–1814.
3. Mayhew, P.D., McLear, R.C., Ziemer, L.S. et al. (2004). Risk factors for recurrence of clinical signs associated with thoracolumbar intervertebral disk herniation in dogs: 229 cases (1994–2000). *J. Am. Vet. Med. Assoc.* 225: 1231–1236.
4. Levine, J.M., Levine, G.J., Kerwin, S.C. et al. (2006). Association between various physical factors and acute thoracolumbar intervertebral disk extrusion or protrusion in Dachshunds. *J. Am. Vet. Med. Assoc.* 229: 370–375.
5. Dugat, D.R., Bartels, K.E., and Payton, M.E. (2016). Recurrence of disk herniation following percutaneous laser disk ablation in dogs with a history of thoracolumbar intervertebral disk herniation: 303 cases (1994–2011). *J. Am. Vet. Med. Assoc.* 249 (12): 1393–1400.

6. Bartels, K.E., Higbee, R.G., Bahr, R.J. et al. (2003). Outcome of and complications associated with prophylactic percutaneous laser disk ablation in dogs with thoracolumbar disk disease: 277 cases (1992–2011). *J. Am. Vet. Med. Assoc.* 222 (12): 1733–1739.

7. Dickey, D.T., Bartels, K.E., Henry, G.A. et al. (1996). Use of the holmium yttrium aluminum garnet laser for percutaneous thoracolumbar intervertebral disk ablation in dogs. *J. Am. Vet. Med. Assoc.* 208: 1263–1267.

8. Irizaryy, I.N., Dugat, D.R., Sippel, K.M., and Payton, M.E. (2021). Evaluation of the intervertebral disk, vertebral body, and spinal cord for changes secondary to percutaneous laser disk ablation. *Vet. Surg.* 1–12. https://doi.org/10.1111/vsu.13684.

9. Gangi, A., Basile, A., Buy, X. et al. (2005). Radiofrequency and laser ablation of spinal lesions. *Semin. Ultrasound CT MRI* 26: 89–97.

10. Choy, D.S., Altman, P.A., Case, R.B. et al. (1991). Laser radiation at various wavelengths for decompression of intervertebral disk: experimental observation on human autopsy specimens. *Clin. Orthop.* 267: 245–250.

11. Choy, D.S. and Altman, P. (1993). Fall of intradiscal pressure with laser ablation. In: *Laser Discectomy* (ed. H.H. Sherk), 23–29. Pennsylvania: Hanley & Belfus.

12. Prodoehl, J.A., Lane, G.J., Black, J. et al. (1993). The effect of lasers on intervertebral disk pressure. In: *Laser Discectomy* (ed. H.H. Sherk), 17–21. Pennsylvania: Hanley & Belfus.

13. Choy, D.S., Hellinger, J., Hellinger, S. et al. (2009). 23rd anniversary of percutaneous laser disc decompression (PLDD). *Photomed. Laser Surg.* 27: 535–538.

14. Choy, D.S., Ascher, P.W., Ranu, H.S. et al. (1992). Percutaneous laser disc decompression: a new therapeutic modality. *Spine* 17: 949–956.

15. Lee, S.H., Ahn, Y., Choi, W.C. et al. (2006). Immediate pain improvement is a useful predictor of long-term favorable outcome after percutaneous laser disc decompression for cervical disc herniation. *Photomed. Laser Surg.* 24: 508–513.

16. Ichimura, Y. (1997). Percutaneous laser disk decompression for the cervical disk herniation: experimental studies and early clinical results. *Jpn J. Laser Surg. Med.* 18: 11–20.

17. Krishnamurthy, S. and Powers, K.P. (1994). Lasers in neurosurgery. *Lasers Surg. Med.* 15: 126–167.

18. Gottlob, C., Kopchok, G.E., Peng, S. et al. (1992). Holmium: YAG laser ablation of human intervertebral disc: preliminary evaluation. *Lasers Surg. Med.* 12: 86–91.

19. Dillingham, M.F., Price, J.M., and Fanton, G.S. (1993). Holmium laser surgery. *Orthopedics* 16: 563–566.

20. Jacques, S.L. (1992). Laser-tissue interactions: photochemical, photothermal, and photomechanical. *Surg. Clin. North Am.* 72: 531–558.

21. Tonami, H., Yokota, H., Nakagawa, T. et al. (1997). Percutaneous laser discectomy: MRI findings within the first 24 hours after treatment and their relationship to clinical outcome. *Clin. Radiol.* 52: 938–944.

22. Bernd, L., Schiltenwolf, M., Mau, H. et al. (1997). No indications for percutaneous lumbar discectomy? *Int. Orthop.* 21: 164–168.

23. Gastambide, D., Peyrou, P., and Lee, S.H. (2003). Percutaneous cervical discectomy. In: *Surgical Techniques in Orthopaedics and Traumatology* (ed. G. Bentley, N. Bohler, H. Dorfmann, et al.). Paris: Elsevier; 55-095-A-10.

24. Ahn, Y., Lee, S.H., and Shin, S.W. (2005). Percutaneous endoscopic cervical discectomy: clinical outcome and radiographic changes. *Photomed. Laser Surg.* 23: 362–368.

25. Aikawa, T., Fujita, H., Shjibaba, M. et al. (2012). Recurrent thoracolumbar intervertebral disc extrusion after hemilaminectomy and concominant prophylactic fenestration in 662 chondrodystrophic dogs. *Vet. Surg.* 41: 381–390.

26. Fry, T.R., Bartels, K.E., and Henry, G.A. (1994). Holmium: YAG laser discectomy in dogs: a pilot study. *Biomed. Opt.* 2128: 42–48.

27. Cvitanic, O.A., Schimandle, J., Casper, G.D. et al. (2000). Subchondral marrow changes after laser discectomy in the lumbar spine: MR imaging findings and clinical correlation. *Am. J. Res.* 174: 1363–1369.

28. Delamarter, R.B., Howard, M.W., Goldstein, T. et al. (1995). Percutaneous lumbar discectomy. *J. Bone Joint Surg. Am.* 77-A: 578–583.

29. Tonami, H., Yokota, H., Nakagawa, T. et al. (1997). Percutaneous laser discectomy: MR findings within the first 24 hours after treatment and their relationship to clinical outcome. *Clin. Radiol.* 52: 938–944.

30. Kahn, I.A., Vaccaro, A.R., and Zlotolow, D.A. (1999). Management of vertebral diskitis and osteomyelitis. *Orthopedics* 22: 758–765.

31. Vangsness, C.T., Watson, T., Sadatmanesh, V. et al. (1995). Pulsed Ho: YAG laser menisectomy: effect of pulse width on tissue penetration rate and lateral thermal damage. *Lasers Surg. Med.* 16: 61–65.

9

The Cranial Thoracic Spine: Approach via Dorsolateral Hemilaminectomy

Yael Merbl and Annie Vivian Chen-Allen

Washington State University, Pullman, WA, USA

Indications

Cranial thoracic compressive spinal lesions are less frequently encountered in veterinary medicine compared to the thoracolumbar spine [1]. This difference partially arises from the cranial thoracic spine being more stable than the thoracolumbar spine. Additionally, traumatic injuries of the spine at this region are less common; however, this region of the spine is being approached more frequently in the last decades for diseases such as caudal cervical spondylo-myelopathy and cranial thoracic disk protrusions as well as resection of tumors (Figure 9.1).

The surgical approach to the cranial thoracic (T1–T9) spine is also less commonly reported in veterinary medicine and is described mainly in case reports and small case series [2–6]. Several reports describe the surgical approach to the caudal cervical and cranial thoracic region through a lateral incision [7–9]. Another report recently described a dorsolateral hemilaminectomy approach for treatment of neoplastic [1] and intervertebral disk disease [1, 10], and other disease processes causing spinal cord compression. Lastly, a case report described a ventral approach to stabilize T2–T3 luxation via sternotomy [11]. The appropriate/chosen approach depends on the disease process, goals

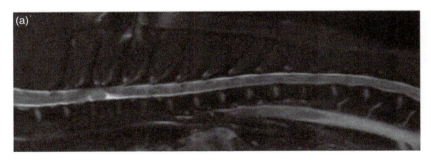
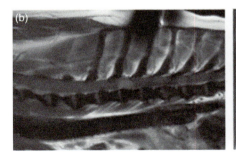
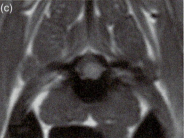

Figure 9.1 Magnetic resonance imaging. (a) Sagittal T2 weighted image depicting the intradural extramedullary oval shaped, well defined, space occupying mass, at the level of T3. (b) Sagittal T1 weighted image post gadolinium showing moderate homogenous contrast enhancement. (c) Transverse T1 weighted image post gadolinium showing the lesion occupying at least 80% of the spinal canal.

Advanced Techniques in Canine and Feline Neurosurgery, First Edition. Edited by Andy Shores and Brigitte A. Brisson.
© 2023 John Wiley & Sons, Inc. Published 2023 by John Wiley & Sons, Inc.
Companion site: www.wiley.com/go/shores/advanced

of surgery, as well as the surgeon's level of comfort for that procedure. A dorsolateral hemilaminectomy is at the focus of this chapter as it is the most common procedure at this region.

Surgical Anatomy

The articular processes of all the cranial thoracic spine (up to the tenth thoracic vertebra) are in a nearly dorsal plane so that the cranial articular process is dorsal (Figure 9.2a) and the caudal articular process is ventral [12]. The plane differentiation is very different from the thoracolumbar spine making the articulation less recognizable at the cranial thoracic region compared to the thoracolumbar region (Figure 9.2b). Close attention should also be paid to the regional arterial blood supply. The course of the arteries located in this region have been previously described [12]. The arteries the surgeon should be familiar with are the dorsal scapular artery (Figure 9.3, white arrowhead) that

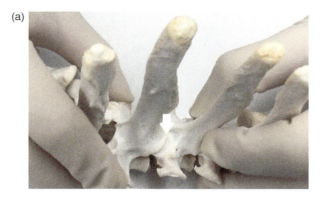

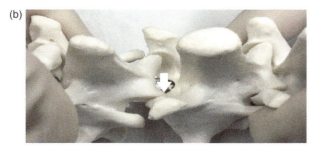

Figure 9.2 Dorsolateral view of a canine model of the cranial thoracic vertebral column (a) and the thoracolumbar (b) vertebral column. Articulation of the cranial thoracic vertebras is oriented dorsoventrally (white arrows) as opposed to the thoracolumbar vertebras in which the articulation is lateralized and more palpable and prominent. The cranial thoracic and thoracolumbar articulations were distracted in the picture to allow better visualization.

arises from the cranial surface of the costo-cervical trunk, approximately the middle of the medial surface of the first rib. Then, this artery continues dorsally and leaves the thoracic cavity cranial to the first rib. The dorsal scapular artery at the proximal end of the first rib inclines dorsocaudally, crosses the lateral surface of the first costotransverse joint, and branches in the dorsal part of the thoracic portion of the serratus ventralis muscle. The second artery is the thoracic vertebral artery (Figure 9.3, black asterisk). This artery continues medially to the first rib and passes through the costotransverse foramen dorsal to the neck of the rib. Caudal to the second and third ribs that it crosses, the thoracic vertebral artery sends a small intercostal artery ventrally, which anastomoses with the intercostal branches (Figure 9.3, black arrows). Lastly, when performing the facetectomy of the thoracic vertebra, the inter-arcuate branches of the internal vertebral venous plexus can be found within the inter-arcuate ligament. It may be necessary to cauterize or ligate prior to transecting these branches [13]. While retracting the muscles to expose the vertebras at this level, special consideration should be given to the anatomy and blunt dissection and retraction should be conducted with care. If an artery is accidentally injured, bipolar cautery can be used to achieve hemostasis for the smaller vasculatures. If bleeding continues, digital pressure utilizing gauze and gel foam can be used as well. Sometimes it will not be possible to locate the bleeding site as the ruptured artery will retract into the deeper muscle layers. Attempts should be made to find the retracted artery if bleeding is significant. If the artery is accidentally torn and larger in size, hemostats can be used to achieve hemostasis and ligation with sutures or hemoclips may be needed.

Patient Positioning

Several positions have been described in the literature to allow for better exposure and visualization. For a hemilaminectomy, the dog should be positioned in sternal recumbency with the head in a neutral position. Some surgeons prefer extending and crossing of the front limbs in an x-sign cranially (Figure 9.4) to allow retraction of the scapula laterally. Other surgeons prefer sternal recumbency with the torso elevated to enable the thoracic limbs in an orthostatic posture [1]. Clipping should extend from the caudal cervical region to the mid thoracic area depending on the site intended. The thoracic limbs are tied cranially, and tape is used over the thoracic region caudally to secure the positioning of the dog on the table.

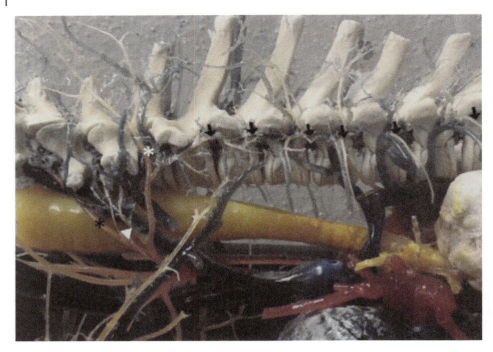

Figure 9.3 Model of a dog at the level of the cranial thoracic region showing the spine and blood vessels. Dorsally, the dorsal intercostal arteries (black arrows) are noted. The dorsal scapular artery (white arrowhead), the thoracic vertebral artery (black asterisk), and deep cervical artery (white asterisk) are depicted as well.

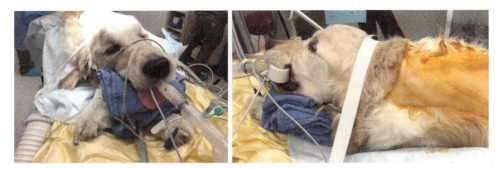

Figure 9.4 Positioning for approaching the cranial thoracic region via hemilaminectomy. The dog is in a dorsal recumbency. The head is in a neutral position (not flexed or extended) and the thoracic limbs are crossed over.

Surgical Technique

A skin incision is made on the dorsal midline from the caudal cervical to the cranial thoracic region, depending on the site of interest, from the C6 vertebrae to the level of T5 vertebrae. The distinct T1 spinous process compared to a much shorter C7 spinous process is palpated as an anatomical landmark. Alternatively, fluoroscopy can be used to obtain the correct surgical site using a "pin shot" by inserting a needle through the spinous process. The dorsal midline tendinous raphe is seen after incision of subcutaneous tissues on the midline. An incision is made in the tendinous raphe on the borders of the spinous processes, either on the left or right depending on the lesion side. Periosteal elevator, osteotome, and or fine dissection tools are used to remove the muscles attached to the spinous process and the articular facet up to the level of the rib attachment to the vertebrae. Careful attention is needed to not accidentally enter the thorax when elevating musculature off the rib heads. A high-speed drill is used to create the hemilaminectomy site. Due to the plane differentiation and the articulation being less recognizable at the cranial thoracic region (mentioned prior), using the costovertebral junction located lateral to the articulation as a landmark

(Figure 9.5a) is helpful in determining the margins of the hemilaminectomy. Additionally, a drill hole to appreciate the level of the spinal canal has been suggested as a part of the surgical technique in a previous paper [1].

It may be helpful to have the hemilaminectomy intentionally longer than the lesion site so that normal spinal cord tissue can be visualized both cranially and caudally to the lesion, particularly in spinal tumor resection. (Figure 9.5b). This will allow better visualization and demarcation of where the lesion is relative to the spinal cord and may be very helpful when removing a tumor and trying to appreciate normal versus diseased tissue. When trying to resect a tumor, another key to optimal resection is finding the plane of section between the normal spinal cord and diseased tumor tissue, so good visualization is critical. Once a durotomy is performed, gentle lateral or ventral traction of the dura with stay sutures or fine microsurgical forceps will also improve assessment of the intradural tumor margins.

The dorsolateral approach to the cranial thoracic spine avoids cutting the nuchal ligament and lateral retraction is sufficient for visualization of the lateral spine. However, if partial or complete dorsal laminectomy is also indicated, it is noteworthy that the nuchal ligament attaches to the spinous process of T1–T3 in dogs and, if needed, can be cut without major complications since the nuchal ligament is somewhat continuous with the supraspinous ligament [8].

Once decompression is completed (Figure 9.5c), a thin piece of gel foam (absorbable gelatin sponge, USP, Pfizer) is placed over laminectomy site. Muscles, subcutaneous tissues, and skin incision are positioned and sutured in layers as previously described elsewhere. Tacking of the subcutaneous layers to the deeper layers is recommended to prevent seroma formation.

Postoperative Care

Postoperative care of the hemilaminectomy patient involves cage rest with monitored leash walks using a body harness and sling if needed. Activity should be limited in the first four to six weeks after surgery. Free activity should be allowed once recovery is complete or close to complete, usually by eight weeks postoperatively. Pain control is important in the postoperative period and can be achieved with opioids such as fentanyl as a constant rate infusion and fentanyl patches with or without NSAIDs such as meloxicam or carprofen. Gabapentin is also an option for patients with neuropathic pain. Prednisone can also be used at anti-inflammatory doses for treatment of spinal cord edema and nerve root inflammation, but not in conjunction with NSAIDs. Ice packing can be performed every 4–6 hours for 24–48 hours to reduce post-surgical swelling and seroma formation. If a seroma is noted, warm packing and minimizing movement would be indicated. In severe cases of seroma formation, pressure bandaging with a figure-of-eight pattern around the thoracic limbs may be beneficial. Non-ambulatory patients will benefit from physical rehabilitation, and soft bedding and routine recumbency care are essential in preventing decubital ulcers. Cleanliness is important in preventing incisional infection.

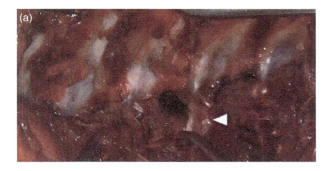
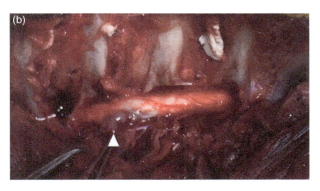
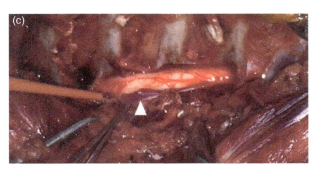

Figure 9.5 Intraoperative pictures showing (a) the dorsolateral approach to the cranial thoracic spine depicting the rib attachment to the vertebrae (white arrow). Spinous processes of T1–T5 are shown. (b) A round grayish mass was noted ventrolateral to the spinal cord after opening the dura. (c) Indentation of the spinal cord is noted after removal of the meningioma, as confirmed by histopathology.

Video clips to accompany this book can be found on the companion website at:
www.wiley.com/go/shores/advanced

References

1. Bray, K.Y., Early, P.J., Olby, N.J., and Lewis, M.J. (2020). An update on hemilaminectomy of the cranial thoracic spine: review of six cases. *Open Vet. J.* 10(1): 16–21.

2. Gilmore, D.R. (1983). Cranial thoracic intervertebral disk extrusion in a dog. *J. Am. Vet. Med. Assoc.* 182: 620–621.

3. Liptak, J.M., Watt, P.R., Thomson, M.J. et al. (1999). Hansen type I disk disease at T1-2 in a dachshund. *Aust. Vet. J.* 77: 156–159.

4. Jäderlund, K.J., Hansson, K., Lindberg, R., and Narfstrom, K. (2002). T3-T4 disc herniation in a German shepherd dog. *Vet. Rec.* 151: 769–770.

5. Gaitero, L. and Anor, S. (2009). Cranial thoracic disk protrusion in three German shepherd dogs. *Vet. J.* 182: 349–351.

6. Gaitero, L., Daniel, R., Nykamp, S., and Monteith, G. (2011). Cranial thoracic intervertebral disc disease in German shepherd dogs: a retrospective comparative MRI study [abstract]. *J. Vet. Intern. Med.* 25: 730.

7. Lipsitz, D. and Bailey, C.S. (1992). Lateral approach for cervical spinal cord decompression. *Prog. Vet. Neurol.* 3: 39–44.

8. Piermattei, D.L. and Johnson, K.A. (2004). The vertebral column. In: *An Atlas of Surgical Approaches to the Bones and Joints of the Dog and Cat*, 4e, 72–77. Philadelphia: Saunders.

9. Rossmeisl, J.H., Lanz, O.I., Inzana, K.D. et al. (2005). A modified lateral approach to the canine cervical spine: procedural description and clinical application in 16 dogs with lateralized compressive myelopathy or radiculopathy. *Vet. Surg.* 34: 436–444.

10. Hearon, K., Berg, J.M., Bonczynski, J.J. et al. (2014). Upper thoracic disc disease (T1-T9) in large-breed dogs. *J. Am. Anim. Hosp. Assoc.* 50: 105–111.

11. Klatzkow, S., Johnson, M., James, M., and Carrera-Justiz, S. (2018). Ventral stabilization of a T2-T3 vertebral luxation via median sternotomy in a dog. *Case Rep. Vet. Med.* 9: 1–6.

12. Bezuidenhout, A. (2013). The heart and arteries. In: *Miller's Anatomy of The Dog*, 4e (ed. H.A. Evans and A. DeLahunta), 460–466. Missouri: Elsevier Saunders.

13. Fauber, A. and Bergman, R. (2017). Spinal procedures. In: *Current Techniques in Canine and Feline Neurosurgery* (ed. A. Shores and B.A. Brisson), 495–510. New Jersey: Wiley.

10

Principles in Surgical Management of Locked Cervical Facets in Dogs

Andy Shores[1] and Ryan Gibson[2]

[1]*Mississippi State University, Mississippi State, MS, USA*
[2]*Auburn University, Auburn, AL, USA*

Introduction

The description of locked cervical facets (subaxial cervical articular process subluxation and dislocation) is relatively new in the veterinary field. It was first described by Gibson at Mississippi State in 2018 [1] and later by Woelfel at North Carolina State in 2021 [2]. A previous report in 1986 [3] described a similar condition, but this was not referred to as "locked facets." In all there are 14 cases described as unilateral locked cervical facets (ULCF) in dogs and all have been at either C5–C6 or C6–C7. In addition, all but two have been a consequence of big dog/little dog confrontations; the exceptions being a result of automobile trauma. The likely mechanism for the malady is a combination of flexion and rotation of the cervical spine. In this chapter, we will describe the surgical management of locked cervical facets in the dog. The incidence is likely much higher than has been reported.

Unilateral Locked Cervical Facets in Humans

This condition is well described in the human literature [4]. In addition, there are also descriptions of bilateral locked cervical facets. In ULCF the treatment remains controversial and is somewhat case dependent. A nonsurgical reduction, a more conservative therapy, uses a halo apparatus; however, anatomical results are reported as poor. In most cases, closed reduction is attempted and, if successful, is followed by surgical stabilization (anterior approach). When closed reduction fails, open reduction is performed using a posterior approach.

Clinical Presentation

Reported cases are overwhelmingly in small or toy breeds and as a result of big dog/little dog encounters [1, 2]; however, one patient was medium sized (Llewelin Setter – 15.9 kg) and was presented after automobile trauma [1]. In addition, other coexisting cervical injuries are possible. In the two dogs in the original report there was also atlantoaxial subluxation [1]. The 2021 report described some axial rotation of the more cranial segments and a variety of fractures including a transverse process, articular process, and a lamina fracture [2]. These findings emphasize the need for advanced imaging of the entire cervical spine to display all components of the spinal/vertebral injury.

The majority of the dogs will present as severely tetraparetic and many can be described as having a central cord syndrome, since the thoracic limbs are often more severely affected than the pelvic limbs and the injury involves the more caudal cervical vertebrae. In addition, some patients will present with respiratory compromise, likely as a consequence of damage to the C5 segment's contribution to the phrenic nerve [5]. Based on this, it is ideal that the respiratory function of these patients – to include an arterial blood gas analysis – be performed before any sedation/anesthesia is started.

Most ULCF patients are considered emergent and thus require immediate attention, including referral to a specialty hospital. After initial evaluation (usually including complete physical and neurologic exam plus cervical

---

Advanced Techniques in Canine and Feline Neurosurgery, First Edition. Edited by Andy Shores and Brigitte A. Brisson.
© 2023 John Wiley & Sons, Inc. Published 2023 by John Wiley & Sons, Inc.
Companion site: www.wiley.com/go/shores/advanced

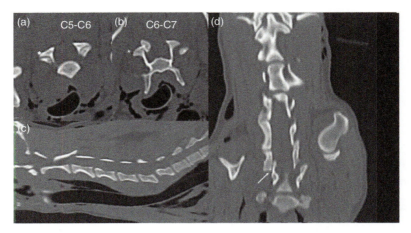

Figure 10.1 Computed tomography (CT) images of a canine patient with unilateral locked facet at C6–C7. (a) Transverse image through C5–C6 articulation. The asterisk shows intact left articulation at C5–C6. (b) Transverse image through C6–C7 articulation. The asterisk shows the cranial left C7 facet locked over the top of the left C6 caudal facet. (c) Sagittal CT reconstruction showing dorsal deviation of the C7 vertebral body. (d) Arrow points to the override of the cranial left C7 facet locked over the top of the left C6 caudal facet.

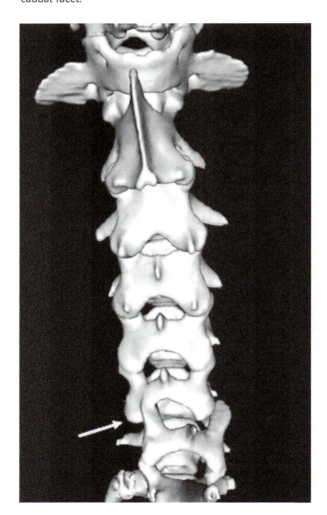

Figure 10.2 3D reconstruction of CT image showing override of the cranial left C7 facet locked over the top of the left C6 caudal facet (arrow).

radiographs) a computed tomography (CT) scan is performed (Figure 10.1). A 3D reconstruction of the CT scan is helpful in surgical planning (Figure 10.2). Depending on the severity of the neurologic condition, immediate or next day surgical intervention is recommended.

Surgical Techniques

From the authors' experience, a dorsal approach is recommended. This allows direct visualization of the locked facet and direct visualization of the correction. Intraoperatively, the dorsally displaced cranial facet of the more caudal vertebra is removed with rongeurs or a high-speed surgical drill. At the same time, the more caudal vertebra is held in position with point-to-point forceps (Figure 10.3) to prevent further rotation. After removal of the locket facet, the opposing facets are realigned and temporarily fixed into position using a K-wire placed through the facets. With the vertebra aligned, dorsal fixation of the two vertebrae is performed. And while a variety of fixation techniques have been used, many consider the use of bilateral locking (SOP™)[1] plates as the most secure fixation in this area (Figure 10.4). Other options include wire fixation techniques, pins and PMMA, ventral fixation techniques, or a combination of dorsal and ventral fixation (Figure 10.5). The authors feel this method of reduction of the locked facets has the advantage of not placing undue stress on an already compromised caudal cervical spinal cord. Admittedly, the limited literature on this condition does contain case reports where reduction has been successfully employed, leaving the locked facet intact both with and without surgical stabilization.

---

[1] SOP/String of Pearl Plates; Orthomed, Huddersfield, West Yorkshire, UK.

10 Principles in Surgical Management of Locked Cervical Facets in Dogs | 93

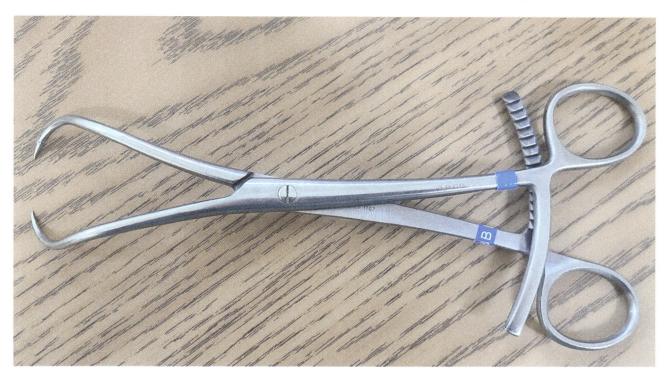

Figure 10.3 Point-to-point forceps used to rotate the luxated vertebra into alignment after removal of the locked (overriding) facet.

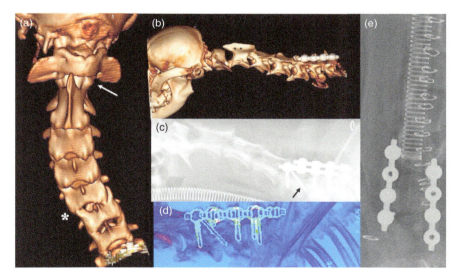

Figure 10.4 Use of bilateral SOP locking plates is generally considered the most reliable and stable fixation. In this patient, there was a unilateral locked facet at the C5–C6 junction. (a) Three-dimensional reconstruction of the initial (preop) CT scan. Note the overriding cranial left facet of C6 (asterisk) and the malalignment (subluxation) of the atlanto-axial joint (arrow). (b) 3D reconstructed postoperative CT scan of the dorsal fixation using two SOP locking plates. Note the two small holes in the spinous process of C2; these were placed when performing a dorsal suture fixation of C1–C2 to correct the malalignment. (c) Lateral postoperative radiograph showing the locking plate fixation. Note the small K-wire (black arrow) that was initially placed through the right C5–C6 articulation to maintain temporary stabilization and realignment/reduction in preparation for the locking plates. (d) A colorized volume rendering reconstruction of the CT scan to better demonstrate placement of the plates. (e) Ventrodorsal postoperative radiograph of the fixation.

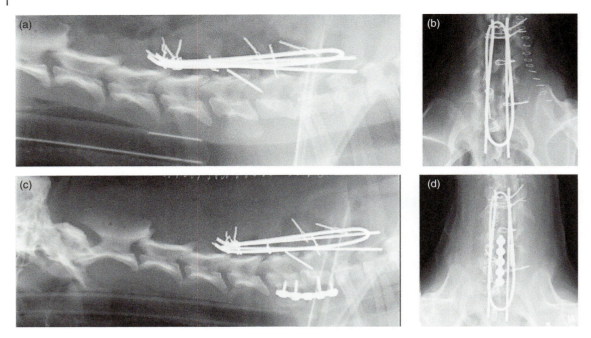

Figure 10.5 Other forms of fixation include pins and wires and ventral plating. (a) Lateral and (b) ventrodorsal radiographs showing a dorsal fixation technique described by the authors as paperclip fixation, a form of segmental fixation. The K-wires are bent into a u-shape and the length is adjusted to incorporate one vertebra cranial and one caudal to the locked facet. This fixation method would be considered adequate for smaller (less than 10 kg) patients; however, the size of this patient (16 kg), and the need for more rigorous postoperative physical therapy, dictated additional fixation ventrally. Also notice the holes In the C2 spinous process – this patient also required realignment of the atlanto-axial joint. (c) and (d) lateral and ventrodorsal views of the additional (ventral) fixation using a five-hole SOP locking plate.

Postoperative Care

Intraoperative stability and patient's neurologic status and respiratory status largely govern the postoperative plan. Arterial blood gas analysis is usually performed. Patients having difficulty maintaining SpO_2 or that have any suggestion of hypoxia should be placed on supplemental oxygen. In addition, some patients will have difficulty maintaining a sufficiently low pCO_2 and may require some ventilatory support during the immediate postoperative period. Often these patients are maintained in a neck brace for one to two weeks. The brace may consist of soft-roll cotton, roll gauze, and a self-adherent wrap (Figure 10.6). Intravenous analgesics are used for at least the first 24 hours and oral medications can be started as the patient is being weaned off the intravenous therapy.

Physical therapy is often another component of the postoperative care. In the initial postoperative period, passive range of motion and e-stem are used. After adequate time for the fixation to begin to heal, water treadmills and cart therapy can be used.

Summary/Conclusions

Locked cervical facets are not common occurrences but are unique, and veterinary neurosurgeons should have a heightened awareness of this condition as therapeutic measures may differ considerably from other neck injuries. Clearly, a procedure that has less chance of placing additional stress/injury potential on the caudal cervical spinal cord deserves the strongest consideration. Multiple cervical injuries may also be present with this condition and the diagnostics should address this concern (i.e., imaging the entire cervical spine). Fixation techniques vary.

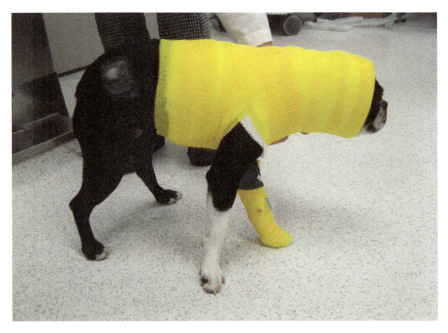

Figure 10.6 A brace applied to support stabilization of the caudal cervical spine. Patients are maintained in a neck brace for one to two weeks. The brace consists of soft-roll cotton, roll gauze, and a self-adherent wrap.

References

1. Gibson, R., Shores, A., Beasley, M., and Hatfield, J. (2018). Diagnosis and surgical management of unilateral cervical locked facets in the canine. *Proceedings of the SEVEN Conference October 2018*, Athens, GA.
2. Woelfel, C.W., Bray, K.Y., Early, P.J. et al. (2022 Jan). Subaxial cervical articular process subluxation and dislocation: cervical locked facet injuries in dogs. *Vet. Surg.* 51 (1): 163–172. https://doi.org/10.1111/vsu.13746.Epub 2021 Nov 24. PMID: 34820884.
3. Basinger, R.R., Bjorling, D.E., and Chambers, J.N. (1986). Cervical spinal luxation in two dogs with entrapment of the cranial articular process of C6 over the caudal articular process of C5. *J. Am. Vet. Med. Assoc.* 188 (8): 865–867. PMID: 3710877.
4. Shapiro, S.A. (1993). Management of unilateral locked facet of the cervical spine. *Neurosurg.* 33 (5): 832–837. https://doi.org/10.1227/00006123-199311000-00007; discussion 837. PMID: 8264879.
5. De Troyer, A.D. (1998). The canine phrenic-to-intercostal reflex. *J. Phys.* 508 (Pt 3) (Pt 3):: 919–927. https://doi.org/10.1111/j.1469-7793.1998.919bp.x.

11

Spinal Stabilization: Cervical Vertebral Column

Bianca F. Hettlich

University of Bern, Bern, Switzerland

Introduction

Cervical stabilization might be indicated for vertebral column instability resulting from trauma, anomalies, or pathologic conditions such as diskospondylitis. In these scenarios, orthopedic fixation principles are used to achieve functional alignment and apply rigid fixation. Stabilization has also become increasingly popular for the treatment of cervical spondylomyelopathy (CSM). For CSM, the goal of surgery is to eliminate motion at the affected vertebral articulation, thereby decreasing tissue responses secondary to instability such as ligamentous or annular hypertrophy as well as articular facet proliferation.

Distraction of the intervertebral disk space is beneficial for traction responsive lesions, such as soft tissue compression by thickened dorsal longitudinal ligament (DLL) or ligamentum flavum. While distraction per se may not lead to improvement of bony compression by facet prolifera-tion, it may improve compression by proliferative soft tissues. The use of a disk spacer in a neutral or slightly distracted position maintains distraction and is beneficial for load sharing between the affected vertebrae, thereby improving implant longevity. Interbody fusion is desired to provide long-term stability and prevent implant failure. This chapter will focus on ventral stabilization techniques of the cervical vertebral column used primarily to treat dogs with CSM. The principles presented here can be applied to many other conditions of the cervical spine requiring stabilization.

Preoperative Planning

Well positioned orthogonal radiographs of the cervical ver-tebral column are obtained to gain a general idea of vertebral body and disk space dimensions. To be used for measurements, radiographs must be calibrated with an appropriated positioned calibration tool (i.e. metal ball of known diameter). For plate fixation, radiographs help determine plate size and length and screw location. Knowledge of the latter is important to avoid screw place-ment in intervertebral disk spaces. Computed tomography provides excellent bony detail and is considered the most useful modality for preoperative planning of vertebral col-umn stabilization. Vertebral body dimensions, in particu-lar height, should be determined via CT at several locations to assist with selection of screw lengths. If an intervertebral spacer is used, endplate height and width and disk space depth need to be calculated to obtain an appropriate size spacer. Disk space dimensions should be obtained from unaffected sites (if available) to determine "normal" dimensions. While MRI is considered the gold-standard imaging modality for spinal cord evaluation and invaluable for overall assessment of disease, the osseous detail it pro-vides can be challenging for preoperative planning.

Anatomical Considerations

Cervical vertebral anatomy is challenging for rigid fixation due to limited compact bone stock and the proximity of important neurovascular structures (Figure 11.1). Dorsal approaches for stabilization of the cervical vertebral col-umn in large dogs are uncommon. The vertebral body offers the most bone for fixation and is easily approached via a standard ventral approach. However, even this part of the vertebra offers on average only 6–12 mm in bone depth in most large dogs until the vertebral canal is breached. Due to the hour glass shape of the vertebral body, the greatest bone depth is near the vertebral endplate and the thinnest

---

Advanced Techniques in Canine and Feline Neurosurgery, First Edition. Edited by Andy Shores and Brigitte A. Brisson.
© 2023 John Wiley & Sons, Inc. Published 2023 by John Wiley & Sons, Inc.
Companion site: www.wiley.com/go/shores/advanced

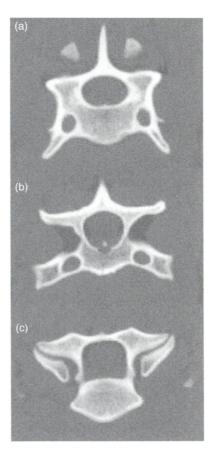

Figure 11.1 Axial CT images at different levels of C5 vertebra in a large breed dog. (a) Just caudal to the cranial endplate of C5; the pedicles and the vertebral body dimensions are relatively large; the transverse foramina are prominent. (b) Mid body of C5; pedicle dimensions are minute and the body depth has decreased significantly; note the limited space within the transverse processes when avoiding the transverse foramina. (c) just cranial to the caudal endplate of C5; the vertebral body enlarges again, offering more bone for implant purchase; pedicle dimensions are minute.

portion over the mid-body. Intervertebral disk orientation is oblique in a craniodorsal to caudoventral direction; therefore, most bone will be purchased if implants are directed parallel to the endplates. The presence of the sternum and the limited exposure of the caudal cervical vertebral column can make implant placement parallel to the endplate in C6 and C7 challenging. The transverse processes offer additional fixation sites; however, bone is quite thin and care must be taken to avoid penetration into the transverse foramen (present C1–C6), which houses the vertebral artery. While some spinal locations (i.e. lumbar spine) offer additional bone purchase by also utilizing the vertebral pedicle, this is not recommended in the cervical vertebral column. Pedicle width is limited and not uniform throughout the individual cervical vertebra, making it challenging to be engaged with a pin or screw (Figure 11.1).

Implant Selection

Evidence in the veterinary literature strongly supports that bicortical implant placement in the cervical vertebral bodies is associated with a high risk of injury to important neurovascular structures such as spinal cord, nerve roots, or vertebral vasculature [1–3]. Therefore, bicortical vertebral body implants are not recommended for cervical fixation. Despite less bone purchase and concern for implant stiffness, monocortical screw fixation seems to compare favorably to bicortical pin fixation and eliminates the potential for major iatrogenic injury [3, 4]. Monocortical screw fixation has become the standard in current techniques publications [5–9]. The use of monocortical screws with Poly(methyl methacrylate) (PMMA) provides the most freedom in regard to screw placement; however, the presence of a large bulk of cement can interfere with adjacent soft tissues and also makes implant removal more time consuming. Plate fixation eliminates bulky implants, improves soft tissue closure and ease of implant removal if required. Depending on the surgeon's comfort level with the technique and available inventory, locking plates with monocortical screws can be applied to the ventral vertebral bodies. In contrast to angle-stable locking plates, polyaxial locking plates allow screw insertion within a given range of variable angles, which gives these plates some degree of flexibility with screw placement. Traditional nonlocking plates should be avoided as they are challenging to apply with appropriate contouring to produce excellent plate/bone contact and friction.

To date, most used veterinary plate systems are made of stainless steel, prohibiting the use of postoperative MRI. Titanium implants significantly reduce artifact development on MRI and are the preferred metal for vertebral instrumentation, regardless of these being titanium alloy screws in conjunction with PMMA or plate systems [10].

Positioning and Approach

The dog is placed in dorsal recumbency with thoracic limbs tied back caudally (Figure 11.2). The cervical vertebral column is supported with towels and a bean bag to level the spine horizontally in a neutral position. Placing a large roll of towels under the neck should be avoided as this overly extends the vertebral column and makes it more difficult to maintain the spine in alignment while traction is applied. Care must be taken to securely tie down the dog's body to prevent displacement, especially if manual traction is applied for distraction. The dog's right side should be placed toward the edge of the surgery table to improve ease of access for the main surgeon during a routine right-sided ventral approach. Both proximal humeri are included in

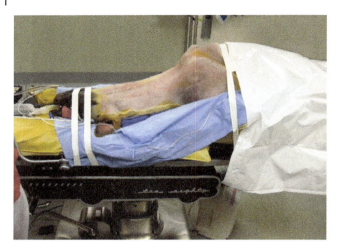

Figure 11.2 Photo of positioning of a dog for cervical distraction and stabilization. The dog is in dorsal recumbency with the neck in neutral and the head extended. The sterile field includes both shoulder joints to allow for bone graft harvesting from the proximal humerus. Both forelimbs are tied back and body is maintained in a straight position by using a vacuum bag. Tape is used to secure the dog to the table. During manual distraction, the tape holding the head will be removed.

the sterile field to allow harvesting of an autologous cancellous bone graft (if desired). Bone graft should be obtained as late as possible during the procedure and stored in a blood-soaked sponge until implantation to improve graft survival.

With the surgeon standing on the right side, a standard ventral midline or right paramedian approach to the cervical vertebral column is performed. With a paramedian approach, the insertion of the right sternocephalicus muscle can be partially tenotomized from the sternum to improve access to the caudal cervical spine. In some cases, it is necessary to split the manubrium sterni [11].

For a single site stabilization, the ventral vertebral bodies adjacent to the affected disk space are exposed but dissection can usually spare the neighboring disk spaces. If PMMA fixation is used, part of the longus colli musculature can be resected to make room for the cement. Otherwise, soft tissues are preserved.

Vertebral Distraction

Distraction of the intervertebral space can be achieved via manual traction or vertebral distractors. Good distraction greatly facilitates diskectomy and decompression of extruded material if present. For manual traction it is important to secure the patient's body sufficiently to the surgical table without interfering with respiration or compromising circulation of blood flow to distal limbs. The pinnae and mandibular rami can be used as extra anchor points while gently pulling the dog's head rostrally. Manual traction usually leads to sufficient disk space distraction to perform the diskectomy, remove extruded disk material from the vertebral canal, and place a disk spacer. It avoids placement of distractors or distractor pins that can interfere with access to the affected disk space(s) and possibly compromise bone needed for fixation. However, manual traction is labor intense and can often only be maintained for a few minutes without losing distraction. The person applying traction must do so in a slow and deliberate way and avoid sudden collapse of the vertebral articulation with possible injury to the spinal cord. A variety of human vertebral distractors are available with the most commonly used one in veterinary surgery being a Caspar-style distractor (Figure 11.3). This instrument uses two fixation pins placed perpendicularly into adjacent vertebral bodies. These pins are then connected to the distractor and the disk space is carefully distracted. If properly placed and assembled, distraction is easily achieved and greatly facilitates diskectomy. However, over distraction is also easily achieved and must be avoided to protect articular facet integrity and prevent nerve root injury. Also, since most distraction and stabilization techniques require implant placement along the ventral aspect of the vertebral bodies, distractor pins can be in the way of and compromise valuable bone stock for instrumentation. A commonly used veterinary instrument to aid in disk space distraction is a modified Gelpi-retractor, where the tips have been shortened to 2–3 mm length. The Gelpi-retractor is placed into small holes that are drilled into the ventral vertebral bodies adjacent to the affected disk space. As with Caspar distractors, use of such retractor – while beneficial for disk space distraction – will occupy and potentially compromise valuable bone needed for fixation. Therefore, the benefits of a distractor need to be weighed against the potential disadvantages.

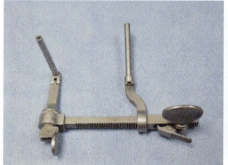 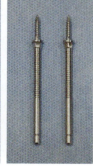

Figure 11.3 Caspar retractor with instrument specific distraction pins. The pins are placed into the ventral aspect of adjacent vertebral bodies. Thereafter, the retractor arms are inserted over the pins. Distraction is then achieved by slowly turning the ratchet.

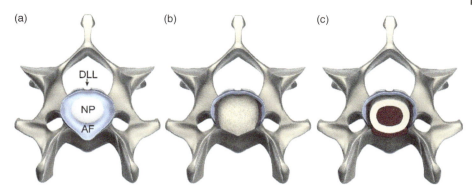

Figure 11.4 Illustration of an intervertebral disk in situ (a); a partial diskectomy with only a thin rim of annulus fibrosus remaining laterally and dorsally (b); and an intervertebral spacer using a cortical ring graft filled with cancellous bone (c). DLL, dorsal longitudinal ligament; NP, nucleus pulposus.

Diskectomy

Diskectomy is performed with the goal of ultimate arthrodesis between the affected vertebral bodies. Both endplates must be cleared of disk material to allow bone fusion as any remaining soft tissue will impede bony bridging. Sharp dissection of the ventral annulus fibrosus with an 11 blade will speed up disk removal. Lempert rongeurs are used to carefully remove the nucleus pulposus and as much of the lateral and dorsal annulus as possible. Distraction is required to allow rongeurs to be inserted sufficiently deep to remove enough disk. The goal is to remove approximately 90% of the disk, leaving a thin rim of annulus along the lateral and dorsal aspect (Figure 11.4). The remaining rim will prevent graft material and the intervertebral spacer from protruding into the vertebral canal or dislodging laterally. Aggressive dorsal and lateral annulus resection should be avoided to prevent inadvertent damage to the spinal cord as well as adjacent vasculature and nerve roots.

If a disk extrusion has occurred, the dorsal annulus must be partially removed to allow extraction of extruded material from the vertebral canal. Once as much disk material as possible has been removed by rongeurs, bone curettes are used to gently clear both vertebral endplates of remaining cartilaginous material. Careful use of a pneumatic drill can assist in clearing of the endplates; however, excessive remove of bone can weaken the endplates and lead to subsidence of the disk spacer (if used).

Intervertebral Spacer

Distraction of an intervertebral articulation ameliorates spinal cord compression by proliferated soft tissues and protruding dorsal annulus fibrosus. As there is no bone on bone contact between the affected vertebrae, stabilizing implants must carry most of the load during normal movement of the cervical vertebral column. The goal of an intervertebral spacer is to maintain the desired disk space depth and provide load sharing between the affected vertebral bodies, thereby increased implant longevity. Addition of an intervertebral spacer significantly increases construct stiffness [12].

Intervertebral spacers can range from simple cement plugs to carbon fiber reinforced polymer cages, cortical rings, and metal cages. While solid materials such as a cement plugs will maintain distraction, they will not allow ingrowth of bone and fusion within the disk space. Cages or cortical ring allografts provide distraction while allowing placement of a fresh cancellous autogenous bone graft in the middle of the cage/ring to encourage bone fusion [3, 5]. In the case of a cortical allograft, the ring will be resorbed and replaced with autogenous bone over time. In the USA, cortical allografts are commercially available in different lengths and diameters (Bergman block – Veterinary Transplant Services, Inc., Kent, WA, USA). A round or slightly oval section of bone is preferred (femur or distal tibia). Patient-specific dimensions of a normal appearing cervical disk space are measured. If all intervertebral disks are affected, the width and height of the vertebral endplates are obtained, and disk space depth is estimated (traction may aid). Based on these measurements, a cortical allograft is ordered. Block segments are generally 2–5 cm long and several rings can be made from one length of bone for the same patient. Most large breed dogs undergoing cervical distraction and stabilization have similar disk space dimensions and, if the case load is high enough, several cortical ring allografts can be stored in hospital. At the time of surgery, the allograft is thawed to room temperature in warm sterile saline. A sagittal saw is used to cut a cortical ring of sufficient depth (Figure 11.5). It is recommended to cut the ring slightly larger and do final adjustments by removing more bone with a bone rasp to avoid a ring that is of insufficient size. Fresh cancellous autograph is obtained from the proximal humerus just prior to placement of the disk spacer. The ring allograph is packed tightly with this fresh graft. The disk space is distracted and the ring

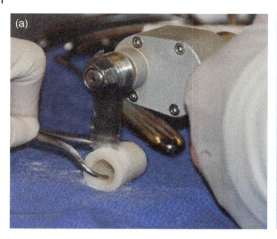 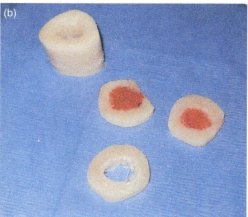

Figure 11.5 (a) A sagittal saw is use to cut a cortical allograft segment into a ring of appropriate depth to be used as an intervertebral spacer. (b) Several cortical rings have been cut and two are packed with fresh cancellous bone graft. One of the rings has been modified for improved fit by carefully cutting part of the cortex. It is, however, preferred to order a cortical segment that fits the patient specific disk space dimensions rather than compromising the structure of the ring.

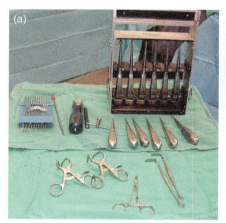 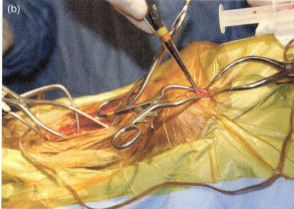

Figure 11.6 (a) Instrumentation used to obtain a fresh cancellous autograph from the proximal humerus. The greater tubercle is approached and a large Steinmann pin is used to create a hole in the cortical bone. Curettes of increasing sizes are used to remove cancellous bone, which is collected in a sterile container. Keeping the graft in a blood-soaked sponge or adding some fresh blood, as well as harvesting the graft as late in the procedure as possible, increases graft survival. (b) Intraoperative photograph of a dog undergoing cervical distraction/stabilization. Both forelimbs are pulled caudally (toward the right) and both shoulder joints are included in the sterile prep and drape. A standard approach to the caudal cervical spine has been performed and large drop-handle Gelpi retractors are in place. The right proximal humerus has also been approached and a cancellous bone graft is currently being harvested.

allograph is inserted along the endplate orientation. Care must be taken to insert the ring sufficiently dorsal. The concavity in the endplate of the cranial vertebral body can act as a trap for the ring, preventing its full insertion and leading to poor fit and inappropriate distraction of the disk space. If allograft ring dimensions fit with disk space dimensions and the diskectomy has been performed appropriately, the ring allograft should be flush with the ventral aspect of the vertebral bodies. Any remaining cancellous graft is placed around the ventral aspect of the disk space and fixation of the affected vertebrae commences (Figure 11.6).

Alternatives to a cortical ring allograft include cortical autograft (potential harvest sites include rib, distal ulna, iliac crest) or synthetic spaces made of various materials (i.e. polyetheretherketone: PEEK; polyetheretherketoneetherketone: PEEKEK; titanium; acrylic). Most commercially available spacers are for human spine surgery, positing challenges regarding their size and cost.

Indication for Additional Decompression

The two main indications for decompressive procedures in addition to cervical stabilization in dogs with CSM are compression of extruded nuclear material or severe dorsolateral compression by articular processes. In case of disk extrusion, removal of sequestered nuclear material can usually be achieved through the disk space after diskectomy. If needed, a narrow ventral slot can be performed; however, any breach in vertebral endplate may compromise the stability of a disk spacer, if used. If no spacer is inserted, the ventral slot space can be filled with cancellous bone graft prior to closure to aid bony fusion. Care must be taken when filling the slot with bone graft to avoid displacement into the vertebral canal. A small piece of gel foam can be placed at the dorsal aspect of the slot, although usually enough DLL remains to act as a natural barrier, unless the bone graft is too aggressively packed into the slot.

Of more clinical significance is the need for removal of dorsolateral compression by hypertrophied articular processes (Figure 11.7). While distraction/stabilization is aimed at alleviating compression by soft tissues as well as slowing or halting bony proliferation of articular facets, it does not remove existing bony compression. The surgeon must decide whether the degree of bony compression in dogs with osseous-associated CSM warrants additional decompression. Such decompression is best achieved by removal of one of the hypertrophied facet joints via cervical facetectomy. The affected vertebral articulation will first be distracted and stabilized via a ventral approach followed by repositioning and facetectomy. As both procedures are considered major surgeries, they are sometimes performed separately with a few days of recovery in-between. In some cases, facetectomy might be performed as the sole procedure without additional stabilization. Performing a dorsal laminectomy with removal of compressive articular process bone from within the vertebral canal carries a higher risk of iatrogenic spinal cord injury and is not as effective as direct decompression via hemilaminectomy. Rarely, a dorsal laminectomy is performed in addition to distraction/stabilization, if significant dorsal soft tissue compression is present that cannot be improved by distraction.

Surgical Stabilization

Monocortical Screw/PMMA Fixation

The vertebral body of large breed dogs easily accommodates 3.5 mm cortical screws for monocortical implantation. Cancellous screws are not recommended due to their smaller core diameter and decreased stiffness compared to their cortical counterparts.

Nonself-tapping screws might be beneficial for this fixation as these screws have a larger area of threads at the screw tip and can engage the limited bone stock more readily. Also, self-tapping screws have the potential of inadvertent penetration of the transcortex into the vertebral canal, since the cortical bone toward the vertebral canal tends to be thinner. The use of titanium screws is advantageous over stainless steel as it allows postoperative spinal cord evaluation via MRI.

The fixation construct consists of six 3.5 mm cortical screws that are placed into the adjacent vertebrae of the affected vertebral articulation. In the cranially located vertebral body, 1 screw is positioned mid-body on midline and 2 screws next to one another in the caudal metaphyseal region. In the caudally located vertebral body, 2 screws are placed parallel to each other in the cranial metaphyseal region and 1 mid-body on midline. This configuration allows for 2 screws in each vertebral body to engage the area of the bone with the most bone height (adjacent to the vertebral endplates) (Figure 11.8). If more fixation points are desired, an additional screw can easily be planned parallel to the mid-body screw (4 screws per vertebral body).

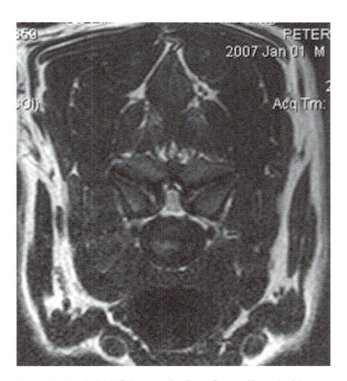

Figure 11.7 Axial MR image of a Great Dane affected with osseous-associated CSM. There is severe dorsolateral spinal cord compression by proliferated articular processes. In addition to stabilization to halt progression of proliferation, this dog requires direct decompression via cervical facetectomy.

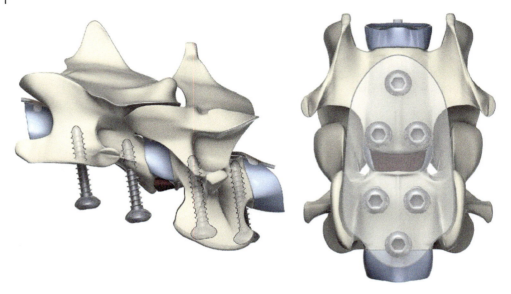

Figure 11.8 Illustration of the monocortical screw/PMMA construct. Three screws are placed per vertebra with 2 screws in the metaphyseal bone closest to the endplates. Screws are placed parallel to the vertebral endplate orientation to avoid interference with the disk space.

For each screw, a hole is drilled into the ciscortex with a 2.5 mm drill bit. Drill bit orientation should be parallel to the vertebral endplates in a caudoventral to craniodorsal direction to engage the furthest depth of bone. Endplate angles can be reviewed on the lateral radiographic projection of the patient. The two screws positioned parallel to each other in the metaphysis can be slightly angled away from midline to avoid interference of one screw with the other during placement. To prevent over drilling into the transcortex, a drill stop (Animal Orthopedics, Bishop Auckland, UK) or a depth-limiting drill guide (DePuye Synthes, West Chester, PA, USA) can be used. Otherwise, drilling should be performed with careful pressure and attention to change in drill bit position once the ciscortex is breached. A depth gauge or small, blunt probe is then used to carefully evaluate integrity of the transcortex prior to tapping and screw placement. This is a vital part of the procedure of placing monocortical screws, as it assures an intact transcortex. Depth gauge measurement is also used for selection of screw length – 10–15 mm in length are added to allow for incorporation of the screw head into PMMA. An inventory of 3.5 mm screws of 18–24 mm length should be sufficient for this type of fixation in large and giant breed dogs. Screws are then carefully placed and advanced until increased resistance indicates that the screw tip is contacting the transcortex (Figure 11.9). If self-tapping screws are used, screws are placed after the drill hole is made without the need for tapping. Care must be taken to stop advancement of the screw once the transcortex is reached or once the measured depth has been inserted, as self-tapping screws have an increased potential for breaking through into the vertebral canal. Due to the relatively small amount of available vertebral body bone, care must be taken when drilling and tapping for screw placement as bone threads may strip. When using screws with PMMA, a stripped screw can be more easily replaced by a new screw in a different position compared with plate fixation.

The musculature around the monocortical screws needs to be sufficiently retracted to allow enough room for PMMA to fully engage all screw heads. If needed, musculature may be partially resected to accommodate the PMMA; however, overly aggressive resection should be avoided. Cement mantle height should be approximately 10–15 mm and should not exceed the ventral border of the longus colli muscles to prevent compression of adjacent soft tissues such as esophagus or trachea.

Vertebral Body Plates

Several locking plate systems have been reported in clinical use and some have been evaluated biomechanically in canine cadavers [4–6, 8, 9, 13]. Most plate sizes ranged from 2.4 to 3.5 mm for medium to large breed dogs. Locking plates rigidly couple screws to the plate via a variety of locking mechanisms. To appropriately lock, most mechanisms require the screw to be inserted at a fixed angle trajectory, which dictates screw orientation (Figure 11.10). There are several important advantages of locking plates over traditional plates. Because screws are locked, plates do not need

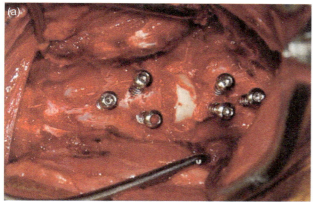
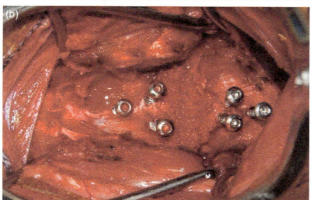
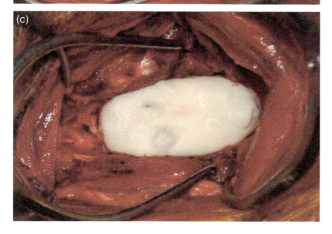

Figure 11.9 Intraoperative photographs of monocortical screw/PMMA fixation. (a) Three screws each have been placed into two adjacent vertebral bodies in a triangular pattern. Approximately 10 mm of screw is protruding to allow incorporation into PMMA. The intervertebral disk has been removed and a cortical ring allograft is in place. The graft is filled with fresh cancellous autograft and is flush with the ventral aspect of the endplates. (b) Remaining cancellous autograft is placed over the ring allowgraft. (c) Twenty grams of PMMA has been applied and covers all screw heads.

to be contoured to the undulating bone of the ventral vertebral bodies but can be laid on the bony surface with a potential offset of several millimeters. As any contouring would

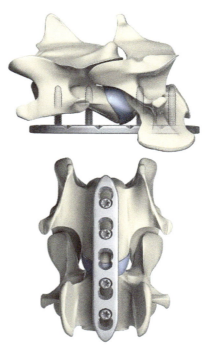

Figure 11.10 Illustration of a 3.5 locking compression plate (LCP®, Synthes, Westchester, PA, USA) applied to C5–C6 vertebral bodies. Due to the locking mechanism, the plate does not require contouring and can sit proud on the bone. Screws engage the vertebral bodies in a monocortical fashion. Due to the dimensions of the plate, usually only 2 screws can be placed per vertebral body.

change the fixed angle screw trajectory, contouring should be avoided unless a change of screw orientation is desired. The second benefit is that locking plates can be used with monocortical screws, as rigid fixation does not rely on friction between the implant and the bone. This greatly reduces potential damage to the spinal cord, nerve roots, and vessels by bicortical implants. Most biomechanical studies on monocortical locking plate fixation are based on long-bone models, therefore care must be taken to extrapolate data to the bony structure of the vertebral column. One study using canine cadaveric cervical spines assessed stiffness of an LCP (Locking Compression Plate® by DePuy Synthes, West Chester, PA, USA) with 2 screws in each vertebra, but only compared it to a ventral slot, preventing comparison of construct stiffness [5]. Another study compared 2 locking plates (3.5 SOP, String of Pearls™, Orthomed Ltd., West Yorkshire, UK; 2.4 cuttable titanium reconstruction plate, DePuy Synthes, Westchester, PA, USA) to screw/PMMA fixation and found comparable construct stiffness among the three implant types (Figure 11.11) [4]. Of note is the fact that two plates with a total of 3 or 4 screws per vertebra were used, which is different to the reported LCP fixation with only 2 screws per vertebra. It is not known how the LCP compares

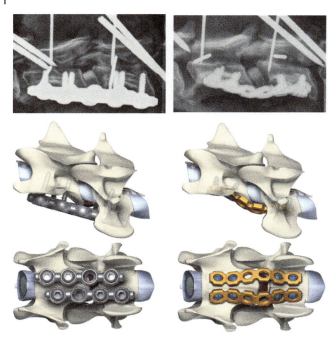

Figure 11.11 Illustration and lateral radiographic projection of two locking plates (3.5 SOP, String of Pearls, Orthomed Ltd., Huddersfield, UK; 2.4 titanium reconstruction plate, Synthes, Westchester, PA, USA) used in double configuration to stabilize the cervical vertebral column. Both plate constructs, with 6 and 8 screws, respectively, had comparable stiffness to screw/PMMA fixation. Note also that the reconstruction plates could be contoured nicely to the ventral vertebral bodies, but also how contouring changes screw trajectories.

biomechanically to these double-plate constructs. The titanium reconstruction plate can be contoured well to the ventral vertebral bone surface. As with any locking plate, screw trajectory changes with plate contouring.

Technical challenges with the application of locking plates arise from the predetermined screw location based on hole position within the plate and the fixed screw trajectory. The dimensions of most plates allow 2 consecutive screws per vertebral body but care must be taken not to inadvertently violate the slanted intervertebral disk space. Monocortical drilling and careful tapping (unless self-tapping screws are used) commences as with regular screw placement. Measurement for screw length is performed prior to tapping and must be done through the locking plate, keeping in mind that many of these plates will sit proud on the bone and screws will traverse open space before engaging bone. The plate should be held as close to the bone with digital pressure, while maintaining it in the desired position during screw application. Accurate placement of the first screw is paramount as this single screw, once locked, will determine the path for all subsequent screws.

Polyaxial locking plates offer the advantage over fixed-angle locking plates that screws can be inserted with an angle up to 15° depending on the implant used. This offers some flexibility regarding screw placement, but it does not, however, eliminate the challenge of inappropriate screw hole position over undesirable anatomic structures. Therefore, regardless of type of locking plate, impeccable preoperative planning using calibrated imaging is required and careful attention and precise execution during plate application.

Other Techniques

As an alternative or augmentation to monocortical screw/PMMA fixation of the vertebral bodies, bicortical screws can be placed in the prominent transverse processes of the cervical vertebral column (Figure 11.12). For medium to large breed dogs, 3.5 mm cortical screws are placed bilaterally perpendicular to the ventral surface into the center of each transverse process. Screws must be long enough to fully engage the transcortex while still protruding 10–15 mm toward the ventral midline to be

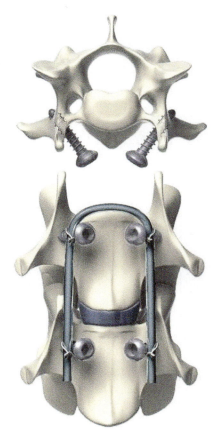

Figure 11.12 Illustration of bicortical transverse process screw/PMMA fixation with a rebar [7]. A Steinmann pin has been contoured to fit around the screws and is secured to the screws with cerclage wire to act as a reinforcement bar. The screws and bar are then incorporated into PMMA.

incorporated into PMMA. Care must be taken to avoid screw placement near the base of the process to prevent injury to the transverse foramen and vertebral artery. Reinforcement of such screw fixation with a contoured Steinmann pin and cerclage wire has been reported and biomechanically assessed [2]. Twenty grams of PMMA are then placed around screws and reinforcement bar for fixation.

So called spinal fusion implants have been established for use in human cervical fixation. Implants typically consist of an interbody spacer of variable height and angle and an interbody plate (typically made of titanium alloy), which fixes the spacer/plate to the adjacent vertebral endplates/bodies. Feasibility for use of three human spinal fusion implants in dogs and biomechanical comparison to the screw/PMMA construct was evaluated, with disappointing results [14]. The study demonstrated that none of these three implants could be recommended for use in medium to large breed dogs.

A canine specific spinal fusion implant, constructed based on the concept of interbody spacer with direct fixation to adjacent bone, has been evaluated in vitro and in vivo [15, 16].

Stabilization of Multiple Spaces

CSM often affects multiple intervertebral articulations. Single space stabilization is generally appropriate for an individual site with obviously worse compression compared to adjacent spaces. However, sometimes there is no single space that would benefit the most from surgery but neighboring spaces are similarly compressed. Stabilization with or without distraction can be performed across multiple disk spaces with the techniques described above. If monocortical screw/PMMA fixation is used, the centrally located vertebral body can house 4 screws with 2 each in the cranial and caudal metaphyseal bone (Figure 11.13). As a longer lever arm is created with the increased distance spanned by rigid internal fixation, concerns of implant failure become more prominent. In the screw/PMMA construct, failure would likely occur by fracturing of the cement, while plate fixation may fail by screw breakage through shear forces or failure of the screw/bone interface. Anecdotal reports indicate a decrease in cement breakage after multiple space fixation with the use of intervertebral spacers. It is likely that the increase in load sharing by the vertebral column via intervertebral spacers has a protective effect on implants and should improve implant longevity for both PMMA and plate fixations. Another method that may strengthen the fixation with PMMA is inclusion of a Steinman pin as a rebar within the cement. As with single site distraction/stabilization, adjacent segment disease can occur with fixation of one or multiple spaces; however, the implication of such is difficult to assess as severity may vary and may not contribute significantly to clinical signs in affected dogs.

Postoperative Assessment

To evaluate overall implant position and assess proper placement of the intervertebral spacer (if used), standard orthogonal radiographs should be obtained, centering over the stabilized vertebral articulations. While radiographs

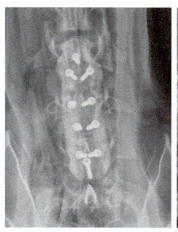
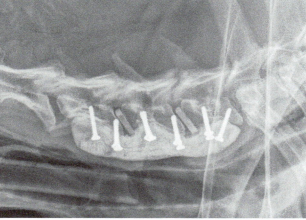

Figure 11.13 Postoperative radiographs of a Great Dane with two-level cervical distraction and stabilization at C5, C6, and C7 using monocortical screw/PMMA fixation and disk spacers. Three screws were placed into C5 and C7, four screws were placed into the cranial and caudal aspect of C6. The most caudal screw in C7 was angled caudally instead of parallel to the endplate due to interference with the sternum. Cortical ring allografts are well positioned within the two disk spaces; however, they are slightly undersized in depth (note the gap between ring and endplates).

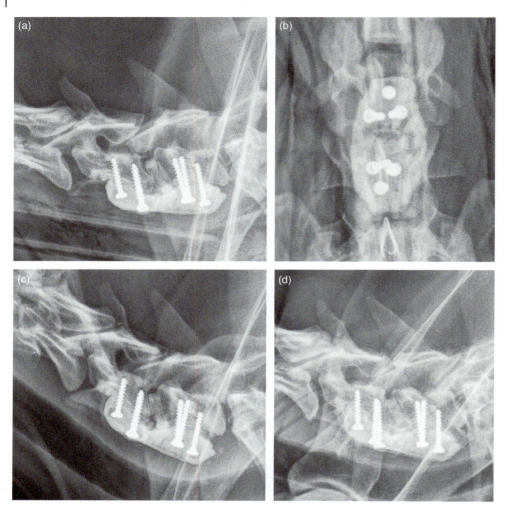

Figure 11.14 Radiographic follow-up of a Great Dane after distraction/stabilization at C6–C7 with monocortical screw/PMMA fixation and cortical ring allograft disk spacer. (a, b) Immediate postoperative orthogonal radiographs showing the fixation with triangular screw pattern and placement parallel to the endplates. (c) Two months postoperative lateral radiograph – the cortical ring has shifted slightly within the disk space compared to A; however, fit of the ring appears excellent at this time. (d) Two years postoperative lateral radiograph – there is evidence of bony fusion across the mid to ventral aspect of the disk space. Implants are intact and appear stable.

have a very low accuracy in predicting the position of bicortical cervical implants in relation to the vertebral canal, they are acceptable for monocortical implants placed ventrally into the vertebral body [3, 10]. Monocortical screws should not protrude beyond the floor of the vertebral canal on a lateral projection. Postoperative CT is excellent in assessing implant position.

Long-term, radiographs can be used to assess implant stability, overall vertebral alignment, and to some degree bony fusion across the disk space; however, it is difficult to adequately judge the degree of arthrodesis on radiographs and even advanced imaging such as CT (Figure 11.14). Due to the common use of stainless steel implants in vertebral column stabilization, postoperative MRI is usually not possible. Titanium implants are MR-compatible and are the implant material of choice to allow immediate and long-term follow-up advanced imaging [10]. This is particularly important for CSM dogs to assess development or progression of signal changes within the spinal cord as the disease progresses.

Complications

The potential injury to immediately adjacent neurovascular structures is decreased by the use of monocortical implants. However, inadvertent drill bit advancement or screw penetration into the vertebral canal can still occur. Familiarization with the patient specific vertebral body dimensions and use of a drill stop can help decrease over-drilling and subsequent screw placement into the canal. Damage to the vagosympathetic trunk, carotid artery, esophagus, or trachea can occur during aggressive approaches or negligent use of tissue retractors to access the ventral aspect of the vertebral column. Implant failure typically occurs through failure of the bone/screw interface, shearing of locking screws, or by cracking of the cement. It is unusual for screws to sheer at the screw/cement interface. While an intervertebral spacer aids in maintaining disk space distraction and helps with load-sharing, it can be improperly placed, leading to continued chronic pain and dysfunction, or it can acutely dislodge causing sudden onset pain, radiculopathy, or myelopathy. Deep infection after surgical fixation is rare and would require implant removal. In the case of screw/PMMA fixation, cement is removed around screws via a pneumatic drill. Filling screw heads with sterile bone wax prior to PMMA application will make screw removal easier. Also, considering the amount of work

required to remove PMMA, strict adherence to aseptic techniques is of paramount importance when using bone cement. Postoperative seroma formation can occur if drill debris is not properly removed via flushing and the dead space not carefully closed. Seromas are typically treated conservatively with warm compresses and time.

Long-term complications usually relate to chronic cycling and fatigue failure of implants when fusion of the stabilized vertebral articulations is delayed or does not occur. Subsidence of the disk spacer indicates insufficient implant rigidity or subclinical implant failure and may be the cause of continued chronic pain and neurologic deficits.

Finally, adjacent segment disease with degenerative disk changes, soft tissue hypertrophy, and bony changes can develop. Whether these changes occur due to the progression of preexisting disease or secondary to biomechanical stress from the longer lever arm of the stabilized vertebral articulation is still debated.

References

1. Corlazzoli, D. (2008). Bicortical implant insertion in caudal cervical spondylomyelopathy: a computed tomography simulation in affected Doberman pinschers. *Vet. Surg.* 37: 178–185.

2. Hicks, D.G., Pitts, M.J., Bagley, R.S. et al. (2009). in vitro biomechanical evaluations of screw-bar-polymethylmethacrylate and pin-polymethylmethacrylate internal fixation implants used to stabilize the vertebral motion unit of the fourth and fifth cervical vertebrae in vertebral column specimens from dogs. *Am. J. Vet. Res.* 70: 719–726.

3. Hettlich, B.F., Allen, M.J., Pascetta, D. et al. (2013). Biomechanical comparison between bicortical pin and monocortical screw/polymethylmethacrylate constructs in the cadaveric canine cervical vertebral column. *Vet. Surg.* 42 (6): 693–700.

4. Hettlich, B.F., Fosgate, G.T., and Litsky, A.S. (2017). Biomechanical comparison of 2 veterinary locking plates to monocortical screw/polymethylmethacrylate fixation in the cadaveric canine cervical vertebral column. *Vet. Surg.* 46: 95–102.

5. Agnello, K.A., Kapatkin, A.S., Garcia, T.C. et al. (2010). Intervertebral biomechanics of locking compression plate monocortical fixation of the canine cervical spine. *Vet. Surg.* 39: 991–1000.

6. Bergman, R.L., Levine, J.M., Coates, J.R. et al. (2008). Cervical spinal locking plate in combination with cortical ring allograft for a one level fusion in dogs with cervical spondylotic myelopathy. *Vet. Surg.* 37: 530–536.

7. Shamir, M.H., Chai, O., and Loeb, E. (2008). A method for intervertebral space distraction before stabilization combined with complete ventral slot for treatment of disc-associated wobbler syndrome in dogs. *Vet. Surg.* 37: 186–192.

8. Steffen, F., Voss, K., and Morgan, J.P. (2011). Distraction-fusion for caudal cervical spondylomyelop thy using an intervertebral cage and locking plates in 14 dogs. *Vet. Surg.* 40: 743–752.

9. Trotter, E.J. (2009). Cervical spine locking plate fixation for treatment of cervical spondylotic myelopathy in large breed dogs. *Vet. Surg.* 38: 705–718.

10. Jones, B., Fosgate, G.T., Green, E. et al. (2017). MRI artifacting of monocortical screw/polymethylmethacrylate constructs in canine cadaveric cervical vertebral columns. *Am. J. Vet. Radiol.* 78 (4): 458–464.

11. Mateo, I. (2020). Median manubriotomy for ventral access to the caudal cervical and cranial thoracic spine. *Vet. Surg.* 49: 923–929.

12. Hettlich, B.F., Allen, M.J., Glucksman, G. et al. (2014). Effects of an intervertebral spacer on stiffness in a cadaveric

cervical monocortical screw/polymethymethacrylate construct. *Vet. Surg.* 43 (8): 988–994.

13. Solano, M.A., Fitzpatrick, N., and Bertran, J. (2015). Cervical distraction-stabilization using an intervertebral spacer screw and string-of pear (SOP™) plates in 16 dogs with disc-associated wobbler syndrome. *Vet. Surg.* 44: 627–641.

14. Morrison, E.J., Litsky, A.S., Allen, M.J. et al. (2016). Evaluation of three human cervical fusion implants for use in the canine cervical vertebral column. *Vet. Surg.* 45 (7): 901–908.

15. Schöllhorn, B., Bürki, A., Stahl, C. et al. (2013). Comparison of the biomechanical properties of a ventral cervical intervertebral anchored fusion device with locking plate fixation applied to cadaveric canine cervical spines. *Vet. Surg.* 42 (7): 825–831.

16. Rohner, D., Kowaleski, M.P., Schwarz, G., and Forterre, F. (2019). Short-term clinical and radiographical outcome after application of anchored intervertebral spacers in dogs with disc-associated cervical spondylomyelopathy. *Vet. Comp. Orthop. Traumatol.* 32 (2): 158–164.

12

Stabilization of the Thoracolumbar Spine

Simon T. Kornberg[1] and Brigitte A. Brisson[2]

[1] *ACVIM, Southeast Veterinary Neurology, Miami, Florida, USA*
[2] *ACVS, University of Guelph, Guelph, Ontario, Canada*

Vertebral column fractures and luxation pose a unique challenge due to their variability in location, severity of instability, and various associated lesions within the injury site. Often, fractures will occur alongside luxation, traumatic disk extrusions, and other systemic injuries. Due to these variations and potential co-morbidities, careful decision-making aided by cross-sectional imaging, sound surgical principles, and proper implant selection is essential in assuring good, lasting outcomes.

In traumatic cases, whether it be from a fall, vehicular accident, bite wounds, projectile injuries, or other, it can be assumed that the patient may be systemically unstable. Proper triage and systemic stabilization should be performed as necessary. If deemed safe to do so, a complete neurologic examination to localize the lesion accurately and to provide a prognosis should be performed prior to providing sedation/analgesia. Cranial nerves should also be examined to ensure there is no evidence of head trauma. Initial patient assessment may include abdominal and thoracic focused assessments using ultrasound and thoracic, abdominal, and spinal radiographs or awake trauma CT to assess for pulmonary lesions, bladder rupture, and potential spinal instabilities that may require immediate intervention or considerations when handling the patient. Adequate pain control should be provided, and in the case of open fractures, antibiotic coverage may also be prudent.

Preoperative Planning

Standard orthogonal radiographs of the spine or trauma CT should be obtained to assess location, and severity of injury. This may also help with further selection of cross-sectional imaging modalities. Ideally, both magnetic resonance imaging (MRI) and computerized tomography (CT) should be utilized when assessing spinal injuries. MRI allows for enhanced assessment of the spinal cord, adjacent soft tissue injury, and traumatic disk extrusions. CT allows superior assessment of bone, 3D reconstruction, and is sensitive in detecting the instability even if the lesion is nondisplaced. It should be utilized to aid implant selection by assessing patient specific anatomy, implant corridors, insertion angles for safe placement, and optimal cortical bone purchase [1] (Figure 12.1).

The three-compartment concept [2] should be utilized in the decision-making process when assessing where or whether spinal instability is present. This concept divides the vertebral column into dorsal, middle, and ventral compartments. The dorsal compartment comprises the spinous process, dorsal ligamentous structures, lamina, articular processes, and pedicles. The middle compartment comprises the dorsal longitudinal ligament, dorsal annulus, and dorsal aspect of the vertebral body. The ventral compartment comprises the remaining vertebral body, nucleus pulposus, remainder of annulus, and the ventral longitudinal ligament. When two or more compartments are compromised, the lesion should be considered unstable (Figure 12.2). The need for stabilization can be assessed by utilizing this concept; however, other considerations such as neurologic status, chronicity, concurrent injuries, and imaging findings should also be considered in the decision-making process (Figure 12.3).

Advanced Techniques in Canine and Feline Neurosurgery, First Edition. Edited by Andy Shores and Brigitte A. Brisson.
© 2023 John Wiley & Sons, Inc. Published 2023 by John Wiley & Sons, Inc.
Companion site: www.wiley.com/go/shores/advanced

110 | *Advanced Techniques in Canine and Feline Neurosurgery*

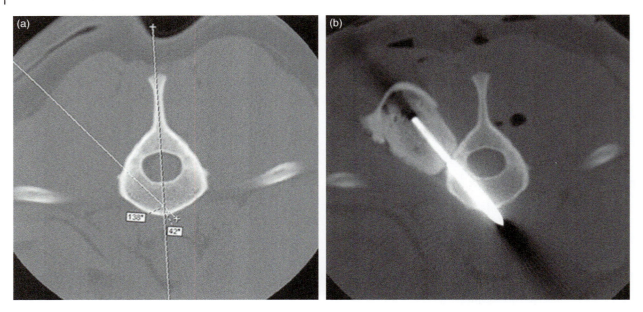

Figure 12.1 (a) Axial CT with superimposed pin insertion angle and location. (b) Postoperative axial CT of the same dog with a bicortical pin placed.

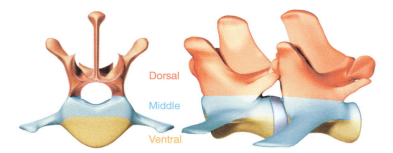

Figure 12.2 Illustration of the three compartments in the lumbar vertebrae. The dorsal compartment in RED includes the spinous processes, dorsal ligamentous structures, lamina, articular facets, and pedicles. The middle compartment in BLUE consists of the dorsal longitudinal ligament, the dorsal annulus, the floor of the vertebral canal, and the transverse processes. The ventral compartment in YELLOW includes the vertebral body, the annulus fibrosus, the nucleus pulposus, and the ventral longitudinal ligament.

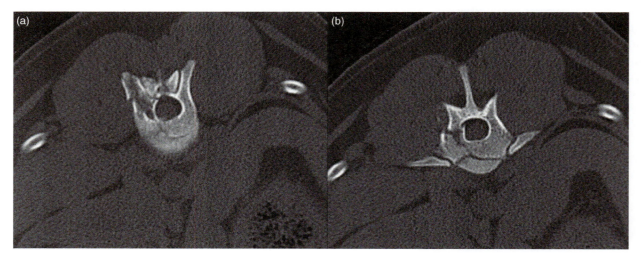

Figure 12.3 Axial CT of thoracic vertebrae, two sequential CT slices (a is cranial to b) showing nondisplaced fractures of the vertebral body (ventral compartment), floor of the vertebral canal (middle compartment), and pedicle and articular facet (dorsal compartment). This is an example of an unstable but nondisplaced fracture evidenced by multicompartmental involvement.

Decompression with Stabilization

Due to the unpredictable nature of traumatic injury, concurrent compression with bone fragments, disk material, or hemorrhage may be present. It may therefore be necessary to combine stabilization of the spine with spinal cord decompression techniques. Cross-sectional imaging with both MRI and CT is the most reliable method to determine whether decompression is needed in addition to spinal stabilization. Other indications for spinal stabilization include certain iatrogenic interventions that can unavoidably cause theoretical destabilization of the spine. Examples of this include bilateral hemilaminectomy over multiple vertebrae, radical dorsal laminectomy, and hemilaminectomy with corpectomy [3]. These procedures may be necessary in certain patients who require surgery for IVDD, tumor removal, or correction of a vertebral malformation. It is essential to apply the three-compartment concept to determine whether stabilization is required and carefully plan surgical approaches and fixation placement in these patients. When considering reduction, while complete anatomical alignment is preferable, on occasion it may not be possible due to chronicity or extent of the injury. In these cases, stabilization is still beneficial and should be performed even with suboptimal alignment.

Technique

Pre-drilling is necessary for the implantation of cortical screws. A 1.5-mm drill bit is used prior to inserting a 2.0-mm bone screw. A 2.0-mm drill bit is used prior to inserting a 2.7-mm screw, and a 2.7-mm drill bit is used prior to inserting a 3.5-mm screw (Table 12.1). High-speed drilling and low-speed screw insertion is recommended to prevent thermal necrosis. Stacked drill guides, drill stops, and – more recently – 3D printed custom drill guides can be used to safely drill to the ideal depth and insertion angle [4, 5]. Pre-drilling is also recommended for insertion of positive-profile threaded pins. It has been shown to decrease microfractures during pin insertion and to allow

Table 12.1 Suggested screw and pin sizes with corresponding drill bit size for pre-drilling.

Dog size	Recommended cortical screw size	Recommended pin size	Drill bit size for pre-drilling
Small	2.0	5/64	1.5
Medium	2.7	3/32	2.0
Large	3.5	1/8	2.7

the removal of loose bone dust that could otherwise become impacted in the insertion corridor and could lead to instability of the implant over time. Pre-drilling is achieved using a drill bit of a slightly smaller gauge than the intended pin followed by low speed power (150 rpm) pin insertion. Smaller dogs' spines can generally accommodate 5/64th or 3/32nd inch pins, while 1/8th inch pins are typical for larger dogs. The sharp pin tip can be cut prior to insertion into the pre-drilled bone to prevent inadvertent iatrogenic injury to soft tissues at the point of exit (Table 12.1) (Figure 12.4).

Implant Selection

When selecting an implant, it is important to consider surgical experience, anatomical considerations, and type of stability needed. The most commonly used implants include screws and plates and screws/pins and PMMA.

Bone plates come in two major types: conventional and locking. Conventional, nonlocking plates require precise contouring and friction so they must sit flush against the surface of the bone to maintain fixation. These also require bicortical purchase which can be technically challenging to achieve in the spine. Due to the undulating anatomy precluding consistent contact of the bone plate, impracticality of bicortical fixation in some locations, and high motion causing shear forces in multiple directions, conventional plates are generally suboptimal for spinal fixation compared to newer locking plates and PMMA constructs in both versatility, implant stability, and ease of application.

Conversely, locking plates do not require friction or bone contact in order to provide rigid fixation. These work by various mechanisms that lock the screws into the plate, creating a rigid construct that does not require bone to plate contact. Locking plates allow for a monocortical fixation that is low profile but without the drawbacks of a conventional plate. Locking plates, with some specific exceptions, require screws to be placed perpendicularly through the holes in order to engage the locking mechanism. This can prove a challenge when placing implants in predefined vertebral corridors and provides limited flexibility in this regard. Although not theoretically necessary, it is preferable to contour a locking plate as close as possible to the vertebral body to reduce the torque applied to the screw head and neck and reduce the risk of failure due to screw pull-out or shear.

There are a variety of proprietary locking implants available. Examples include the locking compression plate (LCP) plate by Synthes, the polyaxial locking plate system (PAX) system by Securos, the string of pearls (SOP) plate and the newer Pedicle Screw System, both by Orthomed. While LCP plates require the plate to be

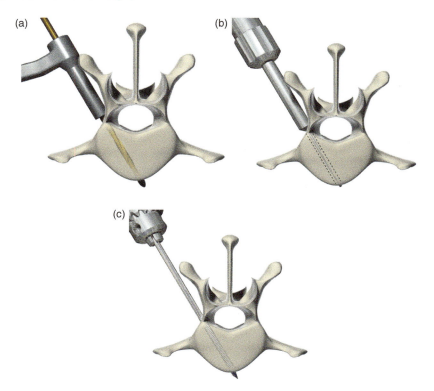

Figure 12.4 Illustration of the application of a positive-profile pin bicortically in a lumbar vertebra. (a) The vertebral body is pre-drilled at a pre-measured angle and depth using anatomical landmarks. Care should be taken to avoid advancing the drill bit past the transcortex. (b) A depth gauge is used to probe the corridor to determine the length and integrity. This ensures that adequate depth and purchase can be obtained with the implant. (c) A positive-profile pin is placed using low power (150 rpm) insertion. This should be advanced to the predetermined depth, measured from preoperative imaging.

perpendicular to the screw insertion into the bone, the latter three mentioned offer various degrees of flexibility with insertion angles by either contouring the plate (SOP), providing screw angle flexibility through the plate holes (PAX), or allowing the screws to be placed first and the rods to be attached and tightened at the nodes (Pedicle Screw System). Discussions on which system is best is beyond the scope of this chapter, and the decision to use either of the systems should be made with the individual case in mind and by the comfort and familiarity of the surgeon with the system (Figure 12.5).

Positive profile pins and polymethyl methacrylate (PMMA) constructs offer greater flexibility in implant placement, as the pins can be placed in a desired location and angle with the PMMA molded over to incorporate the construct. Positive-profile threaded Steinmann pins are preferred over cortical screws when incorporated in PMMA, due to their more substantial core diameter which resists shear forces and reduces thread failure [6]. Bicortical pin placement is recommended for PMMA constructs.

PMMA should be mixed thoroughly according to directions provided by the manufacturer. Although it can be molded manually by hand and placed into the construct, syringe application allows for more homogeneous mixing and leads to greater uniformity of the structure through the PMMA bridge, creating a more stable construct [7]. This can be achieved through a large catheter tip syringe, with perforations placed by the surgeon to allow air to be evacuated. The plunger of the syringe should be removed and the tip of the syringe should be blocked while the viscous mixture is poured into the proximal end of the syringe. The plunger should then be replaced and with the catheter tip still blocked, air should be evacuated with light depression of the plunger, avoiding the mixture escaping through the perforations. The PMMA should then be applied with the syringe and molded using either an osteotome, freer periosteal elevator, or similar. Care should be taken to incorporate all screw heads or pins and ensure that the construct is evenly distributed without air pockets or gaps. During the curing process, an exothermic reaction occurs. This can damage adjacent soft tissue structures so copious amounts of sterile saline should be flushed while the curing process takes place; this is especially important if spinal cord decompression was performed. Once cooled and hardened, it is important to assess the structure for rigidity. Some surgeons advocate adding antibiotics into the PMMA mixture. This is controversial as it may disrupt the strength of the PMMA construct [8]. PMMA constructs can be challenging to remove in the event of complications or infection (Figure 12.6).

12 *Stabilization of the Thoracolumbar Spine* | 113

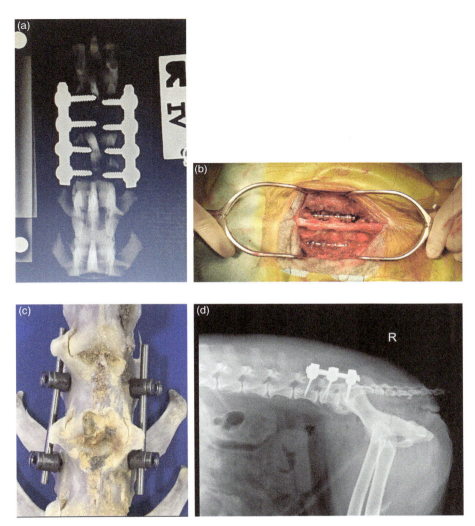

Figure 12.5 Examples of available locking plate systems (a and b) bilateral application of SOP plates in the lumbar spine. (c) Model depicting bilateral application of the Pedicle Screw System in the lumbar spine. (d) Postoperative lateral radiograph of Pedicle Screw System application in the lumbosacral spine. *Source:* Courtesy of Dr. Oscar Thamar-Torres, DVM.

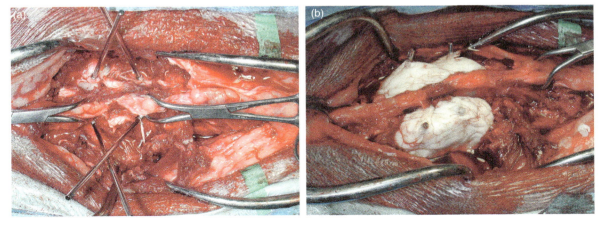

Figure 12.6 Intraoperative images of two different pin and PMMA constructs (a) prior to placement of PMMA and (b) following placement of PMMA. Note that the pins in (b) could have been cut shorter prior to PMMA application.

When applied correctly, both the PMMA construct and various locking plate constructs are appropriate methods for spinal fixation [9, 10]. Theoretically, stainless steel has a much greater fatigue resistance compared to PMMA. This is further supported by the tendency of PMMA constructs to fail where the screw enters the PMMA, when compared to plates which fail at the neck of the screw, likely due to a stress concentration effect [7]. in vivo, it is difficult to ascertain which one of these methods is more effective, and it is likely dependent on anatomy and operator experience. Using the largest possible core diameter screws or positive-profile pins and ensuring adequate bone engagement is the most important aspect of selecting a fixation method.

Thoracolumbar Spine

The thoracolumbar spine is the most common location for spinal stabilization, with T13–L1 being most affected as it is the interface between the more stable thoracic and the more flexible lumbar spine, creating a natural stress riser at this location. Unstable high thoracic fractures and luxations are uncommon due to the stabilizing nature of the ribs and more prominent thoracic limb musculature. Hyperflexion injuries are more commonly seen and typically result in caudal endplate fractures at the associated disk space. This can also lead to concurrent intervertebral disk extrusion.

Thoracolumbar vertebral anatomy varies, posing challenges depending on the area in need of fixation. As one moves cranially along the thoracic spine, the articular processes become less distinct, more dorsally located relative to the spinal cord, and the rib heads become more prominent. The proximal curvature of the rib can also obscure the approach to the vertebral body. This can be overcome by burring down the rib head, by disarticulating the rib, or by incorporating the rib heads and the articular facets using cerclage wire when applying certain dorsal fixation devices. The risk of iatrogenic trauma, such as breach of the pleural space or major vessel injury while drilling, must also be considered. Average insertion angles vary depending on the area of the injury (Table 12.2). It is recommended to determine ideal insertion angles and depth from cross-sectional imaging measurements. It is also important to recognize that the musculature and surgical approach or incision length may hinder ideal angles and a range of safe angles should therefore be determined prior to surgery using diagnostic images [1].

Positioning and Approach

Patients are typically positioned in sternal recumbency for a standard dorsal approach. The patient is stabilized using tape, sandbags, and/or bean bags with suction to maintain the desired position and facilitate appropriate implant angles. It is important to be liberal with your incision to facilitate correct insertion angles and implant placement. If planning bilateral fixation, both sides of the epaxial muscle should be elevated and the cranial transverse processes and/or rib heads should be exposed. It is preferable to keep the dorsal interspinous ligament intact when possible to optimize stability in the dorsal compartment. When performing this approach, it is of the utmost importance to be aware of any trauma-related bone fragments or exposed spinal cord, and to practice careful dissection to prevent inadvertent iatrogenic injury.

Implant Selection

Implant size should be based on the width of the vertebral pedicles and bodies. Generally, 3.5-mm screws or 1/8th-inch positive-profile pins can be accommodated in larger dogs and 2.7-mm screws and 3/32nd-inch positive-profile pins can be accommodated in smaller dogs (Table 12.2).

PMMA constructs provide freedom of insertion across a wide variety of angles, this is especially useful in areas with challenging anatomy or widely varying insertion angles that would cause difficulty due to the lack of

Table 12.2 Recommended insertion angles and landmarks for spinal implants.

Location	Insertion angle from vertical	Landmarks
T10	22° (20–25)	Tubercle of rib and base of accessory process
T11	28° (25–35)	Tubercle of rib and base of accessory process
T12	30.5° (25–35)	Tubercle of rib and base of accessory process
T13	44.5° (40–45)	Tubercle of rib and base of accessory process
L1-L6	60° (55–65)	Junction between pedicle and transverse process.
L7	20° (0–20)	Caudal to the base of the cranial articular process.
S1	0° (0–20)	Fossa caudo-medial to the articular process of L7–S1

Ranges in parentheses. *Source:* Adapted from Watine et al. [1].

flexibility of metal plates. For PMMA constructs, positive-profile, end-threaded pins are preferred over screws as they have improved pull-out resistance and their larger core diameter increases construct stiffness [9, 11]. While potentially more challenging and providing less freedom regarding insertion angle of screws, locking plates have a vastly lower profile than PMMA constructs facilitating closure of the epaxial muscles, and can be removed easily relative to PMMA in the event that implant removal is required. Additionally, if the spinal cord is exposed, plate fixation may reduce the risk of iatrogenic damage secondary to thermal injury from the curing of the PMMA. Implants should span 1–2 vertebrae cranial and caudal to the injury depending on the degree of stabilization required. Plate and screw fixation should incorporate multiple screws per segment, and is preferably bicortical; however, monocortical fixation may be sufficient when using locking screws. Bilateral fixation is generally recommended, particularly if the plate hole alignment does not allow for ideal screw purchase. For PMMA and pin constructs, bilateral fixation is preferred. One pin per segment on each side is ideal for fixation. Eight-pin constructs are generally more stable than four-pin constructs. When using eight-pin constructs, further stability is provided by angling pins away from the area being stabilized; however, with four-pin constructs, pins should be angled toward the site to provide optimal stability [12] (Figure 12.7). Using a goniometer is helpful to determine insertion angles, and using a drill stop as well as pre-measuring pins to allow accurate depth is recommended to prevent iatrogenic spinal cord or vascular injury.

Reduction of vertebral fractures should be performed carefully. While reduction is usually important in acute injuries, it may not be feasible in chronic injuries and may not be necessary when treating mild subluxations. It is important to weigh the benefit vs risk of reduction when stabilization may be sufficient.

In most hyperextension injuries, the affected segment is generally displaced cranially and ventrally. Depending on the size of the patient and the degree of instability, various techniques can be used to reduce a luxation. Occasionally, patient positioning alone may reduce the fragments. Point-to-point forceps or towel clamps placed in the spinous processes may be used to carefully obtain reduction. Strategic screw placement with a loop of heavy gauge nylon suture and gentle retraction may also be useful. Once reduction is achieved, K-wires can be placed through the reduced articular facets with or without figure-of-eight cerclage wire to keep the segment reduced while stabilization is achieved. These additional implants can be incorporated into the PMMA construct or removed prior to placement of PMMA. When planning to leave in situ, bending the K-wire can reduce the risk of pin migration. Manual or clamp reduction may still be required while the segment is stabilized. In some cases, additional intraoperative assistance is necessary to achieve this.

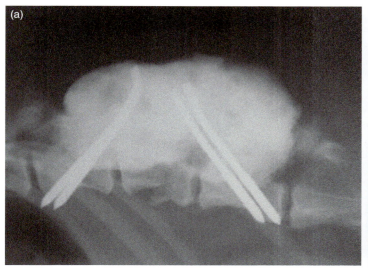
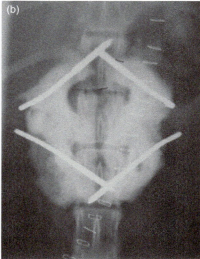

Figure 12.7 Postoperative radiographs of a pin and PMMA construct for L1 vertebral body fracture fixation. Note the pins being angled inward; this is preferable in four-pin constructs.

Closure of the epaxial musculature may be challenging; however, using mattress or cruciate sutures bridging the spinous processes is usually adequate to provide apposition of muscular layers. Standard subcutaneous and skin closure should be performed.

Spinal Stapling/Segmental Fixation

Spinal stapling (also referred to as segmental spinal stabilization) is a less rigid type of fixation that can be considered in smaller dogs to treat relatively stable vertebral column injuries that are expected to heal quickly. This technique is not appropriate if there are bilateral fractures of the vertebral arch or spinous processes [13]. The largest possible Steinmann pin that can be bent to shape to fit the patient should be used. Using a single pin to span the desired length of fixation is ideal to resist distraction while the spine is in flexion. In some cases, pins may be too short to incorporate the required area. The fixation should span two to three vertebrae cranial and caudal to the site of injury. Two pins (one on each side) are generally used; however, in smaller patients, unilateral fixation may be sufficient. A standard bilateral approach should be taken, with care to spare the dorsal interspinous ligament if possible. If this is transected, it should be sutured back in place with thick nylon suture, in a loop and pulley fashion. In the smallest patients, an appropriately sized drill bit can be used to drill a hole through the base of the spinous process at the cranial and caudal-most vertebrae to be included in the fixation. The pins should be placed through these holes and bent at 90°. This may only be feasible in the lightest of patients, as higher gauge pins may be too difficult to bend appropriately in situ. In most patients, however, the pins should be pre-contoured, and placed cranially and caudally to the desired area to be fixed. These pins should be contoured as closely as possible to the base of the spinous processes. Once placed, the open ends should be facing each other with overlap. From here, a small drill bit should be used to place small holes through the base of each incorporated spinous process and cerclage wire threaded through. The cerclage wire should be tightened around the pins, securing them into place, and tightening the fixation to contour as close to the spinous processes as possible. Additional holes can be drilled through the articular processes to place cerclage wire anchored to each side of the construct. Finally, cerclage wire can be looped underneath rib heads and tightened to further enhance stability (Figure 12.8).

Lubra plates are paired, curved plastic plates that are fitted on either side of the spinous processes, bridging the area to be stabilized and providing additional dorsal stabilization. These plates are fitted with surgical bolts applied between the spinous processes. Lubra plates are relatively inexpensive, do not require a steep learning curve, and can provide stability with some flexibility in patients with sufficiently large spinal processes. In contrast, Lubra plates do not provide adequate stability for fractures in larger and more muscular dogs, they can reportedly cause pressure necrosis of the spinous processes and require an intact dorsal column to be effective. Lubra plates have now

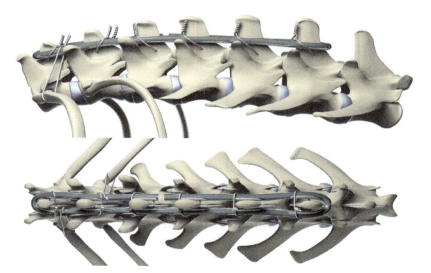

Figure 12.8 Lateral (a) and dorsoventral (b) radiographic projections of spinal staple of the thoracolumbar spine. A Steinmann pin is bent and contoured to fit closely around the most cranial and caudal spinous processes. Cerclage wire is placed through the base of the spinous processes and tightened to the Steinmann pin to hold it in place. Additional cerclage wire can be looped under rib heads to provide further anchor points and maintain further stability of the construct.

been mostly replaced by newer and more stable methods of fixation (Figure 12.9).

External fixation of the spine is less commonly performed but has some distinct advantages over internal fixation that include a wider range of insertion angles into the vertebral bodies, as the fixation is not confined to the limitations of an internal fixation device and the surrounding musculature dictating the angles of insertion and adjustment of construct. Furthermore, the implants can be removed once healing has occurred without the need for a second surgery. Threaded pins can be applied by either an open approach or percutaneously using fluoroscopy without the need for a large incision. External fixator pins should be placed bicortically, one in each vertebra spanning two vertebrae cranially and caudally to the site of instability. These pins are then bridged with a rigid structure such as PMMA or carbon fiber arches. External fixation requires strong owner compliance with daily aseptic pin care to keep the apparatus clean. In addition, external devices will impede certain aspects of postoperative rehabilitation, which can have a negative effect on recovery time [14].

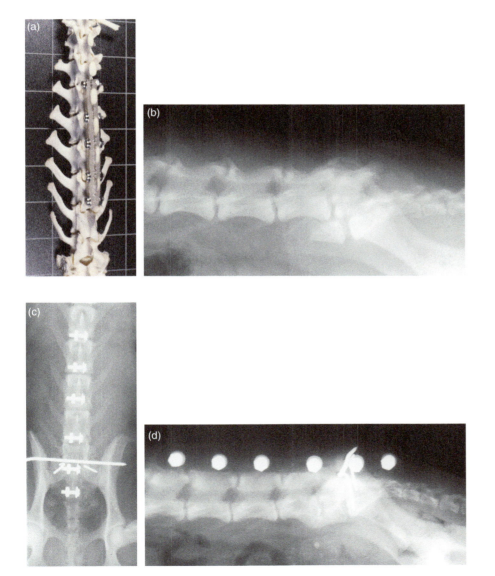

Figure 12.9 (a) Image of lubra plates applied on a spine model. Note the compression on the spinous processes and the way the plate "press fits" around them. (b) Lateral radiographic projection of an L7 fracture-luxation. (c and d) Dorsoventral and lateral radiographic projections of an L7 fracture-luxation. This has been reduced and stabilized with lubra plates, transilial pin, and K-wires through the articular facet joints.

Lumbosacral Spine

Lumbosacral injuries generally result from severe hyperflexion and high energy trauma. Fracture of the caudal endplate of L7 and ventral subluxation of the sacrum is the most encountered injury affecting the lumbosacral articulation in the dog. This is generally the result of severe hyperflexion and compression forces, often as a result of vehicular trauma. Additional injuries such as abdominal trauma, pelvic fractures, and caudal vertebral fractures are common comorbidities.

Anatomy

The illial wings and sacroiliac joints limit the approach to dorsal and dorsolateral. The L7–S1 articular processes are significantly wider than those of other lumbar vertebrae and are vitally important stabilizers in this area. The wide shape of the pedicles and their large mass of bone allow for an almost vertical placement of screws with excellent boney purchase. In contrast, the wide and flat sacrum offers limited area for implant placement. Insertion angles should be 0–20° from vertical angled dorsolaterally to ventromedially. The implant insertion point on L7 is slightly caudal to the base of the cranial articular process. If angled medially, insertion should occur slightly laterally to this landmark at approximately the base of the L7 transverse process. For S1, the insertion point should be in the fossa, slightly caudal to the cranial articular process. Implant insertion must avoid the cauda equina and exiting nerve roots (Figure 12.10).

Positioning and Approach

Patients should be positioned in sternal recumbency, with the hindlimbs placed in flexion, avoiding abduction of the coxofemoral joints. It is recommended to place the patient as far back as safely possible on the surgical table to facilitate bilateral access as well as access to the caudal aspect of the surgical site. Patients should be secured using a combination of tape, vacuum positioning system, or sandbags. A table with a tilt mechanism may also be convenient to facilitate insertion angles and maintain a perpendicular approach. A large approach is recommended to gain adequate exposure. Wood-handled periosteal elevators are recommended here, as they allow for quicker and more effective elevation when exposing the dorsal aspect of the lumbosacral joint.

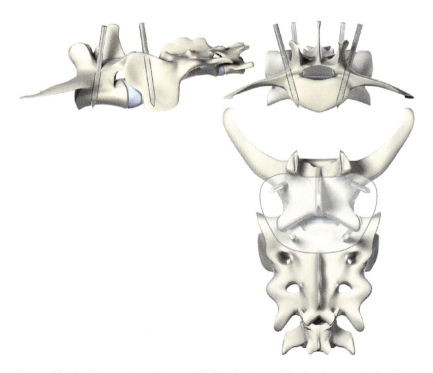

Figure 12.10   Illustration of pin and PMMA fixation of the lumbosacral joint. Bicortical positive-profile fixation pins are placed L7 and S1. These should be placed at between vertical and 20° based on preoperative planning. The insertion landmark for L7 is slightly caudolateral to the base of the cranial articular process. The insertion landmark for S1 is the fossa caudo-medial to the articular process of L7–S1.

Reduction

Bone reduction forceps can be used and anchored to the spinous processes to improve alignment. The ileal wings can also be used as a point of reduction, particularly with the aid of a surgical assistant. For chronic injuries, anatomical reduction may be difficult or impossible and fixation without full reduction may be needed. If the injury causes compression of the cauda equina, a dorsal laminectomy can be performed in addition to the stabilization to relieve nerve root compression. Once reduction is achieved, much like in other areas of the lumbar spine, temporary or permanent transarticular pins or screws can be placed to hold reduction in place while the remainder of the construct is applied.

Implant Selection

The lumbosacral joint is one of high motion and due to its location, a large fulcrum is created with a tremendous amount of torque, particularly with flexion and extension. Implants should be strong to counteract this motion, particularly in flexion, and should be placed in a fashion that avoids shear and implant loosening. It should be noted that even though implants fail, this may not necessarily preclude fracture healing or a successful outcome; however, the implant should be designed to counteract these strong forces until the fracture is healed. Pins of 1/8th inch diameter or 3.5-mm cortical screws are used in most medium to large dogs (Table 12.1).

While transarticular screws are the least technically demanding option, these are prone to failure by loosening or may lead to fracture of the articular facets in this area of high motion. Fixation is achieved by encouraging arthrodesis of the articular processes. Due to the size of these articulations, cartilage can be removed using a curette or drill and fresh cancellous bone graft or substitute packed into the area to promote joint fusion. Screws should be inserted from the mid body of the caudal articular facet of L7 at approximately 45° in a craniodorsal to caudoventral direction and 30° to the dorsomedial to ventrolateral plane through the articular facet of the sacrum (Figure 12.11).

Compared to standard plates, which require perfect contouring with the vertebral bones, locking plates, while more technically challenging than other methods, can be used to provide a stable, monocortical, and low-profile fixation. The newer Pedicle Screw System (Orthomed) is specifically designed with this in mind. Using pre-placed screws and a node/rod attachment system, the screws can be inserted prior to attaching the nodes with the bar and locking in place. Fixation should

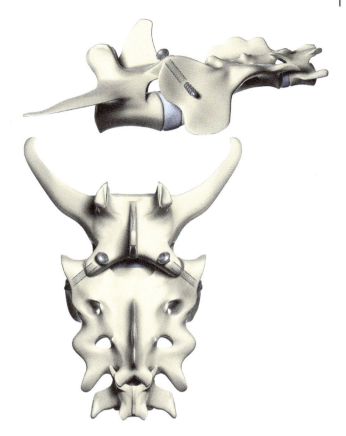

Figure 12.11 Illustration of transarticular screw placement across the L7–S1 articular facets. The articular cartilage should be debrided prior to fixation and a bone graft placed to encourage arthrodesis of this high motion joint. Without successful arthrodesis, failure of the implant is more likely. Note the screw insertion angle from the mid body of the caudal articular facet of L7 at approximately 45° in a craniodorsal to caudoventral direction and 30° to the dorsomedial to ventrolateral plane through the articular facet of the sacrum.

be bilateral to accommodate sufficient fixation points. These are more technically challenging than PMMA constructs as screw angles and plate contouring must match to ensure engagement of the locking mechanism.

Like in other areas of the spine, pins or screws with PMMA provide versatility, relative ease of use, and strong resistance to mechanical stress. Positive-profile pins are favored over screws due to the larger core diameter, which increases construct stiffness and greater resistance to shear forces and pull-out. Previously described implant corridors (Table 12.2) should be used and additional implants can be placed in L6, the ilial body, or transarticular if desired. Pins placed in L7 can be bent carefully in the caudal direction and those placed in the sacrum can be bent cranially. This allows greater pin incorporation into the PMMA through a variety of angles which may improve construct strength.

Cerclage wire may also be incorporated in a figure-of-eight pattern to act as "rebar" and improve resistance to flexion of the lumbosacral joint.

Postoperative Imaging

Immediate postoperative imaging is necessary to ensure adequate reduction and safe and effective screw placement, and can prevent complications by allowing the surgeon to identify and correct any concerns prior to recovering the patient. In some cases, full reduction is not possible, and a stable construct that allows an unobstructed spinal canal is sufficient to allow healing and a successful outcome. Similarly, mildly malpositioned implants may not require surgical revision. However, at a minimum, postoperative imaging provides feedback and valuable knowledge for future imaging in case of complications.

Standard orthogonal radiographs while the patient is still under anesthesia can be used to assess correct reduction and approximate implant corridors. They also provide a baseline for future follow up, should questions on implant migration or failure arise. It should be noted that, while providing valuable information, plain radiography is inadequate in assessing breach of the spinal canal [15]. CT provides all the advantages of radiographs, with far superior detail to precisely determine implant positioning, penetration through cortices, and bone purchase. It is also excellent in identifying screws or pins that have violated the canal, the intervertebral foramen, or a disk space. It can also identify implants that have been inadequately embedded in PMMA constructs. Furthermore, it allows for three-dimensional reconstruction of images which can be useful in determining adequate reduction (Figure 12.12).

MRI is generally inadequate for assessing postoperative implants and reduction as the stainless steel used in most implants creates susceptibility artifacts, which severely limit the assessment capability of this modality. Titanium implants may help alleviate some of these limitations; however, the speed, accuracy, and spatial fidelity of the CT makes it a superior modality for this purpose.

Complications

Due to complicated anatomy and proximity to vital neurovascular structures, iatrogenic injury to the spinal cord, nerve roots, intervertebral disks, and vascular structures as well as invasion of the thoracic cavity are possible. Excellent knowledge of anatomy combined with meticulous preoperative planning and precise execution in surgery should mitigate risks of catastrophic iatrogenic injury. As outlined previously, postoperative imaging at minimum provides feedback to the surgeon, assessing what went right and what could be improved upon. This is one of the most valuable tools to help improve surgical technique, minimize iatrogenic complications, and improve outcomes as one progresses throughout their career.

If implant placement is adequate and reduction is acceptable, most complications are caused by implant failure or infection. Implant loosening can be due to inappropriately sized implants, poor placement of implants within the bone, poor bone holding properties, lack of fundamental surgical technique such as not pre-drilling, selecting the wrong sized drill bit, or not using a drill guide. Catastrophic failure may occur with some of the former, but can also be due to poor decision-making regarding implant type and size of fixation – leading to fracture or sudden failure, misdiagnosis of comorbidities such as fractures, inadequate accommodation of implants within PMMA, or not mixing PMMA appropriately. Lack of appropriate activity restriction in the immediate postoperative period can also lead to implant failure. Infection is less likely due to intraoperative factors, and most often secondary to hematogenous spread or, in the case of open fractures, to the inciting injury. The former is especially pertinent in patients with inadequate bladder function due to neurologic injury as they have a much higher chance of resistant urinary tract infections. Perioperative antibiotics, usually cefazolin, should be used appropriately. Postoperative antibiotic prophylaxis should be done on a case-by-case basis but is rarely recommended except when treating open fractures, especially those resulting from bite wounds. Patients with fractures caused by penetrating injuries should undergo surgery as soon as possible and receive copious intraoperative lavage and postoperative drainage (closed suction drain), at least until the results of culture and sensitivity are available. It may be wise to avoid the use of PMMA in such patients. Patients with a skin infection, urinary tract infection, or other coinfections at the time of surgery should either be treated prior to surgery, if the outcome is not likely to be affected, or be placed on appropriate antibiotics in the perioperative and postoperative period based on targeted selection or preferably culture and sensitivity. Depending on the nature of the infection, clinical signs, or compromise in stability, implant removal may be necessary once the fracture has healed, unless implant loosening and fracture complications develop prior to this occurring. Replacing implants in

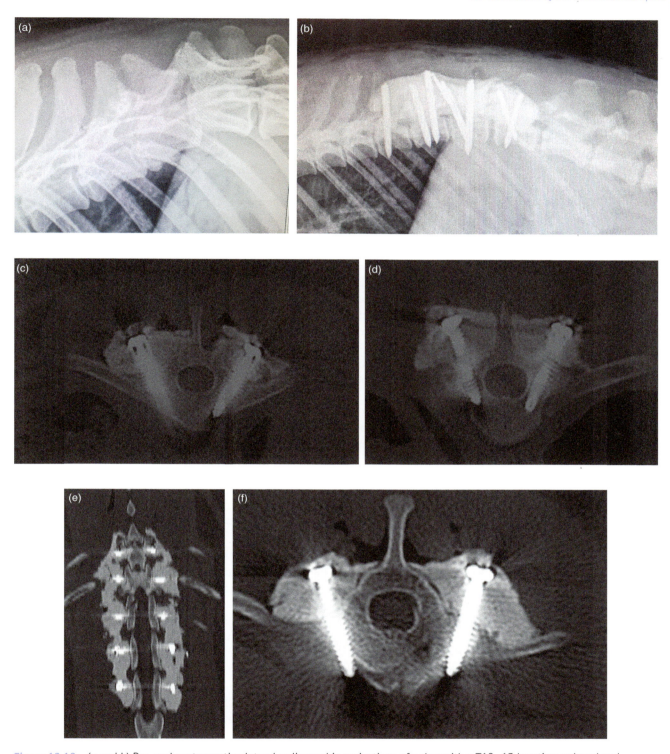

Figure 12.12 (a and b) Pre- and postoperative lateral radiographic projections of a dog with a T12–13 luxation reduced and stabilized with pins and PMMA construct. (c–e) Postoperative CT, axial and dorsal images to assess appropriate screw placement in the thoracic vertebrae. (f) Postoperative CT to assess placement of screws used to engage fragments of a vertebral body fracture.

the face of infection can be complicated given the high likelihood of recurrent infection. Low grade, "smoldering" infection may not necessitate immediate implant removal, but is important to monitor as this may cause bone lysis and loosening of implants. PMMA lends itself poorly to antibiotic penetration in vivo, but various antibiotics can be added to it during mixing. Addition of antibiotics to the PMMA is controversial as it may lead to weakening of the construct [8]. Stainless steel implants, while less likely to harbor infection and more easily removed if infection arises, are prone to developing a bacterial biofilm which can also hinder effective antibiotic action and lead to chronic infection.

Seroma formation is one of the more commonly encountered postoperative complications reported by owners. This benign, sterile fluid accumulation can be resolved with regular warm compresses. Aspiration of the fluid should be avoided except to rule-out infection, as seromas are usually self-resolving and aspiration can potentially seed infection. Though it can be difficult around bulky implants, meticulous closing of dead space can usually prevent seroma formation.

The goal of stabilization is to lead to fracture healing, stable fibrosis of luxation, and in some cases arthrodesis. As each implant has a predetermined cyclic strength, it is expected that an implant will eventually "fail" if given enough time. Longer term complications include stable nonunion, granuloma formation, and chronic pain from implant loosening or migration or from smoldering infection. If stability is deemed satisfactory based on robust imaging studies, these implants may be removed. Unless there is a complication, the implants typically remain in situ.

Aftercare

The nature of the aftercare depends on the severity of neurologic signs, the magnitude of the instability, the area of fixation, and the type of fixation applied. Immediate postoperative patients should be hospitalized for adequate pain relief and nursing care. This is beyond the scope of this chapter, as it pertains to most spinal surgeries. However, it is important to consider that the implant provides temporary stability and, long term, relies on the body's ability to heal and to permanently stabilize the site of injury. Keeping this in mind, exercise restriction and assistance during the immediate to mid-term postoperative period is crucial. As back braces are ineffective, this is generally not necessary for thoracic, thoracolumbar, lumbar, and lumbosacral injuries. All patients should be confined for a minimum of four weeks to a crate or small fenced-off area, being carefully leash-walked with a supportive sling until strong enough to walk independently. Length of activity should be gradually increased over time. Stairs should be avoided during this period. As the patient improves, a room with good flooring should be provided. The patient is to be eased into a normal schedule; however, rough play and high impact activities, such as jumping on and off furniture, should be avoided. Return to normal activity should take approximately 8–12 weeks, depending on the age of the patient, assumed stability of the fracture repair, and expected healing time. Rehabilitation can be performed once the incision has healed and can include at-home standing exercises and passive range of motion, or more directed professional inpatient or out-patient programs under the supervision of a certified rehabilitation therapist.

Acknowledgments

The authors wish to acknowledge Dr. Bianca Hettlich for the use of several images from Current Techniques in Canine and Feline Neurosurgery, Vertebral fracture and luxation repair.

References

1. Watine, S., Cabassu, J.P., Catheland, S. et al. (2006). Computed tomography study of implantation corridors in canine vertebrae. *J. Small Anim. Pract.* 47: 651–657. https://doi.org/10.1111/j.1748-5827.2006.00070.x.
2. Shores, A. (1992). Spinal trauma, pathophysiology and management of traumatic spinal injuries. *Vet. Clin. North Am. Small Anim. Pract.* 22: 859–888.
3. Revés, N.V., Bürki, A., Ferguson, S. et al. (2012). Influence of partial lateral corpectomy with and without hemilaminectomy on canine thoracolumbar stability: a

biomechanical study. *Vet. Surg.* 41: 228–234. https://doi.org/10.1111/j.1532-950X.2011.00912.x.
4. Elford, J.H., Oxley, B., and Behr, S. (2020). Accuracy of placement of pedicle screws in the thoracolumbar spine of dogs with spinal deformities with three-dimensionally printed patient-specific drill guides. *Vet. Surg.* 49: 347–353. https://doi.org/10.1111/vsu.13333.
5. Fujioka, T., Nakata, K., Nakano, Y. et al. (2020). Accuracy and efficacy of a patient-specific drill guide template system for lumbosacral junction fixation in

medium and small dogs: cadaveric study and clinical cases. *Front. Vet. Sci.* 9 (6): 494. https://doi.org/10.3389/fvets.2019.00494 . PMID: 31998769; PMCID: PMC6964317.

6. Hettlich, B.F., Allen, M.J., Pascetta, D. et al. (2013). Biomechanical comparison between bicortical pin and monocortical screw/polymethylmethacrylate constructs in the cadaveric canine cervical vertebral column. *Vet. Surg.* 42 (6): 693–700. https://doi.org/10.1111/j.1532-950X.2013.12040.x. Epub 2013 Jul 25. PMID: 23888877.

7. Mekavichai, M., Kanjanawong, N., Chattammanat, T., and Soontornvipart, K. (2018). Fatigue study of cancellous and cortical stainless steel screws used with polymethylmethacrylate and the SOP plate system for immobilization of vertebral luxation in canine cadavers. *Thai J. Vet. Med.* 48 (2): 227–234. https://he01.tci-thaijo.org/index.php/tjvm/article/view/139201.

8. Ficklin, M.G., Kunkel, K.A., Suber, J.T. et al. (2016). Biomechanical evaluation of polymethyl methacrylate with the addition of various doses of cefazolin, vancomycin, gentamicin, and silver microparticles. *Vet. Comp. Orthop. Traumatol.* 29 (5): 394–401. https://doi.org/10.3415/VCOT-16-01-0005. Epub 2016 Jul 29. PMID: 27468765.

9. Hettlich, B.F., Fosgate, G.T., and Litsky, A.S. (2017). Biomechanical comparison of 2 veterinary locking plates to Monocortical screw/polymethylmethacrylate fixation in canine cadaveric cervical vertebral column. *Vet. Surg.* 46 (1): 95–102. https://doi.org/10.1111/vsu.12581. Epub 2016 Nov 30. PMID: 27902850.

10. Sandman, K.M., Smith, C.W., Harari, J. et al. (2002). Comparison of pull-out resistance of Kirschner wires and Imex™ miniature interface fixation half pins in polyurethane foam. *Vet. Comp. Orthop. Traumatol.* 15: 18–22. https://doi.org/10.1055/s-0038-1632708.

11. Agnello, K.A., Kapatkin, A.S., Garcia, T.C. et al. (2010). Intervertebral biomechanics of locking compression plate monocortical fixation of the canine cervical spine. *Vet. Surg.* 39 (8): 991–1000. https://doi.org/10.1111/j.1532-950X.2010.00755.x. PMID: 21133955.

12. Garcia, J.N., Milthorpe, B.K., Russell, D., and Johnson, K.A. (1994). Biomechanical study of canine spinal fracture fixation using pins or bone screws with polymethylmethacrylate. *Vet. Surg.* 23 (5): 322–329. https://doi.org/10.1111/j.1532-950x.1994.tb00491.x. PMID: 7839589.

13. Voss, K. and Montavon, P.M. (2004). Tension band stabilization of fractures and luxations of the thoracolumbar vertebrae in dogs and cats: 38 cases (1993–2002). *J. Am. Vet. Med. Assoc.* 225 (1): 78–83. https://doi.org/10.2460/javma.2004.225.78. PMID: 15239477.

14. Walker, T.M., Pierce, W.A., and Welch, R.D. (2002). External fixation of the lumbar spine in a canine model. *Vet. Surg.* 31 (2): 181–188. https://doi.org/10.1053/jvet.2002.31045. PMID: 11884964.

15. Hettlich, B.F., Fosgate, G.T., Levine, J.M. et al. (2010). Accuracy of conventional radiography and computed tomography in predicting implant position in relation to the Vertebral Canal in dogs. *Vet. Surg.* 39: 680–687. https://doi.org/10.1111/j.1532-950X.2010.00697.x.

13

Surgical Management of Congenital Spinal Anomalies

Sheila Carrera-Justiz and Gabriel Garcia

University of Florida, Gainesville, FL, USA

Congenital spinal malformations, specifically hemivertebrae, have been long recognized in veterinary medicine [1, 2]. Hemivertebrae are the most frequently noted vertebral malformation in "screw-tailed dogs," a group that traditionally includes French Bulldogs, English Bulldogs, Pugs, and Boston Terriers [3]. This topic has become more important to the veterinary profession in recent years with the increasing popularity of screw-tailed dogs, the French Bulldog in particular. The prevalence of thoracic hemivertebra in neurologically normal French and English Bulldogs has been reported to be as high as 93.5% and 73.2%, respectively [4]. A large proportion of hemivertebrae are subclinical and never require intervention [5] (Figure 13.1). French Bulldogs were shown to have a significantly higher incidence of hemivertebrae than English Bulldogs and Pugs [6]. The same study noted that Pugs are more likely to have ventral hypoplasia and kyphosis, putting Pugs into a different category of hemivertebrae than English and French Bulldogs.

Most dogs affected by vertebral body malformations tend to show clinical signs in the first year of life [7]. Clinical signs are reflective of a myelopathy and are dependent on the specific location of the malformation; signs can include ataxia, paresis, scoliosis, lordosis, kyphosis, and incontinence. The cause of the myelopathy in these dogs remains unknown and is thought to be secondary to findings that cause intermittent compression and ischemia of the spinal cord, including stenosis of the spinal canal, spinal cord tethering, and microinstability.

In Pug breeds, severe kyphosis, and fewer hemivertebrae have been associated with a higher likelihood

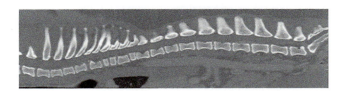

Figure 13.1 A sagittal computed tomography image of a dog spine illustrating the concept that multiple malformations are less likely to cause a severe kyphosis.

of neurological disease. A Cobb angle greater than 35° has been shown to have the highest sensitivity and specificity for predicting clinical signs in dogs [8, 9].

Diagnostics

Congenital vertebral abnormalities can be visualized with various modalities, including radiographs, myelography, computed tomography, and magnetic resonance imaging (MRI). Radiographs serve as a good screening tool for vertebral body malformations and can be used to calculate Cobb angles (Figure 13.2); however, as neural structures cannot be visualized on plain radiographs, advanced imaging is recommended if there is any evidence of a myelopathy. While myelography can highlight spinal cord compression, it cannot show intramedullary changes. As such, cross-sectional imaging is often chosen over traditional myelography.

Computed tomography is an excellent modality for evaluation of bony malformations and allows for the creation

---

Advanced Techniques in Canine and Feline Neurosurgery, First Edition. Edited by Andy Shores and Brigitte A. Brisson.
© 2023 John Wiley & Sons, Inc. Published 2023 by John Wiley & Sons, Inc.
Companion site: www.wiley.com/go/shores/advanced

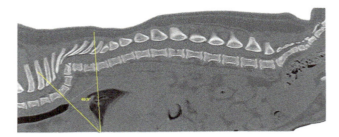

Figure 13.2 A sagittal computed tomography image of a dog spine with a vertebral malformation causing a Cobb angle of 40.9.

of three-dimensional models, digital or 3-D printed (Figure 13.3). MRI is most useful for evaluation of the spinal cord parenchyma and any associated abnormalities. Given their ability to provide clinically significant data regarding the various different aspects of the spinal column, Computed tomography (CT) and MRI are often recommended in combination for complete evaluation of a case prior to surgery.

Considering the high incidence of these malformations in commonly affected breeds, it is important to evaluate the entire neuroanatomic segment affected to prevent overlooking an additional lesion that may be partially or completely responsible for the clinical signs.

Treatment

Various protocols of medical management have been used for treatment of myelopathy due to congenital vertebral malformations. Dogs affected with a mild and non-progressive myelopathy can be treated with conservative management [10]. More recent data suggests that outcomes are quite poor with medical management, with all dogs showing progression of neurological signs despite treatment [11]. It has been suggested that some mildly affected dogs stabilize, and even improve, in their clinical signs when vertebral growth ceases around nine months of age [10]. This concept suggests that surgical intervention in young dogs should be considered after approximately nine months of age.

Surgical intervention in these cases has historically been fraught with complications and variable outcomes. Affected dogs are often skeletally immature animals with limited purchase in soft bone and markedly abnormal anatomy. Traditionally, management with decompressive surgery alone has been considered to hold a guarded to poor prognosis.

Multiple surgical techniques are described for the treatment of congenital vertebral malformations. As the most commonly affected vertebral bodies are thoracic [4, 5], dorsal

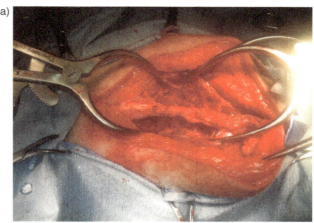

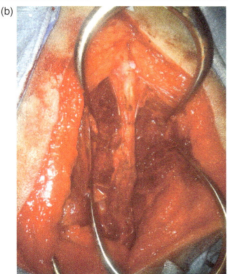

Figure 13.3 (a) Surgical image from the left side of the patient showing a bilateral muscular approach to the thoracic spine for a biologic in situ fusion. (b) Multiple views of the surgical approach required for a biologic in situ fusion. Dorsal midline approach over the mid-thoracic spine showing bilateral paraspinal muscle elevation to the level of the lamina.

surgical approaches have been preferred due to the difficulty and complications associated with a ventral approach to the mid-thoracic spine. A single report describes a ventral approach to the cranial thoracic spine in a Labrador puppy [12]. This report describes a partial ventral corpectomy and stabilization with pins and polymethylmethacrylate. Clinical signs markedly improved, though complications were noted. This is a unique report not only for the approach but given the atypical breed and location for this condition.

Various surgical techniques for this condition are aimed at providing decompression, stabilization, or a combination of the two. A total of 12 dogs were described as having

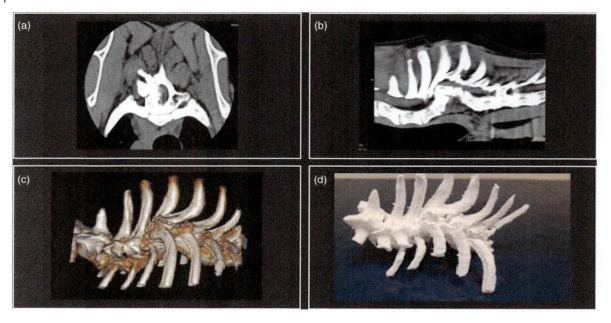

Figure 13.4 A one-year-old female spayed Doberman Pinscher presented for gait abnormalities described as a two-engine gait, predominately pelvic limb deficits, and a progressively declining neurologic status. A high thoracic localization was suspected. (a) Transverse CT (soft tissue window) at the level of the T4 vertebrae. (b) Sagittal CT reconstruction of the upper thoracic spine. (c) A 3-D computer modeling of the upper thoracic spine and (d) a 3-D printed model of the same region. 3-D printed models can be very helpful in planning a surgery.

some form of stabilization, with 11/12 undergoing simultaneous decompression [10, 13]. Stabilization techniques employed included positively threaded profile pins and Poly(methyl methacrylate) PMMA, positively threaded screws and PMMA, and segmental spinal stabilization with PMMA. While one dog remained static, all remaining dogs showed clinical improvement, though one dog never became ambulatory despite improvements. Spinal segmental stabilization has also been successfully reported to improve clinical signs of dorsal hemivertebrae. Nine dogs underwent spinal segmental stabilization, three of which also received decompressive surgery. Three of nine dogs suffered implant complications. Eight of the nine dogs showed long-term improvement, and all eight were ambulatory 1.5–5.5 years after surgery [14]. Multiple surgical techniques have resulted in clinical improvement without a change in the degree of kyphosis [10, 13, 14], which implies that stabilization, not decompression or correction of the kyphosis, may be the main effector of clinical improvement in these dogs.

A novel surgical technique was presented by Gorgi et al. This biological in situ technique for congenital vertebral anomalies in brachycephalic dogs was described in eight young dogs [15]. All dogs were non-ambulatory paraparetic prior to the procedure. The technique involves abrasion of the periosteum over the affected area and application of autogenous and allogenic bone graft to promote ankylosis. The spinal canal is not opened, and no metallic implants are used. All dogs had a minimum of 12 months of follow up and all became ambulatory with the novel procedure. This procedure is appealing as it is less invasive in that it does not open the spinal canal, it does not require permanent surgical implants, and it does not preclude a later surgery in that area of the spine. A larger scale report on this technique is in progress. Preoperative and postoperative imaging are seen in Figure 13.4.

A recent report showed that pedicle screw placement can be safe in dogs with thoracolumbar malformations when using three-dimensional printed patient-specific drill guides [16]. This report showed that placement can be accurate using this technique, though neurological outcome was not described.

Prognosis

Measuring Cobb angles is highly recommended in screw-tail dogs with hemivertebra since an angle greater than 35° has a positive predictive value of 75% for neurological signs [8, 9]. Unfortunately, there is no correlation between severity of the malformation and progression of disease. The prognosis for improvement of myelopathy due to congenital vertebral malformations with medical management is poor. Based on that, medical management should be recommended with caution, especially in the young dog. Surgical intervention has the potential to, at a minimum, halt the progression of clinical signs, and ideally improve status to ambulatory.

Future Directions

It has been suggested that progress can be made to reduce the incidence of vertebral malformations in the French Bulldog through selective breeding [3]. Screening programs of young dogs have the potential to identify high risk individuals at an early stage. Radiographs should be performed by skeletal maturity, 9–12 months of age, from T1 through L7, centered at T8–L1, as suggested by Gutierrez-Quintana et al. [5]. A grading scheme should be applied to vertebral malformations, to allow for the provision of more uniform recommendations on these cases.

Summary

Congenital vertebral malformations are becoming a more commonly encountered clinical syndrome given the increase in popularity of screw-tailed breeds of dogs. Dogs are often affected at a young age and may not be skeletally mature at first presentation. Diagnosis is made by imaging, and a combination of imaging modalities may be necessary to obtain enough information to make treatment recommendations. Given that medical management has not been shown to provide a good long-term outcome, surgical intervention is recommended. Though there is no definitive data to support one surgical technique over the other for the treatment of congenital vertebral malformations, it appears that stabilization may be the most important element of surgical intervention.

 Video clips to accompany this book can be found on the companion website at:
www.wiley.com/go/shores/advanced

References

1. Morgan, J.P. (1968). Congenital anomalies of the vertebral column of the dog: a study of the incidence and significance based on a radiographic and morphologic study. *Vet. Radiol.* https://doi.org/10.1111/j.1740-8261.1968.tb01082.x.
2. Done, S.H., Drew, R.A., Robins, G.M., and Lane, J.G. (1975). Hemivertebrae in the dog: clinical and pathological observations. *The Vet. Record* 96 (14): 313–317.
3. Schlensker, E. and Distl, O. (2013). Prevalence, grading and genetics of hemivertebrae in dogs. *Eur. J. Comp. Anim. Pract.* 23: 119–123.
4. Ryan, R., Gutierrez-Quintana, R., Ter Haar, G., and De Decker, S. (2017). Prevalence of thoracic vertebral malformations in French bulldogs, pugs and English bulldogs with and without associated neurological deficits. *Vet. J.* 221: 25–29. https://doi.org/10.1016/j.tvjl.2017.01.018. Epub 2017 Jan 31. PMID: 28283076.
5. Gutierrez-Quintana, R., Guevar, J., Stalin, C. et al. (2014). A proposed radiographic classification scheme for congenital thoracic vertebral malformatiosn in brachycephalic "screw-tailed" dog breeds. *Vet. Radiol. Ultrasound* 55 (6): 585–591.
6. Ryan, R., Gutierrez-Quintana, R., Gertter, H., and De Decker, S. (2019). Relationship between breed, hemivertebra subtype, and kyphosis in apparently neurologically normal French bulldogs, English bulldogs, and pugs. *Am. J. Vet. Res.* 80: 189–194.
7. Dewey, C.W., Davies, E., and Bouma, J.L. (2016). Kyphosis and kyphoscoliosis associated with congenital malformations of the thoracic vertebral bodies in dogs. *Vet. Clin. Small Anim.* 46: 295–306. Http://dx.doi.org/10.1016/j.cvsm.2015.10.009.
8. Guevar, J., Penderis, J., Faller, K. et al. Computer-assisted radiographic calculation of spinal curvature in brachycephalic "screw-tailed" dog breeds with congenital thoracic vertebral malformations: reliability and clinical evaluation. *PLoS One* 9 (9): e106957. https://doi.org/10.1371/journal.pone.0106957.
9. De Decker, S., Packer, R.M.A., Capello, R. et al. (2019). Comparison of signamlemtn and computed tomography findings in French bulldogs, pugs, and English bulldogs with and without clinical signs associated with thoracic hemivertebrae. *J. Vet. Intern. Med.* 33: 2151–2159. https://doi.org/10.1111/jvim.15556.
10. Jeffery, N.D., Smith, P.M., and Talbot, C.E. (2007). Imaging findings and surgical treatment of hemivertebrae in three dogs. *J. Am. Vet. Med. Assoc.* 230: 532–536.
11. Wyatt, S., Goncalves, R., Gutierrez-Quintana, R., and De Decker, S. (2018). Outcomes of nonsurgical treatment for congenital thoracic vertebral body malformations in dogs: 13 cases (2009–2016). *J. Am. Vet. Med. Assoc.* 253: 768–773.

12. Meheust, P. and Robert, R. (2010). Surgical treatment of a hemivertebra by partial ventral corpectomy and fusion in a Labrador puppy. *Vet. Comp. Orthop. Traumatol.* 23: 262–265.

13. Aikawa, T., Kanazono, S., Yoshigae, Y. et al. (2007). Vertebral stabilization using positively threaded profile pins and polymethylmethacrylate, with or without laminectomy, for spinal canal stenosis and vertebral instability caused by congenital thoracic vertebral anomalies. *Vet. Surg.* 36: 432–441.

14. Charalambous, M., Jeffery, N.D., Smith, P.M. et al. (2014). Surgical treatment of dorsal hemivertebrae associated with kyphosis by spinal segmental stabilization, with or without decompression. *The Vet. J.* 202: 267–273.

15. Gorgi, A.A., Wininger, F.A., Fox, D.B. et al. (2012). Biological in situ technique for congenital vertebral anomalies in brachycephalic dogs. Abstract presented at the ACVIM Forum 2012 New Orleans, Louisiana (30 May to 2 June 2012).

16. Elford, J.H., Oxley, B., and Behr, S. (2020). Accuracy of placement of pedicle screws in the thoracolumbar spine of dogs with spinal deformities with three-dimentionally printed patient-specific drill guides. *Vet. Surg.* 49: 347–353. https://doi.org/10.1111/vsu.13333.

14

Lumbosacral Decompression and Foraminotomy Techniques

Stef H. Y. Lim[1] and Michaela Beasley[2]

[1] Bush Veterinary Neurology Service, Leesburg, VA, USA
[2] Mississippi State University Mississippi State, MS, USA

Pathophysiology and Anatomy

Degenerative lumbosacral stenosis (DLSS), also commonly known as cauda equina syndrome or disease or lumbosacral compression, is commonly seen in canine patients causing pain and neurological dysfunction secondary to the compression of the seventh lumbar (L7) nerve roots, local vasculature, and cauda equina [1–5]. It is prevalent among large male dogs, with German Shepherd, military, and working dogs seemingly predisposed [6, 7]. Manifestation of clinical signs include lumbosacral pain, paresis, lameness, reluctance to jump, and in severe cases neurological deficits including urinary and fecal incontinence and dysesthesias (abnormalities of skin sensation) [1–5, 8, 9].

The anatomy of the connectors and stabilizers of the LS joint consist of the intervertebral disk (IVD), facetal synovial joints, dorsal and ventral longitudinal ligaments, interarcuate ligaments, interspinous ligaments, and perispinal fascia and muscles [1–5, 9–11]. Change to the forces of the LS joint can be exacerbated by additional anatomical malformations, such as sacralization of the seventh lumbar vertebrae, malarticulation of the diarthrodial joints at L7–S1 junction, lumborization of the first sacral vertebrae, or other breeds such as Airdale Terriers, Belgian Shepherds (Malinois), German Shepherds, Greyhounds, and Labrador Retrievers that have inherited abnormal motion pattern at L7–S1 [12–14].

The cause of DLSS is multifactorial. The high mobility of the LS joint, especially in a dorsolateral extension, places a high amount of stress on the LS disk space which is responsible for connecting a flexible lumbar spine to the rigid sacrum and pelvis [1–5]. Though the specific progression of events is unknown, DLSS is a combination of LS IVD protrusion, subluxation of the facet joints, thickening of the joint capsule of the articular facets, and hypertrophy of the ligament flavum. However, additional changes – including lumbosacral transitional vertebrae and osteochondrosis of the sacral endplate – may also predispose animals to DLSS [8]. It is speculated that chronic repetitive microtrauma and aging causes the nucleus pulpous to desiccate, thereby leading to changes to the biomechanical ability for the disk to absorb impact. Thus, greater forces are then being absorbed by the annulus fibrosus, which weakens as a sequela, and the dorsal aspect of the annulus develops small tears. This allows the disk to protrude: a Hanson Type II disk. This in turn causes compression along the cauda equina but also subsequent instability, which can result in subluxation between L7 and S1. The body counters the instability by way of the dorsal longitudinal ligament, the interarcuate ligaments, and facetal synovial capsule hypertrophy, and spondylosis deformans forms on the ventral aspect of L7–S1. The combination causes cauda equina compression secondary to the IVD protrusion and dorsal longitudinal ligament ventrally with dorsal compression from interarcuate ligaments with subsequent foraminal stenosis from the facetal joint hypertrophy and spondylosis causing the clinical signs of DLSS [1–5, 9, 11, 13].

L7–S1 Foramina Anatomy

In humans, terminology of "entrance," "middle," and "exit" zones has been applied to the location of the L5–S1 neurovascular foramen according to their location with relation to the pedicle and articular processes of L5–S1. The entrance zone is located closest to the vertebral canal and is the medial portion of the L5 vertebral pedicle.

Advanced Techniques in Canine and Feline Neurosurgery, First Edition. Edited by Andy Shores and Brigitte A. Brisson.
© 2023 John Wiley & Sons, Inc. Published 2023 by John Wiley & Sons, Inc.
Companion site: www.wiley.com/go/shores/advanced

The middle zone is the center of the pedicle and the exit zone is the intervertebral foramen [15, 16]. Canines differ anatomically with more oblique angles and the lateral recess is longer and narrowing in shape compared to humans [16–18]. With this in mind, unless there is an extremely lateralized protruding disk, the L7 nerve roots will be spared with DLSS with concurrent intervertebral disk herniation (IVDH). As vertebral spacing is lost, the sacral articular process will telescope into the intervertebral neurovascular foramina, which will create dynamic impingement of L7 at the exit zone. Thus, it is important when performing imaging diagnostics to be mindful of which zone(s) L7 nerve root entrapment occurs in to consider appropriate surgical approach and treatment (Figure 14.1) [17].

Diagnosis

Diagnosis of DLSS can be difficult, but should always begin like any other examination: thorough history; physical, neurologic, and orthopedic examinations.

History and Clinical Signs

One of the most common complaints for patients with DLSS is pain and weakness. Once neurological abnormalities are noted, clinical signs include mild paresis, decreased to loss of tail function, proprioceptive ataxia, and incontinence (urinary, fecal, or both) [1–5, 8, 9]. These deficits are secondary to the sciatic nerve involvement (caudal thigh and muscles distal to the stifle) and pelvic and pudendal nerves causing lower motor neuron urinary incontinence and fecal incontinence secondary to poor anal sphincter tone [1–5, 9].

Physical Examination Findings

Physical examination should include a thorough neurological and orthopedic examination on top of the baseline physical examination. Common findings on physical exams include atrophy of gluteal or stifle flexor muscles, pain when pressure is applied over the lumbosacral space – which can be elicited with a lordosis test, and "tail jack" (Figure 14.2) [1, 9]. Direct palpation of the sciatic nerve at its exit zone can be accomplished with what we have described as the "sciatic nerve entrapment test"; however, concurrent iliopsoas pain can also be triggered with this movement (Figure 14.3).

Orthopedic Examination Findings

Orthopedic examination is crucial as hip dysplasia and cranial cruciate ligament ruptures can complicate DLSS or appear similar without a thorough exam. Pain elicited on extension of the hip is not specific enough to distinguish between DLSS from primary orthopedic disease [5].

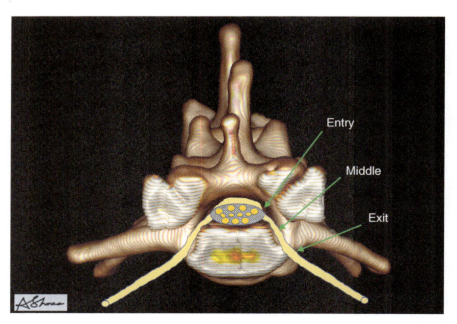

Figure 14.1 Illustration of the foraminal zones for the L7 nerve roots (entry, middle, exit). When performing imaging diagnostics, evaluation of the zones of L7 nerve root entrapment may aid in the surgical planning.

14 Lumbosacral Decompression and Foraminotomy Techniques

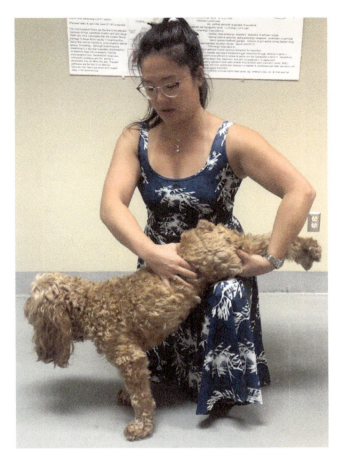

Figure 14.2 Both the lordosis test and tail jack have been described as methods to elicit pain associated with the lumbosacral joint. In this photo, the lordosis test is being performed. Thumb pressure is placed over the lumbosacral joint as the joint is being extended. A painful response is considered positive.

Neurologic Examination Findings

Common neurological abnormalities include ataxia, depressed cranial tibial, gastric, and withdrawal reflexes. Pseudo-hyperreflexia of the patellar reflex can also be appreciated from the secondary lack of contralateral muscle tone of the flexor muscles of the stifles [5, 19]. Neurologic diseases that can mimic DLSS include degenerative myelopathy (DM); however, pain is typically not concurrent with degenerative myelopathy and early DM cases usually present with a thoracolumbar localization. It is advised that prior to performing any surgery or invasive procedures, genetic testing be performed for degenerative myelopathy to ensure that it will not compound your attempts to improving DLSS [19].

Radiography

As DLSS is multifactorial with involvement of soft tissues including IVD and multiple ligaments, plain radiography and contrast studies are not ideal. Radiographs can provide quick investigation of the lumbosacral joint and rule out boney neoplasias, trauma, diskospondylitis, and possible vertebral abnormalities [20–24].

Radiographs are not accurate as they can produce false-positive (presence of degenerative changes without clinical signs) and false-negative (inability to show soft tissue changes) results [19, 25]. Positional radiography has revealed that L7–S1 is the most mobile of all the vertebral segments in dogs with DLSS [15]. As DLSS includes instability as part of the contributing factors to the disease process, it was once thought that extension and flexion of the pelvic limbs were important; however, because radiographs

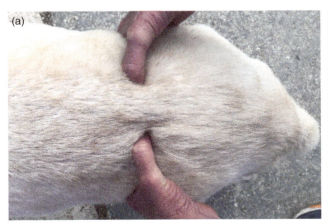
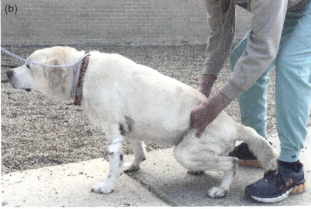

Figure 14.3 We routinely use what we describe as a "sciatic entrapment test" to evaluate patients for lumbosacral pain and discomfort. To perform the test, both hands are used with the thumbs placing pressure over the lumbosacral joint. Then the hands are rotated outward causing the thumbs to roll across the paraspinal muscles. Patients with lumbosacral pain and discomfort will almost immediately flex the stifles and go into a sitting position. Photo (a) shows the position of the hands and (b) shows a patient with a positive response. This can also be seen in some dogs with iliopsoas pain.

are two-dimensional imaging, instability is difficult to assess [25]. Dogs with LS disease have an increased LS angle when positioned in neutral position, increased angle in flexion, and decreased angle in extension comparatively to dogs who do not have DLSS [26, 27]. In another paper by Suwankong et al. [28], step lesions between L7 and S1 have been reported in 69% of dogs with DLSS, and can be appreciated in normal dogs free of clinical signs associated with DLSS [25, 28, 29].

For correct positioning for a lateral radiograph of the lumbosacral joint of the dog, a small foam pad is placed under the lumbar spine and a foam block between the hindlimbs to prevent oblique views of the LS joint (Figure 14.4).

Both extended lateral and flexed radiographs should be performed. However, note that lumbosacral articular facets positioned dorsolateral to the vertebral canal at the lumbosacral intervertebral space summate dorsally over the vertebral canal, and should not be mistaken for a compressive boney lesion [25, 30].

It is important to note that the presence of radiographic changes suggestive of DLSS does not always correlate with clinical signs [25, 26, 31]. It is also true that the absence of abnormalities on radiographs does not preclude the diagnosis of DLSS. Radiographs may be more useful for diagnosing other orthopedic diseases, such as canine hip dysplasia and changes secondary to cranial cruciate ligament ruptures.

Myelography (Contrast Study)

If MRI and CT are unavailable, myelograms can be utilized; however, these have fallen out of favor in comparison to the previously mentioned advanced imaging modalities. The contrast agent should be given via cisternal puncture only to prevent inadvertent epidural injection of contrast. Myelograms should be performed in neutral, flexion, and extension. Flexion is recommended to precede extension to allow for the flow of contrast to disperse [32]. Dogs that have DLSS show dorsally displaced and compressed contrast columns [25].

Limitations are similar to radiographs, which include the inability to reveal compression of the L7 nerve root within the foramen, that stenosis may be present despite a lack of abnormalities seen on myelogram, and that artifacts can be caused secondary to the dural sac extending over the LS joint appreciated in most large breed dogs [25].

Computed Tomography (CT)

CT allows for cross-sectional evaluation of the vertebral canal and for the ability to 3D reconstruct and evaluate the LS joint. Transverse views can help identify thickened or entrapped nerve roots [5]. Dynamic CT (extension and flexion) should be performed as disk protrusion and telescoping of S1 can be overlooked without extension views [15]. There is a negative linear relationship between

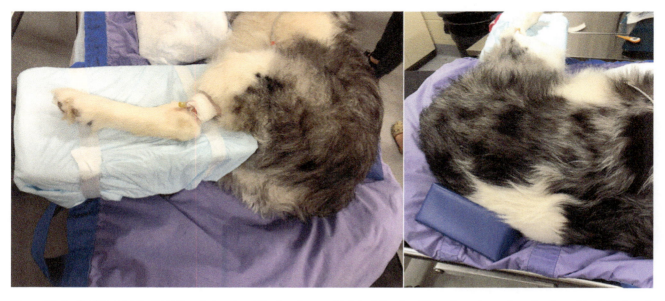

Figure 14.4 Positioning for lateral radiographs of the lumbosacral joint of the dog. These two views show the foam block is placed between the pelvic limbs, and a small foam pad is placed under the lumbar spine to prevent obliquity.

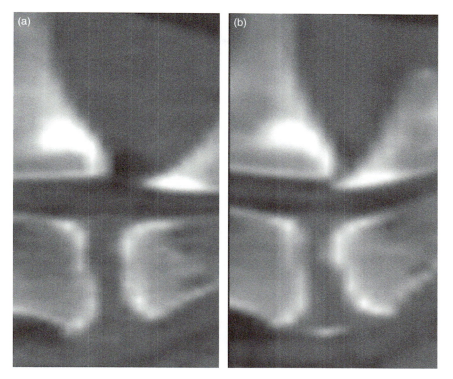

Figure 14.5 (a) Bone window showing image of L7–S1 in flexion vs (b) bone window showing image of L7–S1 in extension. The interarcuate space appears wider in flexion than extension. *Source:* Jones JC et al. [2008] / American Veterinary Medical Association.

the angle of the LS junction and intervertebral foraminal area whereby the intervertebral foramen and lumbosacral interarcuate space appear wider on flexion than extension (Figure 14.5) [15, 25].

CT images also allow for the evaluation of the entrance, middle, and exit zones of the intervertebral foramina, and the width of the intervertebral foraminal area [15, 16]. With this knowledge, the appropriate surgical approach can be considered for the particular area of stenosis causing impingement of the L7 nerve root [15]. Other changes indicating DLSS on CT include the increased opacity of soft tissue within the intervertebral foramina, narrowing of vertebral canal and loss of epidural fat, IVD protrusion, diskospondylitis/diskospondylosis, thickened or osteophytosis or articular processes, and subluxations [25, 33].

Magnetic Resonance Imaging (MRI)

Soft tissue is most accurately assessed by MRI [27]. Similar to CT, MRI allows for the collection of images that can be assessed on multiple planes. However, the one significant advantage is the ease of visualizing the L7 nerve root as it can be followed throughout its journey through from the entrance zone to the exit zone and its course visualized as it travels from the foraminal exit ventral to the SI joint [16]. As DLSS has a dynamic component on the size of the lumbosacral foramina, utilizing MRI's imaging sensitivity for soft tissue and adjusting the body's position during the scan is key for successful diagnosis. It is recommended that the LS joint be imaged in extension, as this allowed for improved diagnosis of subclinical compressive lesions and IVD protrusion. Patients placed in neutral and hyperextended positions during MRI exhibit exaggerated differences with the neuroforaminal dimension. The exit zones are larger than the entrance zones in neutral position and smaller than the entrance zone in hyperextension. It is suspected that hyperextension position is more dynamic for the compression of the exit zone secondary to ligaments and IVD protrusions [16].

Traditional diagnosis of DLSS on MRI involves looking at the spine from parasagittal, transverse, and dorsal planes. MRI images in oblique planar images show smaller neuroforamina than in standard parasagittal planar images [16]. In those images, the middle zone was noted to be the narrowest zone. This has been supported by past studies utilizing CT scans that measured the middle and exit zones as being the narrowest on cross-sectional images compared to that of the entrance zone [33].

Thus, oblique planes may provide increased sensitivity for the diagnosis of lumbosacral stenosis and nerve root compression [16]. It has also been suggested that a 1–2 mm slice protocol should be avoided due to partial-volume artifacts and false-positive findings [25, 33, 34].

Force Plate Analysis

Force plate analysis (FPA) can detect changes in the propulsive forces of the pelvic limbs in dogs that are affected with DLSS. It is a noninvasive measurement of canine locomotion. In dogs with DLSS, the propulsive forces are significantly lower than that of healthy dogs. However, this can be a difficult diagnostic modality to interperate in dogs with DLSS, as it is typically utilized for patients with a mono-limb lameness vs a bilateral pelvic limb ataxia [36–38].

Electrodiagnostics

Electromyography (EMG) can be used to support the diagnosis of DLSS, but it is not specific for the source of the abnormality or lesion. Thus, somatosensory evoked potentials (SEPs) are more sensitive toward the detection of L7 nerve compression associated with DLSS – as is an increase in F-wave onset latency and the F-ratio. However, these tests are extremely time consuming and demanding, and are not utilized often as they do not assist in evaluating potential surgical planning [39–40].

Treatment: Conservative and Medical Therapy

Medical treatment can be useful for some patients with a mild manifestation of DLSS; however, 32% may still require surgery. A more aggressive conservative therapy involves epidurals utilizing methylprednisolone acetate, which is a slow-release depot corticosteroid with an elimination half-life of 139 hours [41]. This allows for local delivery of steroids while minimizing the systemic side-effects of corticosteroids. Signs of systemic absorption of corticosteroids include polyphagia, polydipsia, and polyurea; however, these clinical signs tend to be transient in nature [41, 42]. Epidural injection would be an appropriate treatment option for patients who do not show proprioceptive deficits and have appropriate urinary and fecal continence.

The recommended dose of methylprednisolone acetate (40 mg/ml concentration) is 1 mg/kg, with a minimum volume of 0.5 ml and a maximum volume of 1 ml over three injections suggested at day 1, 14, and 41 [41] or as needed [39, 40]. Once the medication has been given, the

author prefers to flex and extend the LS region with the most affected side ventral to aid in the flow of the corticosteroid into the middle and exit zones of the affected L7 nerve roots; the patient can then be flipped if necessary for bilateral lesions. Studies have shown that with a 0.2 ml/kg injection of iodinated radiographic contrast medium, LS epidurals can travel as far as the TL junction, so an epidural injecton can also be used to treat higher disk protrusions in dogs with multifocal lesions [43]. Guidance of the spinal needle can be performed with fluoroscopy, CT, or ultrasound if needed [40–46].

It should be recognized that conservative treatment alone has a high rate of relapse [4, 7, 9]. In patients who receive epidurals, 79–84% transiently improve; however, 77.2% relapse after six months [42].

Concurrent medical management includes rest, leash-walks to maintain healthy muscle mass, physical rehabilitation to strengthen core muscles that support the lower back and LS junction, weight loss, change in activity levels, and steroids vs nonsteroidal anti-inflammatory drugs [19].

Surgery

Surgical management is indicated if the patient does not respond to conservative management, or the patient has significant neurological deficits. Dogs with more severe neurological deficits preoperatively, such as urinary incontinence, carry a worse prognosis for return to function. The primary goal for surgery for DLSS patients is decompression of the cauda equine, release of entrapped nerve roots, and stabilization of the joint if indicated.

In large breed dogs, the spinal cord ends in the caudal half of L6 and cranial half of L7. It can extend further caudally in some smaller breed dogs [47]. From the conus medullaris arises the cauda equina which is comprised of L6, L7, S1–S3, and CD1–CD5 nerve roots. The interarcuate ligaments and lamina of L7 and S1 border them dorsally, and the dorsal longitudinal ligament, IVD, and vertebral bodies of L7–S1 border them ventrally, while the vertebral foramina and pedicles of L7 and S1 border them laterally. The articulations of L7 and S1 are stabilized by the articular facet joint capsule, dorsal and ventral longitudinal ligaments, interarcuate ligaments, interspinous and supraspinous ligaments, and surrounding spinal musculature and fascia.

As the L7 nerve root can become entrapped in DLSS patients, it is important to ensure that there is adequate decompression of this nerve. The location of the stenosis (entrance, middle, exit zones), will determine the best surgical approach [2, 17].

Dorsal Laminectomy

Dorsal laminectomy is a common surgical procedure, decompressing the cauda equina and allowing the surgeon to evaluate and assess nerve roots entrapped in the entry zone. This requires the removal of the spinous processes and lamina, and possibly includes extending the laminectomy through S2 and S3 [48]. At this time, concurrent dorsal annulectomy or partial discectomy of the LS IVD can be performed simultaneously. However, substantial soft tissue and boney disruption can cause postoperative instability [49]. It has also been reported that dogs with dorsal laminectomies and concurrent partial discectomies had poorer results than dogs with dorsal laminectomies alone.

Dorsal laminectomies have shown 79% improvement without subsequent stabilization surgery. However, recurrence was seen in 33% of patients, and reduction of foraminal volume up to 69% with persistent nerve compression has also been appreciated.

FPA studies showed improved propulsive forces by six weeks, which remained the same six months postoperatively for patients with dorsal laminectomies with concurrent partial discectomies. Thus, although there was improvement, the patients did not return to normal gait despite surgical intervention [36]. Dorsal laminectomies can provide limited access to the entrance zone of L7 foramen; however, if the patient is stenotic at the middle or exit zones, it cannot be treated with the dorsal laminectomy alone, and clinical signs may persist [50].

Patient Preparation and Positioning

The patient is placed in sternal recumbency with pelvic limbs in a "frog-leg" position (neutral) or drawn forward. This allows for the interarcuate ligament to accentuate the dorsal lumbosacral space. The pubis should be supported with rolled towels or sandbags beneath to allow for further opening of the IVD space for the decompressive surgery (Figure 14.6) [48].

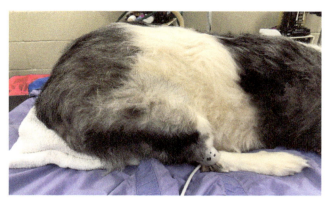

Figure 14.6 Positioning of the patient on the surgery table with the pelvic limbs extended forward with the pubis supported.

Surgical Technique

Landmark the wings of the ilium and the spinous process of L6. Remember, the spinous process of L7 can be shorter than L6, thus making it difficult to palpate. A dorsal midline incision should be made from the spinous process of L5/L6 to the first caudal vertebra. Subcutaneous fat and superficial facias are incised along the midline to expose the deep gluteal and caudal fascia. A fat graft should be harvested from this region and placed aside, wrapped in saline soaked gauze.

Using monopolar cautery, an incision is made through the fascia on both sides of the spinous process from L5/L6 to S1, coming together between the spinous process to give one midline incision. The epaxial muscles are elevated away from the spinous processes, lamina, and articular facets of L6 to S1 and the sacral crests caudally to S3 using blunt dissection with a Freer periosteal elevator or small osteotomes [46, 51, 52]. Gelpi retractors should be utilized at the cranial and caudal edges of the incision to facilitate visualization of the surgical site. The authors find a third pair of Glepi retractors placed in the middle is helpful for best retraction and visualization. Remove the spinous processes of L7–S1 with double action rongeurs. The wide interarcuate space of L7–S1 should be noted and removal of any other associated soft tissue structures (muscle attachments, ligaments) using a scalpel blade or monopolar cautery should be done at this time.

Using a high-speed pneumatic drill, remove the outer cortical and medullary layer from the mid body of L7 to the midbody of S2–S3. Once the inner cortical layer of bone is exposed, continue to drill carefully until the inner cortical bone is soft. Using a small House curette, penetrate and remove the inner periosteum in an area large enough to introduce Kerrison rongeurs, which can then be utilized to complete the laminectomy. Once in the spinal canal, elevate the ligamentum flavum to ensure there are no adhesions and sharply dissect (scalpel blade or Tenotomy scissors) from either the right or left sides. It can then be retracted and incised from the remaining side. Do not dissect deeper than the remaining boney lamina to avoid damage to the cauda equina [9]. At this time, the cauda equina should be exposed along with the nerve roots of L7, S1, S2, S3, caudal nerve roots, vertebral sinus, dorsal longitudinal ligament, and dorsal annulus of LS IVD. S1 nerve roots run lateral to the dural sac while L7 nerve roots are located laterally and run through the lateral recess prior to exiting the entrance zone of the foramina. This means that the middle and exit zones are not visible from this approach [52, 53]. The nerve roots should be explored while utilizing a probe for any adhesions, and while assessing if a partial diskectomy/annulectomy needs to be performed at this time. The L7 nerve should move a few millimeters with minimal traction [9]; however, if this is not possible, further decompression may need to be considered via partial or complete facetectomy/foraminotomy.

Herniated LS IVD can be visualized protruding dorsally within the spinal canal. However, it can also be palpated by running a ball-end probe, nerve retractor, or other blunt object over the floor of the spinal canal just under the cauda equina.

If needed, the cauda equina can be gently retracted laterally using a ball-end probe and the protruding disk visualized. For a diskectomy, using an 18G needle or No. 11 scalpel blade, make an incision into the chronic protruding disk; and with curettes, fenestrate the disk space. It should be noted that some surgeons prefer the pneumatic drill to create a "power fenestration." It is imperative that the cauda equina be protected. This can be accomplished by retracing the cauda equina to one side, and the opposing side of the disk being fenestrated, and then switching sides to accomplish full diskectomy [7, 48]. It should be noted that diskogenic pain can be exhibited during diskectomy, with development of hyperpnea, tachycardia, and an increase in arterial blood pressure [53].

The surgical site should be copiously lavaged with saline. Place the autogenous fat graft harvested during the surgical approach over the laminectomy site to prevent adhesion formation.

Foraminotomy

Foraminal stenosis with concurrent compressive radiculopathy of the L7 nerve root has been reported to be seen in 68% of dogs with DLSS [8]. Foraminotomy can be an extension of a dorsal laminectomy beneath the L7 articular process or a separate lateral approach. It is the removal of the bone that forms the intervertebral foramina whereby the exit zone of the nerve root forms [48, 49, 54]. With concurrent partial diskectomy of L7–S1, a partial collapse of the L7–S1 neurovascular foramen can result, which would not have been present on preoperative imaging [35, 54, 55]. Foraminotomies can increase the risk of an articular facet fracture and hypermobility when performed from a dorsal laminectomy [54, 56].

A lateral approach for a foraminotomy can be performed without concurrent dorsal laminectomy. This would address the middle and exit zone of L7 nerve roots [55]. Utilization of endoscopic assisted lumbosacral foraminotomy has been discussed in current literature, but is currently not designed to replace current surgical interventions for LS disease [57, 58]. Dorsolateral foraminotomy has been shown to increase foraminal volume directly after surgery by 650–800%. However, foraminal volume decreases – up to 335% – with a median follow up of 24 months have been reported following foraminotomies [54, 59]. Enlargement can be lost as soon as 12 weeks postoperatively due to boney regrowth with fibrous tissue generation (Figure 14.7) [35, 55, 57].

The approach for L7–S1 foraminotomy has been described using a lateral approach, transiliac approach, and endoscopic-assisted approach [35, 51, 58]. For this text, the lateral approach shall be discussed as both the transiliac and endoscopic-assisted exploration have only been performed in limited studies and further clinical

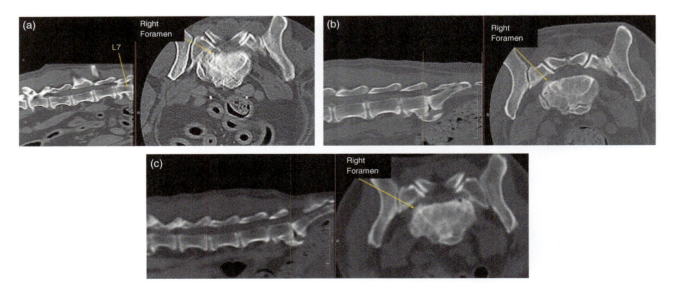

Figure 14.7 CT of a dog with DLSS. Sagittal and transverse images provided. (a) Dog presurgery. (b) Seven month postop dorsal laminectomy and right foraminotomy. (c) Sixteen month postop dorsal laminectomy and right foraminotomy.

research is required to determine if these techniques are appropriate for in vivo patients [35, 51, 58, 60]. As a foraminotomy can be an performed concurrently with the dorsal laminectomy, the patient is placed in the same position as the dorsal laminectomy [33]. Upon completion of the approach through the superficial fascia, an incision is made lateral to the midline facial incision for a dorsal laminectomy approximately halfway between the ileal wing and spinous processes to allow blunt dissection through the connection between the multifidus and sacrocaudalis muscles. The muscular attachments to the caudal L6–L7 articular facets and cranial L7–S1 articular facets are sharply dissected using monocautery and the muscular attachments elevated from the pedicle to the level of the transverse process of L7. This will expose the intervertebral foramen from a dorsolateral oblique angle. A pediculectomy is made using a high-speed bur cranial to the L7–S1 foramen from the transverse process dorsal to the caudal aspect of the caudal L7 articular facet. Once the canal has been exposed, Kerrison ronguers can be used to extend the pediculectomy into the L7–S1 foramen. At this point, the L7 nerve root should be freely movable into its new, more cranially positioned foramen. This approach widens the foramen from the entrance zone through the exit zone.

Facetectomy

Facetectomy is the complete removal of the L7 caudal articular process, which approaches the exit zone of the foramen dorsally. However, due to increased lumbosacral instability, this surgical intervention should be avoided unless a concurrent stabilization is performed [61].

Distraction, Fusion, and Stabilization

One of the greatest controversies regarding DLSS is whether or not instability and subluxation are a pathological process of DLSS or merely abnormal motion [13, 14, 62, 63]. Despite the ongoing debate among veterinary specialists, stabilization (with or without concurrent distraction and fusion) may be required for DLSS patients. This is especially true when partial discectomy or facetectomy may exacerbate preexisting instability [61–63]. Stabilization utilizes string of pearl (SOP) plates, pins, and polymethylmethacrylate (PMMA) or kinematic screw rods. Distraction is to restore the disk width and foramina volume, thereby relieving pressure on neural tissue. Fusion utilizes cancellous bone graft to promote boney growth over the dorsal lamina. The most common complications from these procedures are implant failure.

Pins and PMMA

This technique can be combined with dorsal laminectomies following the decompressive procedure. It functions as an internal fixator along the dorsal aspect of the lumbosacral spine. This method is cost effective and requires no specialized instruments; however, PMMA can be bulky in nature, has an exothermic chemical reaction when setting, can cause a seroma, has increased infection rates, increased wound breakdown, and a fibrotic inflammatory response [65].

Pin placement techniques include the four cross-pinning technique, with two pins in L7 and two pins in S1; or the six-pins technique, with two in the pedicle of L7, two in the sacrum, and two into the ilium [64, 66]. Utilize positive-profile end-threaded pins after pre-drilled holes have been made with a drill bit of smaller diameter. The direction of the pins should be aimed at a 30–45° angle from the sagittal plane to prevent injury to the lumbosacral trunk and entry into the sacroiliac joint [63]. Pins should exit 2–3 mm ventral to the vertebral body. Pins should be cut just below the dorsal edge of the spinous process to allow for overlap and PMMA contact [48, 64].

At this point, if a dorsal laminectomy has been performed and fusion is to be achieved, the placement of autogenous cancellous or commercially available bone graft should be placed into the joint space of the disk space to encourage fusion.

Once the PMMA has been mixed, it should be poured dorsally over the pins, articular facets – including the spinous process of L7 and S1 if a dorsal laminectomy was not performed – and caution used to prevent spreading into the canal with Gelfoam® if a dorsal laminectomy was performed. While the cement cures, constant cool saline lavage should be performed for five minutes to avoid exothermic reaction damage. It has been suggested that for dogs greater than 15 kg in weight, 40 g of PMMA powder mixed in with liquid polymer should be considered [64, 65].

SOP Plating

SOPs are useful due to their ability to bend and twist which allows for a more appropriate interface with L6 and sacroiliac articulation. They can also be utilized in lumbosacral fractures. The utilization of two bilateral SOP plates allows for canal alignment, reduction of instability, and compensation for future diminished plate strength. Due to its low profile, it is less likely to cause a seroma and concurrent dorsal laminectomies can be performed. However, implant failure from mechanical breakage can occur due to over-twisting and screw mispositioning which can cause sequalae such as hemorrhage, fractures, or insufficient bone purchase. SOP is not recommended for patients that are greater than 25 kg [19].

Surgical Technique

The bilateral plates of the SOP plate should be twisted to allow for appropriate engagement of the dorsolateral aspect of the spine at the level of the transverse processes. The SOP plates should be contoured using bending irons and tees and should be twisted caudally to engage the shaft of the ilium with four screws (minimum of three screws) in L7 and the sacrum [64, 66]. It's preferable that two screw holes per vertebra is achieved, a total of at least eight cortices engaged on each side [67].

Screws should be directed at approximately 60° from the mid-sagittal plane into the vertebral body of L6. As the pedicles are wide enough on L7, implantation screws can be placed here. The entry point for the screws should be placed parallel to the sagittal plane at the cranial articular process. For S1, the entry point is a few millimeters caudal to its cranial articular process. The screw for S1 should be 5° laterally relative to the sagittal plane. If possible, screws should be placed into S2 [65].

It should be recognized that placing a pedicle screw in the cranial aspect of L7 and a second screw in the lateral lamina and vertebral body could cause penetration of the vertebral canal, into the intervertebral foramen. Caution with pin placement should be taken [68].

Pedicle Screw and Rod Fixation (PSRF)

Pedicle screw and rod fixation (PSRF) can be useful in realigning and fusing the vertebral bodies to mitigate ventral subluxation. This can be performed concurrently with dorsal laminectomies, and fusion is required to be performed as well. Titanium screws are inserted with fluoroscopy and connected with contoured titanium rods. This system allows for a decreased risk of implant fatigue and subsequent implant failure. The PSRF system is utilized in human medicine. Finding an appropriate size of implantation can be difficult in our canine patients [69]. Novel pedicle screw implantations have been created for the canine lumbosacral joint specifically, but not yet utilized in in vivo patients [18].

The utilization of intervertebral spacers that are commercially available or patient-specific 3D-printed titanium implants are currently being studied, but not yet published with their long-term results in in vivo patients [18, 19, 54].

Prior to pin placements, it is imperative that the implant corridor be calculated appropriately. The implant corridor runs in a dorso-caudo-lateral to ventro-cranio-medial oblique direction from the dorsal cortex of the lamina to the ventral cortex of the vertebral body. The boundaries where perforation is suboptimal include the ventral cortex, medial pedicle wall, and lateral pedicle wall. Therefore, the entry point for L7 should be the caudal border of the facet joint base of the transverse process. The entry point for S1 is halfway between the caudal border of the cranial articular process and intermedial sacral crest [69].

Pre-drilling of the holes can be performed with a K-pin, and should not penetrate the ventral cortex. A depth measurement should be utilized for appropriate pin size selection; 50–80% of the total screw length should be placed into the vertebral bone while the rest of the screw protruding from the vertebra allows for the titanium rod connection. The rod should be bent and adjusted while using a rod bender to allow for appropriate fit with the screws. Once the fit is appropriate, sleeves and nuts should be applied and tightened [18, 69].

The use of intraoperative fluoroscopy to confirm the placement and position of the screws is recommended [69].

Minimally-Invasive Transilial Vertebral (MTV) Blocking

Minimally-invasive transilial vertebral (MTV) blocking is based on human interspinous decompressor implants for the treatment of lower back pain in humans. It is relatively new for the surgical treatment of DLSS in canine patients. A Steinmann pin or 3D-printed pin is implanted from one iliac wing to another while using L7's spinous process as a buttress [70]. The junction is in neutral to slightly flexed position, and prevents dynamic L7 nerve root impingement [54] by increasing the width of the boney frame of the cauda equina and L7 spinal nerves through biomechanical manipulation induced by the implant through reduced extension. This method does not allow for concurrent dorsal decompression, and may not be as effective as a dorsal laminectomy for decompression. Complications include postoperative infection, incorrect implant positioning, stiffness, and pain (Figure 14.8) [70].

For this surgical technique, dissection to the bone is not required, unless other procedures are to be performed concurrently, such as fracture repair or biopsies. The position of this patient should be in a neutral position to maximize the LS flexion. Fluoroscopy is recommended to ensure proper pin positioning intraoperatively.

The length of the MTV should be measured based on the ventro-dorsal radiographs of the pelvis or from CT dorsal views. Measurement is based on the distance from the left

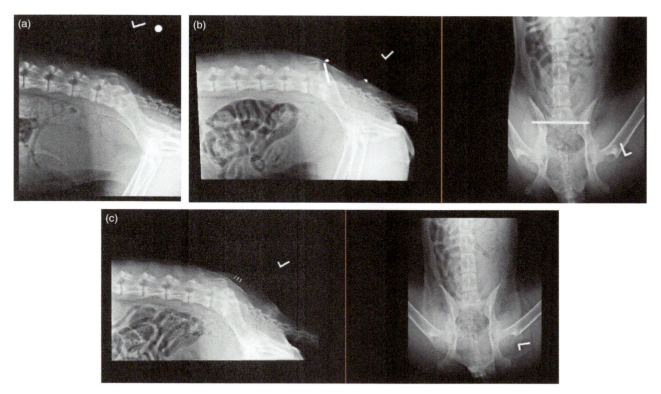

Figure 14.8 Sequential radiograph of a dog with diskospondylitis and secondary LS luxation. Sagittal and transverse images provided. (a) Sagittal view of the patient presurgery. (b) Three month postoperative minimally-invasive transilial vertebral (MTV) blocking pin placement. (c) Images after removal of MTV blocking pin on same day as the images taken from (b).

and right cranial portion of the ileal wings, caudal to the spinous process of L7. A stab incision of 2 cm in length is made on one side of the dog where the incision point on the cranial area of the ileal wing should be placed. A Steinmann pin can be utilized and advanced through the gluteal muscle. Once the placement is confirmed on the ileal wing, the pin can be drilled through the left ileal wing, across the dorsal lamina of L7, and engaging the right ileal wing with the threaded portion of the pin. To prevent migration of the pin, double Kirschner clamps or PMMA should be placed on the pins after incorporating notches to the pins' ends [48].

A custom-designed MTV set has been described in past literature; however, its availability for clinical utilization is unknown [70].

Postoperative Management

A period of four to eight weeks is recommended following any surgical procedure. A gradual return to activity is recommended over four to six weeks following initial postoperative rest. For working dogs, this can be extended.

Physical rehabilitation is recommended for recovery, especially those utilizing underwater treadmills and pools. A patient specific plan should be formulated with their certified physical rehabilitation specialists and the patient's surgeons.

 Video clips to accompany this book can be found on the companion website at: www.wiley.com/go/shores/advanced

References

1. Indrieri, R.J. (1988). Lumbosacral stenosis and injury of the cauda equina. *Vet. Clin. North Am. Small Anim. Pract.* 18: 679–710.

2. De Risio, L., Thomas, W.B., and Sharp, J.N. (2000). Degenerative lumbosacral stenosis. *Vet. Clin. North Am. Small Anim. Pract.* 30: 111–132.

3. Tarvin, G. and Prata, R.G. (1980). Lumbosacral stenosis in dogs. *J. Am. Vet. Med. Assoc.* 177: 154–159.

4. Palmer, R.H. and Chambers, J.N. (1991). Canine lumbosacral diseases. Part I. Anatomy, pathophysiology, and clinical presentations. *Compend. Contin. Edu. Pract. Vet.* 13: 61–68.

5. Meij, B.P. and Bergknut, N. (2010). Degenerative lumbosacral stenosis in dogs. *Vet. Clin. North Am. Small Anim. Pract.* 40: 983–1009.

6. Seiler, G.S., Hani, H., Busato, A.R. et al. (2002). Facet joint geometry and intervertebral disk degeneration in the L5-S1 region of the vertebral column in German Shepherd Dogs. *Am. J. Vet. Res.* 63: 86–90.

7. Moore, G.E., Burkman, K.D., Carter, M.N., and Peterson, M.R. (2001). Causes of death or reasons for euthanasias in military working dogs: 927 cases (1993–1996). *J. Am. Vet. Med. Assoc.* 219: 209–214.

8. Mayhew, P.D., Kapatkin, A.S., Wortman, J.A., and Vite, C.H. (2002). Association of Cauda Equina Compression on magneteic resonance images and clinical signs in dogs with degenerative lumbosacral stenosis. *J. Am. Anim. Hosp. Assoc.* 38: 555–562.

9. Sharp, N.J.H. and Wheeler, S.J. (2005). Lumbosacral disease. In: *Small Animal Spinal Disorders*, 2e (ed. N. Sharp and S. Wheeler), 181–209. Edinburgh: Elsvier Mosby.

10. Braund, K.G., Taylor, T.K., Ghosh, P., and Sherwood, A.A. (1977). Spinal mobility in the dog. A study in chondrodystrophoid and non-chondrodystrophoid animals. *Res. Vet. Sci.* 22: 78–82.

11. Hediger, K.U., Ferguson, S.J., Gedet, P. et al. (2009). Biomechanical analysis of torsion and shear forces in lumbar and lumbosacral spine segments of nonchondrodystrophic dogs. *Vet. Surg.* 38: 874–880.

12. Dewey, C.W. and da Costa, R.C. (2016: 2–5;). Breed-associated neurological abnormalities of dogs and disorders affecting the cauda equina in dogs and cats. In: *Practical Guide to Canine and Feline Neurology*, 3e (ed. C.W. Dewey and R.C. de Costa), 406–412. Ames, IA: Wiley Blackwell.

13. Benninger, M.I., Seiler, G.S., Robinson, L.E. et al. (2004). Three-dimensional motion pattern of the caudal lumbar and lumbosacral portions of the vertebral column of dogs. *Am. J. Vet. Res.* 65: 544–551.

14. Benninger, M.I., Seiler, G.S., Robinson, L.E. et al. (2006). Effects of anatomic conformation on three-dimensional motion of the caudal lumbar and lumbosacral portions of the vertebral column of dogs. *Am. J. Vet. Res.* 67: 43–50.

15. Jones, J.C., Davies, S.E., Were, S.R., and Shackelford, K.L. (2008). Effects of body position and clinical signs on L7-S1 intervertebral foraminal area and lumbosacral angle in dogs with lumbosacral disease as measured via computed tomography. *Am. J. Vet. Radiol.* 69 (11): 1446–1454.

16. Zindle, C., Tucker, R.L., Jovanovik, J. et al. (2017). Effects of image plane, patient positioning, and foraminal zone on magnetic resonance imaging measurements of canine lumbosacral intervertebral foramina. *Vet. Radiol. Ultrasound* 58 (2): 206–215.

17. Worth, A.J., Hartman, A., Bridges, J.P. et al. (2017). Computed tomographic evaluation of dynamic alteration of the canine lumbosacral intervertebral neurovascular foramina. *Vet. Surg.* 46: 255–264.

18. Zindl, C., Litsky, A.S., Fitzpatrick, N., and Allen, M.J. (2018). Kinematic behavior of a novel pedicle screw-rod fixation system for the canine lumbosacral joint. *Vet. Surg.* 47: 114–124.

19. Worth, A., Meij, B., and Jeffery, N. (2019). Canine degenerative lumbosacral stenosis: prevalence, impact and management strategies. *Vet. Med.: Res. Rep.* 10: 169–183.

20. Ramirez, O. III and Thrall, D.E. (1998). A review of imaging techniques for canine cauda equina syndrome. *Vet. Radiol. Ultrasound* 39: 283–296.

21. Morgan, J. and Bailey, C. (1990). Cauda equina syndrome in dog: radiographic evaluation. *J. Small Anim. Pract.* 31: 69–76.

22. Sande, R.D. (1992). Radiograpy, myelography, computed tomography, and magnetic resonance imaging of the spine. *Vet. Clin. North Am. Small Pract.* 22: 811–831.

23. Steffen, F., Hunold, K., Scharf, G. et al. (2007). A follow-up study of neurologic and radiographic findings in working German shepherd dogs with and without degenerative lumbosacral stenosis. *J. Am. Vet. Med. Assoc.* 231: 1529–1533.

24. Scharf, G., Steffen, F., Grunenfelder, F. et al. (2004). The lumbosacral junction in working German shepherd dogs: neurological and radiological evaluation. *J. Vet. Med. A Physiol. Pathol. Clin. Med.* 51: 27–32.

25. Worth, A.J., Thompson, D.J., and Hartman, D.J. (2009). Degenerative lumbosacral stenosis in working dogs: current concepts and review. *N. Z. Vet. J.* 57 (6): 319–330.

26. Schmid, V. and Lang, J. (1993). Measurements on the lumbosacral junction in normal dogs and htose with cauda-equina compression. *J. Small Anim. Pract.* 34: 437–442.

27. Mattoon, J. and Koblik, P. (1993). Quantitative survey radiographic evaluation of the lumbosacral spine of normal dogs and dogs with degenerative lumbosacral stenosis. *Vet. Radiol. Ultrasound.* 34: 194–206.

28. Suwankong, N., Voorhout, G., Hazewinkel, H.A.W., and Meij, B.P. (2006). Agreement between computed tomography, magnetic resonance imaging, and surgical findings in dogs with degenerative lumbosacral stenosis. *J. Am. Vet. Med. A* 229: 1924–1929.

29. DeRisio, L., Thomas, W., and Sharp, N. (2000). Degenerative lumbosacral stenosis. *Vet. Clin. North Am.* 30: 130–133.

30. McKee, M. and Dennis, R. (2003). Radiology corner: lumbosacral radiography. *Vet. Radiol. Ultrasound* 44: 655–666.

31. Gradner, G., Bockstahler, B., Peham, C. et al. (2007). Kinematic study of back movement in clinically sound Malinois dogs with consideration of the effect of radiographic changes in the lumbosacral junction. *Vet. Surg.* 36: 472–481.

32. Lang, J. (1988). Flexion-extension myelography of the canine cauda-equina. *Vet. Radiol.* 29: 242–257.

33. Heninger, W. and Werner, G. (2003). CT examination of the canine lumbosacral spine in extension and flexion. Part 2: soft-tissue window. *Eur. J. Comp. Anim. Pract.* 13: 227–233.

34. Higgins, B.M., Cripps, P.J., Baker, M. et al. (2011). Effects of body position, imaging plane, and observer on computed tomographic measurements of the lumbosacral intervertebral foraminal area in dogs. *Am. J. Vet. Res.* 72: 905–917.

35. Godde, T. and Steffen, F. (2007). Surgical treatment of lumbosacral foraminal stenosis using a lateral approach in twenty dogs with degenerative lumbosacral stenosis. *Vet. Surg.* 36: 705–713.

36. Suwankong, N., Meij, B.P., Van Klaveren, N.J. et al. (2007). Biomechanical flexion-extension forces in normal canine lumbosacral cadaver specimens before and after dorsal laminectomy-discectomy and pedicle screw-rod fixation. *Vet. Surg.* 36: 742–751.

37. Meij, B.P., Suwankong, N., Van Der Veen, A.J., and Hazewinkel, H.A. (2007). Assessment of decompressive surgery in dogs with degenerative lumbosacral stenosis using force plate analysis and questionnaires. *Vet. Surg.* 36: 423–431.

38. Van Klaveren, N.J., Suwankong, N., De Boer, S. et al. (2005). Force plate analysis before and after dorsal decompression treatment of degenerative lumbosacral stenosis in dogs. *Vet. Surg.* 34: 450–456.

39. Meij, B.P., Suwankong, N., Van Den Brom, W. et al. (2006). Tibial nerve somatosensory evoked potentials in dogs with degenerative lumbosacral stenosis. *Vet. Surg.* 35: 168–175.

40. Harcourt-Brown, T.R., Granger, N.P., Fitzpatrick, N., and Jeffery, N.D. (2019). Electrodiagnostic findings in dogs with apparently painful lumbosacral foraminal stenosis. *J. Vet. Intern. Med.* 33: 2167–2174.

41. Janssens, L., Beosior, Y., and Daems, R. (2009). Lumbosacral degenerative stenosis in the dog. *Vet. Comp. Orthop. Traumatol.* 6: 486–491.

42. Gomes, S.A., Lowrie, M., and Targett, M. (2020). Single dose epidural methylprednisolone as a treatment and predictor of outcome following subsequent decompressive surgery in degenerative lumbosacral stenosis with foraminal stenosis. *Vet. J.* 257: 1–7.

43. Kawalilak, L.T., Tucker, R.L., and Greene, S.A. (2015). Use of contrast-enhanced computed tomography to study the cranial migration of a lumbosacral injected in cadaver dogs. *Vet. Radiol. Ultrasound* 56 (5): 570–574.

44. Liotta, A., Sandersen, C., Couvreur, T., and Bolen, G. (2016). Technique, difficulty, and accuracy of computed tomography-guided translaminar and transforaminal lumbosacral epidural and intraarticular lumbar facet joint injections in dogs. *Vet. Radiol. Ultrasound* 57 (2): 191–198.

45. Liotta, A.P., Girod, M., Peeters, D. et al. (2016). Clinical effects of computed tomography- guided lumbosacral facet joint, transforaminal epidural, and translaminar epidural injections of methylprednisolone acetate in healthy dogs. *Am. J. Vet. Res.* 77 (10): 1131–1139.

46. Liotta, A., Busoni, V., Carrozzo, M.V. et al. (2015). Feasibility of ultrasound-guided epidural access at the lumbosacral space in dogs. *Vet. Radiol. Ultrasound* 56 (2): 220–228.

47. Fletcher, T.F. and Kitchell, R.L. (1966). Anatomical studies on the spinal cord segments of the dog. *Am. J. Vet. Res.* 27: 1759–1767.

48. Fossum, T.W. (2007). Surgery of the lumbosacral spine. In: *Small Animal Surgery*, 3e (ed. T.W. Fossum), 1493–1513. St Louis, MO: Mosby Elsevier.

49. Worth, A.J., Hartman, A., Bridges, J.P. et al. (2017). Effect of dorsal laminectomy and dorsal annulectomy with partial lumbosacral discectomy on the volume of the lateral intervertebral neuroforamina in dogs when the lumbosacral junction is extended. *Vet. Surg.* 46: 265–270.

50. Suwankong, N., Meij, B.P., Vorrhout, G. et al. (2008). Review and retrospective analysis of degenerative lumbosacral stenosis in 156 dogs treated by dorsal laminectomy. *Vet. Comp. Orthop. Traumatol.* 3: 285–293.

51. Piermattei, D.L. and Johnson, K.A. (ed.) (2004). The vertebral column: approach to lumbar vertebra 7 and the sacrum through a dorsal incision. In: *An Atlas of Surgical Approaches to the Bones and Joints of the Dog and Cat*, 4e, 92–95. Philadelphia, PA: Saunders.

52. Johnson, K.A. (2014). The vertebral column: approach to lumbar vertebra 7 and the sacrum through a dorsal

incision. In: *Piermattei's Atlas of Surgical Approaches to the Bones and Joints of the Dog and Cat*, 5e (ed. D.L. Piermattei), 94–97. St Louis, MO: Elsvier Saunders.

53. Danielsson, F. and Sjostrom, L. (1999). Surgical treatment of degenerative lumbosacral stenosis in dogs. *Vet. Surg.* 28: 91–98.

54. Smolders, L.A., Knell, S.C., Park, B. et al. (2020). The effects of foraminotomy and intervertebral distraction on the volume of the lumbosacral intervertebral neurovascular foramen: an ex vivo study. *Vet. J.* 256: 1–8.

55. Brickmann, P. and Grootenboer, H. (1991). Change of disc height, radical disc bulge, and intradiscal pressure from discectomy. An in vitro investigation on human lumbar disc. *Spine* 16: 641–646.

56. Moens, N. and Runyon, C.L. (2002). Fracture of L7 vertebral articular facets and pedicles following dorsal laminectomy in a dog. *J. Am. Vet. Med. Assoc.* 221: 807–810.

57. Gomes, S.A., Lowrie, M., and Targett, M. (2018). Long-term outcome following lateral foraminotomy as treatment for canine degenerative lumbosacral stenosis. *Vet. Rec.* 181: 1–6.

58. Wood, B.C., Lanz, O.I., Jones, J.C., and Shires, P.K. (2004). Endoscopic-assisted lumbosacral foraminotomy in the dog. *Vet. Surg.* 33: 221–231.

59. Worth, A.J., Hartman, A., Bridges, J.P. et al. (2018). Medium-term outcome and CT assessment of lateral foramintotomy at the lumbosacral junction in dogs with degenerative lumbosacral stenosis. *Vet. Comp. Orthop. Traumatol.* 31: 37–43.

60. Carozzo, C., Cachon, T., Genevois, J.P. et al. (2008). Transiliac approach for exposure of lumbosacral intervertebral disk and foramen: technique description. *Vet. Surg.* 37: 27–31.

61. Smith, M.E.H., Bebchuk, T.N., Schmon, C.L. et al. (2004). An in vitro biomechanical study of the effects of surgical modification upon the canine lumbosacral spine. *Vet. Comp. Orthop. Traumatol.* 17: 17–24.

62. Meij, B.P., Suwankong, N., Van der Veen, A.J. et al. (2007). Biomechanical flexion-extension forces in normal canine lumbosacral cadaver specimens before nad after dorsal laminectomy-discectomy and pedicle screw-rod fixation. *Vet. Surg.* 36: 742–751.

63. Hankin, E.J., Jerram, R.M., Walker, A.M. et al. (2012). Transarticular facet screw stabilization and dorsal laminectomy in 26 dogs with degenerative lumbosacral stenosis with instability. *Vet. Surg.* 41: 611–619.

64. Weh, J.M. and Kraus, K.H. (2007). Use of a four pin and methylmethacrylate fixation in L7 and the iliac body to stabilize lumbosacral fracture-luxations: a clinical and anatomic study. *Vet. Surg.* 36: 775–782.

65. Nel, J.J., Kat, C.J., Coetzee, G.L., and van Staden, P.J. (2017). Biomechanical comparison between pins and polymethylmethacrylate and the SOP locking plate system to stabilize canine lumbosacral fracture-luxation in flexion and extension. *Vet. Surg.* 46: 789–796.

66. Early, P., Mente, P., Dillar, S., and Roe, S. (2015). In vitro biomechanical evaluation of internal fixation techniques on the canine lumbosacral junction. *Peer J.* 3: e1094.

67. Segal, U., Bar, H., and Shani, J. (2018). Repair of lumbosacral fracture-luxation with bilateral twisted string-of-pearls locking plates. *J. Small Anim.* 59: 1–7.

68. Early, P.J., Mallard, A., and Kraus, K.H. (2017). Stiffness comparisons of SOP interlocking plate configuration in 3D printed canine lumbosacral vertebrae. *Open Access J. Vet. Sci. Res.* 2: 1–9.

69. Smolders, L.A., Voorhout, G., Van de Ven, R. et al. (2012). Pedicle screw-rod fixation of the canine lumbosacral junction. *Vet. Surg.* 41: 720–732.

70. Muller, F., Schenk, H.C., and Forterre, F. (2017). Short-term and long-term effects of a minimally invasive transillial vertebral blocking procedure on the lumbosacral morphometry in dogs measured by computed tomography. *Vet. Surg.* 46: 355–366.

15

Surgical Management of Spinal Nerve Root Tumors

Ane Uriarte

Veterinary Neurology, Southfields Veterinary Specialist, Basildon, UK

Introduction

Spinal cord tumors are described according to their location in transverse section relative to the spinal cord and dura, and are classified as intramedullary (IM), intradural-extramedullary (ID-EM), or extradural-extramedullary (ED-EM). Extramedullary spinal cord neoplasms have been previously described to account for 85% of all spinal cord neoplasms, with IM spinal cord neoplasms comprising the remaining 15% [1, 2]. Spinal cord neoplasms most commonly present in large breed dogs older than five years and the most common primary tumors in dogs are peripheral nerve sheath tumors (PNSTs) and meningiomas. Both pathologies can present with similar but distinctive clinical and imaging findings. This chapter will address these two slow growing, intradural, extramedullary spinal tumors affecting the spinal nerves, then concentrate on the most challenging surgical approach to nerve sheath tumors affecting the spinal canal.

Clinical Presentations

Meningioma

Meningiomas are usually benign, slow-growing neoplasms that arise from the arachnoid cap cells and arachnoid granulations of the meninges. Boxers and Golden Retrievers are the most common breeds reported to be diagnosed with spinal meningiomas and the mean age at diagnosis is 9.8 years [2, 3]. Typically, intraspinal meningiomas cause a chronic, progressive myelopathy with mild to moderate spinal pain. The neurological examination reflects the degree of compression and localization. Spinal meningiomas are more commonly found in the C1–4 area and L1–S1 [2, 4]; therefore, spinal nerve involvement is more likely to occur in the lumbar region.

Peripheral Nerve Sheath Tumors

PNSTs in dogs are malignant mesenchymal tumors that originate from nerve tissue and grow proximally and distally along the affected nerve. No significant breed predisposition has been found in PNSTs. The median age of dogs with PNSTs is 7.7 years [5]. The clinical signs vary from lameness to severe neurological dysfunction and pain depending on degree of invasion and localization. Affected dogs may originally present with a lameness that can be mistaken for orthopedic disease. The signs slowly progress to pain and muscle atrophy of the group of muscles innervated by the affected nerve. In some cases, a palpable mass can be found in the region of the spinal nerve. As the tumor progresses toward the nerve root, the pain increases, and more severe neurological deficits are observed. Once the tumor reaches the spinal canal the contralateral limb might show abnormal proprioception due to the spinal cord compression and, in the C6–T2 localization, proprioceptive deficits of the hind limbs, loss of cutaneous trunci reflex (Figure 15.1), and Horner's syndrome (Figure 15.2) might be observed. Within the spine, the most commonly affect spinal nerve roots are in the C6–T2 area with L4–S1 localization having been less commonly described [6].

Advanced Techniques in Canine and Feline Neurosurgery, First Edition. Edited by Andy Shores and Brigitte A. Brisson.
© 2023 John Wiley & Sons, Inc. Published 2023 by John Wiley & Sons, Inc.
Companion site: www.wiley.com/go/shores/advanced

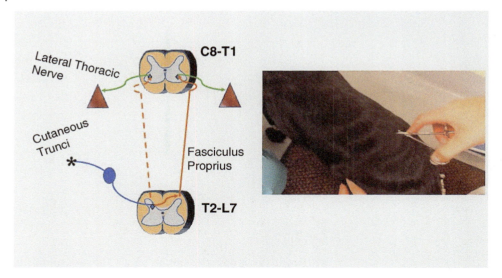

Figure 15.1 Cutaneous trunci reflex: Absent ipsilateral cutaneous trunci (ct) reflex is a common finding on the neurological examination of a dog with a brachial plexus PNST. The illustration demonstrates the pathway of the ct reflex. The photo to the right shows an examiner performing this reflex test. *Source:* redrawn from deLahunta A., Glass E. *Veterinary Neuroanatomy and Clinical Neurology* (edn 3). Saunders-Elsevier, St. Louis. 2009, P86.

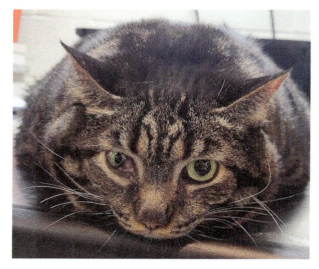

Figure 15.2 This feline patient is exhibiting Horner's Syndrome of the right eye (miosis, enophthalmos, ptosis, and raised 3rd eyelid) and MRI evidence of a mass in the cervical intumescence.

Diagnosis

A tentative diagnosis of intraspinal tumor may be made after advanced imaging, but histologic evaluation of tumor type is essential for definitive diagnosis. Computed tomography (CT) and magnetic resonance imaging (MRI) can be used to identify affected nerves, nerve root involvement, and spinal cord compression. The most common diagnostic findings in intraspinal meningiomas and PNST are briefly describe below.

Imaging

Spinal Meningioma MRI

Meningiomas are generally intradural-extramedullary located within the cranial cervical and lumbar regions of the spine. Meningiomas do not typically grow within the spinal nerves. However, those with a lumbar localization can be found compressing the femoral or sciatic nerve roots.

Typical MRI characteristics of spinal meningiomas include a contrast-enhancing mass with a broad-based dural attachment and variable signal intensity on the pre-contrast T1 and T2 weighted images [2] (Figures 15.3 and 15.4).

Reports of CT imaging are scarce, but contrast-enhancing mass lesions have been described.

PNST MRI

MRI is superior to CT for detecting brachial plexus tumors due to excellent contrast resolution, ability to distinguish nerve bundles from vessels, and primary multiplanar imaging [7]. Small or diffuse tumors that are oriented obliquely may be hard to detect with the limited transverse imaging plane of CT.

15 Surgical Management of Spinal Nerve Root Tumors | 145

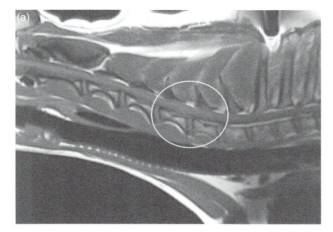

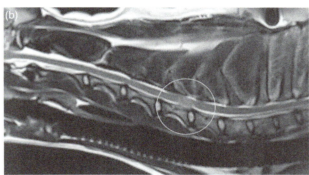

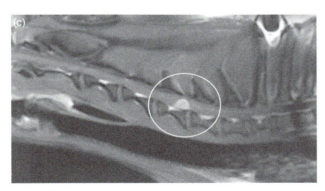

Figure 15.3 Spinal meningioma – typical magnetic resonance imaging (MRI) characteristics of spinal meningiomas include a contrast-enhancing mass with a broad-based dural attachment and variable signal intensity on the pre-contrast MRI T1 and T2 weighted images. (a) T1 sagittal image of a meningioma in a dog at the caudal aspect of the 5th cervical vertebra. (b). T2 sagittal image of the same mass. (c) T1+C image of the mass.

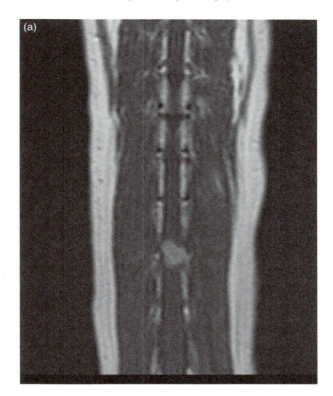

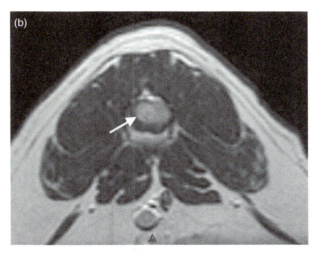

Figure 15.4 (a) Dorsal and (b) transverse MRI T1+(c) images of a lumbar (L4) meningioma in a cat. This mass was extramedullary/intradural.

Assessment of the full anatomic extent of PNST is necessary for decisions regarding appropriate treatment. PNSTs are often anatomically extensive and complex as they arise anywhere along the pathway of these spinal nerve roots or peripheral nerves [7]. Large field of view images should be obtained on MRI when the brachial or lumbar plexus is imaged.

Both the diffuse and mass forms of PNST are typically hyperintense (relative to muscle) on STIR, proton density, and T2-weighted images and isointense on T1-weighted pre-contrast images with minimal to non-uniformly or strong contrast enhancement following gadolinium administration [7]. Vertebral canal involvement can be evident as a focal compressive mass lesion having high signal intensity on STIR, proton density, and T2-weighted

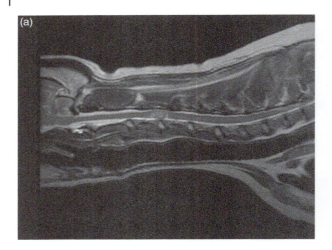
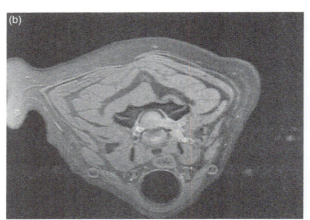
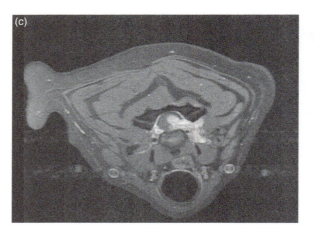

Figure 15.5 MRI of dog with PNST at C3–C4. (a) T2 sagittal; (b) T1–FS transverse; and (c) T1+C images of the mass. Note the strong contrast enhancement and compression of the spinal cord after invasion of the spinal canal

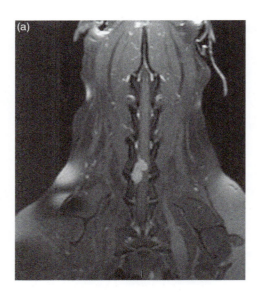
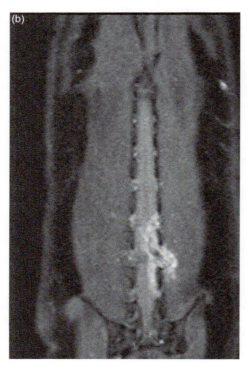

Figure 15.6 (a) Dorsal T1+C image of a cervical PNST in a dog. (b) Dorsal T1–FatSat post contrast image of a lumbar PNST in a dog. In (b) note the contrast enhancement and the extraxial but intradural invasion of the L5 nerve root and invasion of the spinal canal.

images that enhanced on T1-weighted images [7] (Figures 15.5 and 15.6). PNST is present mainly as extramedullary extra or intradural tumors.

Muscle atrophy is often observed with the peripheral nerve involvement in the innervated muscles; hyperintense signal on T2, STIR, and pre-contrast T1 images; and mild contrast enhancement denoting neurogenic atrophy, edema, fatty infiltrate, and fibrosis can be observed [7].

Electrodiagnostics

Intraoperative determination of the affected root and invasion into the foramen by the PNST remains challenging. Electromyography has been described as a sensitive tool for detecting the neuropathic changes associated with these tumors and helps with imaging interpretation. It has been suggested that epaxial muscle electromyography (EMG) studies may predict proximal extension of PNSTs in dogs [8].

Early diagnosis of PNST is challenging due to mild initial clinical signs and common late referral and imaging diagnosis. In the author's experience, achieving a compartmental resection and tumor-free margin is uncommon mainly because most cases are diagnosed when extensive progression of the disease has occurred. In the author's opinion, early recognition of these orthopedic-like cases with thorough clinical examination and electrodiagnosis is fundamental for achieving successful surgical removal.

Cytology/Histology

Meningiomas

The human World Health Organization (WHO) classification and grading system has been adapted for canine meningioma classification. Although several reports have described various histologic subtypes in canine spinal cord meningiomas, tumor grading is rarely used. When this grading has been applied in published reports, grade I and grade II spinal meningiomas in dogs are reported to occur with similar frequency and with no obvious correlation between outcome and tumor grade [2, 9].

The most common histologic subtypes in dogs are shown in Table 15.1.

Canine meningiomas are strongly and uniformly immunoreactive for vimentin and some express focal reactivity to CK (Lu-5). However, the most reliable confirmation of a diagnosis of a canine meningioma still relies on transmission electron microscopy (TEM) with the highly distinctive and consistent features of interdigitating cytoplasmic membranes with normal and abnormal gap and desmosomal junctions [10].

PNST

PNSTs are spindle cell tumors that arise from the connective tissue components of the peripheral nerve and which can infiltrate the subcutis locally. These tumors are thought to arise from perineural fibroblasts, which produce the non-myelinated connective tissues that surround the myelinated nerve fiber. PNSTs appear to be pseudo-encapsulated, are locally invasive, and grow relatively slowly. Histologically PNSTs vary widely in appearance [11].

Cytological evaluation can allow distinction between different brachial plexus neoplasms, which can have a substantial impact on therapy and prognosis. Ultrasound guided cytology can be useful in the diagnosis of distal brachial plexus PNST in dogs [4]. Ultrasonographically, these are hypoechoic, tubular axillary masses with no blood flow [12].

Table 15.1 Classification of histologic subtypes of meningiomas in dogs.

Grade I
- Transitional – common with islands or nests in whorls or crescents and not infrequently with focal accumulations of polymorphonuclear leukocytes
- Meningothelial – common with sheets of cells with no underlying pattern
- Psammomatous – large numbers of psammoma bodies
- Fibrous – streams of elongate cells with prominent extracellular collagen fibers
- Angiomatous – dominant vascular component
- Microcystic – widespread intracellular and interstitial vacuolation

Grade II
- Chordoid – cords or columns of eosinophilic vacuolated cells in a mucoid basophilic matrix
- Atypical – with nuclear atypia, areas of necrosis, sheetlike patterns of cells, more than four mitotic figures per 10 HPF (400X) and increased cellular density with smaller cells

Grade III
- Malignant – characterized by mitotic figures >20 per 10 HPF (400X) and with extreme anaplastic cytological features compared with the atypical subtype
- Papillary subtype – distinctive but rare in the dog

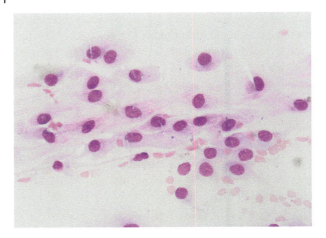

Figure 15.7 Cytological descriptions have a predominance of pleiomorphic stromal to round epithelial cells, with occasional evidence of cartilaginous and osseous metaplasia. In this photomicrograph, there are aggregates of spindle-shaped cells that exhibit modest amounts of anisocytosis and anisokaryosis. The nuclei are round to oval, centrally located, have a granular chromatin pattern, and occasionally have indistinct nucleoli. The cytoplasm is basophilic, moderate in amount, and has spindle-shaped ill-defined borders. Although commonly FNA samples contain stromal cells with features of malignancy, a definitive diagnosis of a MPNST is not possible based on cytology alone. Source: (photomicrograph courtesy of Dr. Matthew Williams).

Cytological descriptions have a predominance of pleiomorphic stromal to round epithelial cells, with occasional evidence of cartilaginous and osseous metaplasia [4]. Although commonly FNA samples contain stromal cells with features of malignancy, a definitive diagnosis of a malignant peripheral nerve sheath tumor (MPNST) is not possible based on cytology alone (Figure 15.7).

Surgery of PNST Within the Spinal Nerves

Local control is the hallmark of treatment of PNST because distal metastasis in dogs is rare. The evidence suggests that greater survival time depends upon achieving a proximal tumor-free margin because recurrence is usually local [6].

Resection of malignant PNSTs followed by radiation therapy is the standard treatment for extraspinal MPNSTs in humans [13]. The surgical technique of en-bloc resection achieving wide margins is an important prognostic factor in achieving local tumor control. However, this can be difficult because of residual tumor cells in such vital structures as the dura, other critical nerves, viscera, or large blood vessels, as well as skip lesions [13].

The most popular therapy for PNST in veterinary medicine has been surgical excision of the tumor combined with limb amputation. However, compartmental resection with preservation of the limb has been described before [14]. Compartmental resection can be achieved if the tumor is encapsulated within the perineurum [15]. If the tumor does not remain within the perineurum, it behaves like a soft tissue sarcoma and limb amputation is recommended [14]

Surgical intervention for PNST tends to be a lengthy procedure, particularly if there is spinal canal involvement. The author advises careful preoperative planning, which will involve neurosurgeon and soft-tissue specialist collaboration, good reconstruction planning, and excellent pain relief protocols.

Below we will discuss the different surgical approaches when operating on a cervical versus lumbar PNST affecting the vertebral canal. The limb sparing technique will be discussed.

Cervical Approach

Positioning

PNST within the cervical region are typically located within the brachial plexus. Approaching the foramen caudal to C5 might be challenging due to the superposition of the scapula.

Lateral Surgical Approach to Caudal Cervical Foramen After Amputation

In the cases where a limb amputation is planned, a hemilaminectomy can be performed on any of the foramina through which the spinal nerves giving rise to the brachial plexus pass. The hemilaminectomy is performed following removal of the scapula. The author would recommend lateral positioning of the dog, in order to facilitate removal of the limb by the soft tissue surgeon to allow the infiltrated nerve to be followed to the intervertebral foramen.

The animal will be clipped and prepared for a limb amputation. It will be placed in lateral recumbency with bean bags under the cervical spine in order to maintain a horizontal position avoiding curvature of the cervical spine. The neck and the chest outside of the surgical field will be securely fixed to the table. Once the limb amputation is finished, tilting the table to place the animal in a more vertical position will ensure better access to the affected intervertebral foramen for the neurosurgeon.

A limb amputation with removal of the scapula will be performed by a soft tissue surgeon, being mindful of skin reconstruction at the end of both procedures. The affected nerve root will be identified, and distinctive sutures will be placed for anatomo-pathological examination. The nerve root will be sharply sectioned, and the limb removed. The affected roots will be proximally dissected toward the affected cervical intervertebral foramen.

The sternothyroideus will be dissected to find the longissimus cervicis muscle which attaches to the cervical vertebrae. The superficial scalenus muscles can be distracted with the help of odd-leg Gelpis and the deep scalenous muscle will need to be removed from its C6 and C7 attachment.

An extended cervical hemilaminectomy will be performed taking great care of the vertebral venous sinus than runs within the ventral part of the spinal canal. The plexus vertebralis internus ventralis will be probably displaced due to the enlarged infiltrated nerve root and should be avoided if possible. Great care needs to be taken of the large vascular foramen located on the floor of each cervical vertebra right in the middle of each vertebral body. Moreover, when approaching C5 and C6, special care needs to be taken with the transverse foramina through which pass the vertebral arteries within the transverse processes. The transverse processes of C7 have no foramina and have a characteristic horizontal orientation.

The hemilaminectomy should be extended enough to permit visualization of macroscopically normal spinal cord. A durotomy can be performed but greater care should be taken when approaching the intraxial cervical spine due to possible respiratory compromise. The surgeon must consider the risks versus the benefits when deciding to perform a rhizotomy versus intradural approach and dissection.

Ideally, if the dura is thick enough, sutures will be placed on each side of the durotomy using a 4-0 nylon suture material. This allows free handling of the tumor and better visualization of the margins. Make sure the dura is elevated from the spinal cord and not ensure that white matter tracts are not caught by the suture material.

Once the sutures are in place, or while elevating the dura with blunt microscopic forceps, a small incision is made in the dura with a number 11 blade or Beaver blade. The incision can be enlarged with neurosurgery micro scissors. A surgical microscope or surgical loops are recommended when opening the dura and handling white matter tracts. The tumor is gently separated from the white matter tracts and bluntly removed with the help of microsurgical loops, surgical spears, flush, and extremely gentle suction.

After resection, in most of the cases, closing the dura might be impossible due to tumor invasion. A DuraGen® or Lyoplant® dural substitute is recommended.

The cervical muscles can be sutured with an absorbable suture following normal surgical reconstruction. In cases where the thoracic wall has been opened, a chest drain must be placed. In cases of large deep muscle reconstruction, active drainage with Jackson Pratt or hemovac drain are recommended, particularly after limb amputation.

Dorsal Surgical Approach for Cervical Hemilaminectomy

If compartmental excision is planned with proximal rhizotomy, a sternal positioning of the dog with the front limbs extended and crossed will allow the best visualization of the caudal cervical articular processes. A dorsal approach to the cervical spine following the cervical hemilaminectomy technique described elsewhere will be followed.

Skin and superficial fascia are incised and retracted to reveal the aponeurosis of the rhomboideus and trapezius muscles. The muscles are divided in the midline. Bleeding from the large neurovascular bundles that penetrate the fascia must be controlled to prevent postoperative hematoma. The nuchal ligament can be palpated at this stage. The fascia overlying the nuchal ligament is divided and cleared. The ligament can be pulled laterally, divided, or freed back to the prominent spinous process of T1 [16]. The muscles are elevated from the spinous process and lamina of the affected vertebra. A dorsal laminectomy with partial dorsal articular process removal may be performed. Tracking of the tumor to and from the canal within the brachial plexus will be challenging. A rhizotomy might help with pain but this will only be a palliative treatment which will require further radiation. The previously described intradural access recommendation can be followed.

The cervical muscles can be sutured with an absorbable suture following normal surgical reconstruction. Active drainage with Jackson Pratt or hemovac drain are recommended on this dorsal approach.

Respiratory Compromise in Cervical Myelopathies

The respiratory system may be compromised by two different mechanisms following cervical spinal cord injury: paresis to paralysis of the respiratory muscles via damage of the phrenic nuclei, or airway hyper-responsiveness subsequent to loss of sympathetic innervation to the airway. The end result of these injuries is either that there is decreased respiratory drive or there is insufficient communication between the respiratory center and the respiratory muscles.

When removing a PNST with caudal cervical spinal cord involvement, care needs to be taken in order to avoid phrenic nerve damage. The phrenic nerve innervates the diaphragm, intercostal muscles, and the extra-thoracic airway muscles. The phrenic nerves course primarily in the C5, C6, and C7 nerves, with some contribution from the C4 nerve. The intercostal muscles also aid in both inspiration and expiration and are innervated by the intercostal nerves that arise from thoracic nerves T1 to T6.

The phrenic nucleus is located cranial to the cervical intumescence. A spinal cord injury cranial to the phrenic nuclei could lead to damage of both the descending respiratory axons and the phrenic motor neurons and it will be more devastating than focal phrenic nerve damage

Lumbar Approach

Access to the foramen on the lumbar spine except for L7–S1 is surgically less challenging. A hemilaminectomy technique described elsewhere should be performed to access all the lateral foramens of the lumbar spine except L7–S1.

Once the affected foramen/foramina have been identified, proximal and distal resection following the macroscopically affected nerve roots may be performed. The author would advise distal approach and resection before access to the spinal canal. A regular hemilaminectomy with pediculectomy of the affected roots should be performed after the tumour is identified. In the case of an intradural or even intraxial extension, the previous recommendation (see cervical approach) for durotomy and dissection should be followed.

If the dura is not opened and the nerve is dissected before entering the spinal cord, local anesthetic (lidocaine 2 mg/kg, 20 mg/ml) infiltration within the nerve before sharp transection has been suggested.

Approach to the L7–S1 Foramen

The presence of the ilium makes an extensive approach to the L7–S1 foramen and spinal canal difficult. Surgical procedures that address foraminal stenosis are challenging. So far, surgical decompression of the L7 nerve root has been achieved by dorsal and medial approaches to the lumbosacral intervertebral foramen, mostly as an extension of a standard L7–S1 laminectomy with or without preservation of the articular facets [17, 18].

Problems and complications of these procedures include limited access to lateralized intraforaminal compressions and postoperative hypermobility and instability and, occasionally, subsequent fractures of the contralateral articular facet.

Surgical procedures that address foraminal stenosis are challenging. So far, surgical decompression of the L7 nerve root has been achieved by dorsal and medial approaches to the lumbosacral intervertebral foramen, mostly as an extension of a standard L7–S1 laminectomy with or without preservation of the articular facets [7].

Lateral foraminotomy has been described for access to the exit and middle zones of the lumbosacral foramen [7]. This technique will only allow regional and limited access to the foramen and should be combined with a dorsal laminectomy of L7–S1 leaving the caudal articular processes and facet joints of L7 intact to preserve stability if access to the spinal canal is required. These approaches are described in detail within this book.

Partial or total hemipelvectomy is an aggressive surgery but has been reported to provide good access to the lumbosacral trunk allowing a foraminotomy, partial sacral spondylectomy, and laminectomy in a case of PNST [19].

Similarly, a lateral approach to the femoral nerve via a ventral ilial osteotomy and subsequent limb amputation has been described elsewhere [20]. Osteotomy of the wing of the ilium has minimal postoperative complications for the dog and is an ideal approach to investigate diseases of the femoral nerve and its roots. It allows inspection of the iliopsoas muscle, femoral nerve, L4–L6 nerve roots, and surrounding structures. The approach also allows good exposure of the lateral aspects of the caudal lumbar vertebral bodies for hemilaminectomy, if required, and the incision can be extended ventrocaudally for hind-limb amputation. If amputation is not necessary, the osteotomy fragment can easily be reattached to the pelvis, using a wire suture [20].

Postoperative Care

Postoperative care consisting of administration of nonsteroidal anti-inflammatory drugs or steroids at 0.5 mg/kg and with ketamine 0.5 mg/kg for 24 hours postoperatively is recommended. Following Glasgow pain scoring, methadone 0.2 mg/kg could be added. Active drains are left until they stop producing fluid and are removed before discharge. Gabapentin at 10 mg/kg three times a day and acetaminophen at 10–15 mg/kg three times a day is recommended in case of pain. Amantadine at 3–5 mg/kg once a day might be used on difficult neurogenic pain cases.

Owners should be advised to strictly confine the dog during the first two weeks and then increase exercise on the leash in a stepwise fashion over six weeks.

Prognosis

The overall prognosis in canines spinal PNST is poor [4] as it is in humans [8]. In human oncology appropriate Enneking removal[1] [21] for MPNST is defined as an en-bloc resection that achieves wide margins. Even with histologically negative margins, wide resections of MPNSTs are complicated by the spread along nerves outside of the gross tumor and the presence of multiple skip lesions. Additionally, spinal MPNSTs often involve several compartments in addition to the nerve, such as epidural and intradural space, bone, and soft tissue. This multicompartment invasion significantly complicates the ability to achieve wide margins and in turn defines microscopic spread compared with non-spinal MPNSTs. While en-bloc resection is technically feasible in some patients, the ability to truly achieve a wide margin is restricted by at-risk structures, such as the spinal cord and major blood vessels [13, 22–24].

In veterinary medicine, several studies have shown that non-infiltrated surgical margins had a statistically significant survival advantage. It has been suggested that dogs which survive the surgical intervention and live for one year will likely experience a long-term survival [17]. Dogs with PNST affecting the spinal canal have a shorter survival time and shorter time to relapse [4] compared to those with distal PNST. Survival time for surgically treated PNSTs ranges from 0.5 to 152.4 months with the median survival time between 5 and 42.8 months depending on the study [3, 4].

Radiation Therapy

Radiation therapy as a sole or adjunctive treatment for spinal meningiomas and PNST has been described in veterinary medicine [2, 3, 25].

Wide resection of these tumors will most likely result in a better long-term recurrence free interval and overall survival for more malignant tumors, whereas marginal excision results in an increased recurrence rate and possible risk of metastases; however, some authors have reported marginal resection either as a sole therapy or combined with radiotherapy [3].

 Video clips to accompany this book can be found on the companion website at:
www.wiley.com/go/shores/advanced

References

1. Pancotto, T.E., Rossmeisl, J.H. Jr., Zimmerman, K. et al. (2013). Intramedullary spinal cord neoplasia in 53 dogs (1990–2010): distribution, clinicopathologic characteristics, and clinical behavior. *J. Vet. Intern. Med.* 27: 1800–1508.
2. Petersen, S.A., Surges, B.K., Dickinson, P.J. et al. (2008). Canine intraspinal meningiomas: imaging features, histopathologic classification, and long-term outcome in 34 dogs. *J. Vet. Intern. Med.* 22: 946–953.
3. Lacassagne, K., Hearon, K., Berg, J. et al. (2018). Canine spinal meningiomas and nerve sheath tumours in 34 dogs (2008–2016): distribution and long-term outcome based upon histopathology and treatment modality. *Vet. Comp. Oncol.* 16: 344–351.
4. da Costa, R.C., Parent, J.M., Dobson, H. et al. (2008). Ultrasound-guided fine needle aspiration in the diagnosis of peripheral nerve sheath tumors in 4 dogs. *Can. Vet. J.* 49: 77–81.
5. Chijiwa, K., Uchida, K., and Tateyama, S. (2004). Immunohistochemical evaluation of canine peripheral nerve sheath tumors and other soft tissue sarcomas. *Vet. Pathol.* 41: 307–318.
6. Brehm, D., Vite, C.H., Steinberg, H.S. et al. (1995). A retrospective evaluation of 51 cases of peripheral nerve sheath tumors in the dog. *J. Am. Anim. Hosp. Assoc.* 31 (4): 349–359.
7. Gödde, T. and Steffen, F. (2007). Surgical treatment of lumbosacral foraminal stenosis using a lateral approach in twenty dogs with degenerative lumbosacral stenosis. *Vet Surg.* 36 (7): 705–713.

---

1 Enneking's classification: based upon the macroscopic findings intraoperatively. The closest margin between the tumor and the resection surface should be assessed. That is, if the tumor is resected mostly with wide margins, but cut in the reactive area around the tumor even in a small part, the margin of this resection is judged marginal. Trovik et al. modified the Enneking's criteria to report adequate (radical or wide) or inadequate (marginal or intralesional) margins.

8. le Chevoir, M., Thibaud, J.L., Labruyère, J. et al. (2012). Electrophysiological features in dogs with peripheral nerve sheath tumors: 51 cases (1993–2010). *J. Am. Vet. Med. Assoc.* 241: 1194–1201.

9. José-López, R., de la Fuente, C., Pumarola, M., and Añor, S. (2013). Spinal meningiomas in dogs: description of 8 cases including a novel radiological and histopathological presentation. *Can. Vet. J.* 54: 948–954.

10. Vandelvelde, M., Higgins, R.J., and Oevermann, A. (2012). *Veterinary Neuropathology Essentials of Theory and Practice*. Wiley-Blackwell.

11. Haagsman, A.N., Witkamp, A.C.S., Sjollema, B.E. et al. (2013). The effect of interleukin-2 on canine peripheral nerve sheath tumours after marginal surgical excision: a double-blind randomized study. *BMC Vet. Res.* 8 (9): 155.

12. Rose, S., Long, C., Marguerite, K., and Hornof, B. (2005). Ultrasonographic evaluation of brachial plexus tumors in five dogs. *Vet. Radiol. Ultrasound* 46 (6): 514–517.

13. Chou, D., Bilsky, M.H., Luzzati, A. et al. (2017). AOSpine Knowledge Forum Tumor Malignant peripheral nerve sheath tumors of the spine: results of surgical management from a multicenter study. *J. Neurosurg. Spine* 26: 291–298.

14. van Stee, L., Boston, S., Teskea, E., and Meij, B. (2017). Compartmental resection of peripheral nerve tumours with limb preservation in 16 dogs (1995–2011). *Vet. J.* 226: 40–45.

15. Kawaguchi, N., Ahmed, A.R., Matsumoto, S. et al. (2004). The concept of curative margin in surgery for bone and soft tissue sarcoma. *Clin. Orthop. Relat. Res.* 419: 165–172.

16. Sharp, J.H. and Wheeler, S.J. (2005). *Small Animal Spinal Disorders Diagnosis and Surgery*, 2e. Elsevier Limited.

17. Gibson, A.D., Davies, E., Lara-Garcia, A., and Lafuente, P. (2016). Palliative epineurotomy for focal radial malignant peripheral nerve sheath tumor in a dog. *J. Am. Anim. Hosp. Assoc.* 52: 330–334.

18. Ruppert, C., Hartmann, K., Fischer, A. et al. (2000). Cervical neoplasia originating from the vagus nerve in a dog. *J. Small Anim. Pract.* 41: 119–122.

19. Niles, J.D., Dyce, J., and Mattoo, J.S. (2001). Computed tomography for the diagnosis of a lumbosacral nerve sheath tumour and management by hemipelvectomy. *JSAP* 42: 248–252.

20. Harcourt-Brown, T.R., Granger, N., Smith, P.M. et al. (2009). Use of a lateral surgical approach to the femoral nerve in the management of two primary femoral nerve sheath tumours. *Vet. Comp. Orthop. Traumatol.* 22 (3): 229–232.

21. Trovik, C.S., Bauer, H.C., Alvegard, T.A. et al. (2000). Surgical margins, local recurrence and metastasis in soft tissue sarcomas: 559 surgically-treated patients from the Scandinavian Sarcoma Group Register. *Eur. J. Cancer* 36: 710–716.

22. Warren, A.L., Miller, A.D., de Lahunta, A. et al. (2020). Four cases of the melanotic variant of malignant nerve sheath tumour: a rare, aggressive neoplasm in young dogs with a predilection for the spinal cord. *J. Comp. Pathol.* 178: 1–8.

23. Poli, F., Calistri, M., Mandara, M.T., and Baroni, M. (2019). Central nervous system metastasis of an intradural malignant peripheral nerve sheath tumor in a dog. *Open Vet. J.* 9 (1): 49–53.

24. Yap, F. and Pratschke, K. (2016). Peripheral nerve sheath tumor of the vagus nerve in a dog. *J. Am. Anim. Hosp. Assoc.* 52: 57–62.

25. Dolera, M., Malfassi, L., Bianchi, C. et al. (2017). Frameless stereotactic volumetric modulated arc radiotherapy of brachial plexus tumours in dogs: 10 cases. *Br. J. Radiol.* 90: 20160617.

16

Surgical Management of Craniocervical Junction Anomalies

Sofia Cerda-Gonzalez

MedVet Chicago, Chicago, IL, USA

Indications

Craniocervical junction (CCJ) anomalies refer to a group of diseases affecting a common area, which include the Chiari-like malformation, elevation of the medulla at the CCJ, atlantooccipital overlapping, atlantoaxial instability, dorsal angulation of the dens, and atlantoaxial fibrous band (also referred to also as a "dural band," a misnomer as dura is not a component of this tissue) [1–5]. Syringomyelia (i.e. an accumulation of fluid in the spinal cord) frequently develops as a component of these diseases, secondary to changes in cerebrospinal fluid flow through the CCJ [2, 6]. Both the CCJ themselves and their secondary syringomyelia, when present, are responsible for the clinical manifestations of these diseases; of note, clinical signs can occur in dogs without syringomyelia [3, 5, 7].

Particularly predisposed breeds include the Cavalier King Charles Spaniel and the Brussels Griffon, although small and toy breed dogs are generally over-represented [7–9]. CCJ anomalies may also be present in cats [10, 11] (Figure 16.1). Clinical signs primarily include hyperalgesia and hyperesthesia along the cranium, CCJ, and cervical spine, although signs consistent with cerebellar/brainstem dysfunction and/or a cervical myelopathy may also develop [12]. There are few clinical descriptions of CCJ anomalies in cats. In addition to cranium and cervical pain and feline-specific manifestations of these, signs of brainstem dysfunction are also described [10].

The CCJ is best evaluated diagnostically using magnetic resonance imaging. This allows for a more comprehensive evaluation of the area for surgical planning than the use of CT imaging or radiographs alone, though CT imaging may be helpful in defining the anatomic relationship between the skull, atlas, and axis. Diagnostic characteristics for each disorder are outlined in Figures 16.2, 16.3 and 16.4.

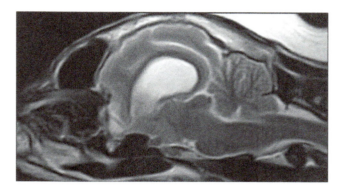

Figure 16.1 T2-weighted sagittal MR image of a Cavalier King Charles Spaniel demonstrating more than one concurrent CCJ anomaly. These include a mild Chari-like malformation (i.e. mild cerebellar herniation, caudal displacement of the brainstem, the absence of CSF at the CCJ), a pronounced atlantoaxial fibrous band (arrow). The cranial-most aspect of the atlas is located immediately caudal to the foramen magnum, suggesting mild AOO (dashed line arrow). Lastly, there is a mild intervertebral disk protrusion at each disk space and syringomyelia (+ sign) is present.

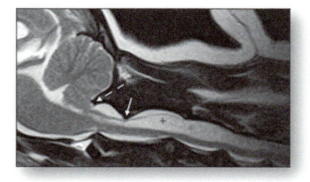

Figure 16.2 T2-weighted sagittal MR image of a Persian cat demonstrating pronounced cerebellar herniation and the absence of CSF at the CCJ, consistent with a Chiari-like malformation. Incidental ventriculomegaly is also evident (lateral ventricle).

Advanced Techniques in Canine and Feline Neurosurgery, First Edition. Edited by Andy Shores and Brigitte A. Brisson.
© 2023 John Wiley & Sons, Inc. Published 2023 by John Wiley & Sons, Inc.
Companion site: www.wiley.com/go/shores/advanced

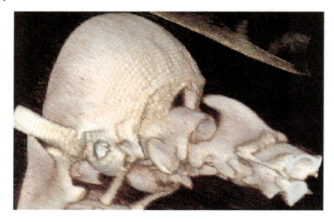

Figure 16.3 3-D-reconstructed image including the caudal half of the skull through mid-C3, demonstrating atlantooccipital overlapping. The craniomedial aspect of the atlas is located within the foramen magnum. Incidental occipital dysplasia is also present.

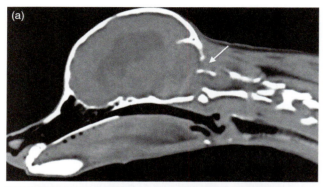

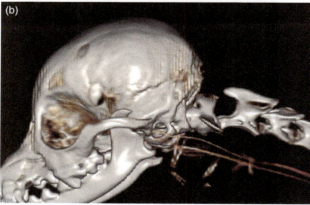

Figure 16.4 This patient, a young Yorkshire Terrier, was originally presented to an atlanto-axial (AA) subluxation because of neurologic signs localized to the upper cervical spine and the spacing (gap) between the cranial tip of the spinous process of C2 and the dorsal arch of C1 on radiographs. However, additional evaluation with a CT scan demonstrated a normal position of the AA joint and severe atlanto-occipital override (AOO) as that cause for the gap between C2 and C1. (a) CT reconstructed sagittal view of the cervical spine and skull showing the severe overlap (arrow); (b) 3-D CT reconstruction demonstrating the AOO.

Medical and surgical management may be used to treat CCJ anomalies. The former is generally employed first, particularly in patients with mild signs and those for whom medical management has not yet been employed [12]. Reports of limited progression of signs in a subset of CCJ anomaly patients and the potential for maintenance of a good to excellent quality of life without surgery, suggest the need to first consider medical management in these groups [12]. This includes the modulation of neuropathic pain (using medications such as gabapentin, pregabalin, amantadine, topiramate, along with acupuncture), the inhibition of cerebrospinal fluid production (e.g. using furosemide, acetazolamide, omeprazole), and the use of corticosteroids for their effects on the pain pathway, CSF production modulation, their anti-inflammatory effects [3, 13, 14]. Indications for surgery, in turn, generally include progressive disease despite medical management, neuropathic pain that is moderate to severe, pain that is not responsive to analgesics, and neurologic deficits attributable to these disorders (e.g. C1–C5 myelopathy secondary to an atlantoaxial fibrous band). Factors such as age and general health/anesthesia risk must also be considered.

Surgical Anatomy

The CCJ refers to the junction between the head and neck, including the occipital bone, foramen magnum, atlas, and axis, along with the ligaments and soft tissues that support this junction (Figure 16.5). A single "occipito-atlas-axis joint cavity" passes through this area [15].

The muscles encountered as part of the dorsal surgical approach to this area include the occipitalis, the semispinalis capitis (biventer cervicis) and the underlying rectus capitis dorsalis muscles, joined by the median fibrous raphe. The cleidocephalicus and sternocephalicus are encountered along the cervical spine superficially [15].

The foramen magnum can vary widely in its size; in patients with occipital dysplasia, the foramen magnum can be "keyhole-shaped" (i.e. narrower dorsal extension of the foramen magnum overlying the cerebellum), circular rather than oval, and/or asymmetrically shaped [15–17]. This is commonly found among brachycephalic and toy/small breed dogs [17]. The shape and size of the foramen magnum should be evaluated prior to surgery and can be assessed with CT and/or MR imaging. Of note, occipital dysplasia is not a pathologic finding but rather individual variation of "normal" [16–18]. The dorsal atlantooccipital membrane is encountered between the craniodorsal lamina of the atlas and the dorsal aspects of the foramen magnum [15].

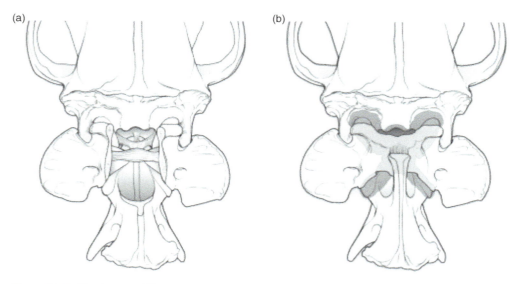

Figure 16.5 The bony and ligamentous anatomy of the craniocervical junction (a) and the single joint space (shaded area) encompassing the atlantooccipital and atlantoaxial junctions (b) [11].

Identifying this and maintaining it as an intact structure during drilling can help protect underlying neural structures. This membrane is often abnormally thickened in patients with CCJ anomalies [4]. The dorsal atlantoaxial membrane is encountered on approach to the dorsal junction of the atlas and axis, in turn [15]. Additionally, the dorsal atlantoaxial ligament spans between the caudal lamina of the atlas and the craniomedial aspect of the lamina of the axis. The nuchal ligament joins the caudal spinous process of the axis with the spinous processes of the first thoracic vertebra (T1) [15].

The cervical vertebral venous system is also to be considered when performing surgery in this area. This valveless venous system is continuous with the cranial venous sinuses and contains external and internal components. When approaching the CCJ dorsally, the veins of the dorsal external vertebral venous plexus are first encountered within the epaxial musculature (i.e. intervertebral and interspinous veins). These traverse ventrally through the ligamentum flavum, to enter the vertebral canal [9, 15]. The interarcuate branches of the internal vertebral plexus are then encountered underlying the ligamentum flavum at the atlantooccipital and atlantoaxial junctions. The bilateral basilar sinuses are located at the lateral aspects of the cervical vertebral column [15].

The paired cervical spinal branches of the vertebral artery perforate the dura, passing into the subarachnoid space at each intervertebral foramen and splitting into dorsal and ventral radicular arteries. The dorsal radicular artery and dorsal spinal artery may be seen if a durotomy is performed; care must be taken to preserve these to maintain adequate irrigation of the spinal cord. The occipital branch of the common carotid courses along the nuchal crest bilaterally. The caudal meningeal arteries branch from these vessels, enter the cranial cavity at the mastoid foramen, and arborize along the dura of the dorsocaudal aspects of the caudotentorial cranial cavity [15].

Patient Preparation and Positioning

Prior to anesthesia for surgery, a comprehensive treatment plan must be made considering the CCJ, generating an individualized surgical plan for each patient. Additionally, as part of anesthetic planning, a guarded endotracheal tube must be used to allow adequate positioning of patients for surgery in this area.

Once anesthetized, the patient is first shaved from the level of the bregma cranially through to the mid-cervical spine (approximately C4/C5) caudally, and laterally overlying the temporal bones, the dorsal half of the pinnae and mid-lateral cervical spine. The tips of the pinnae are restrained ventrally bilaterally in dogs with erect ears, either using a penetrating towel clamp or suture to attach these to the lateral aspect of the head, or by tucking them under the head in patients with downward sloping ears. If a fat graft is to be used, then an area overlying the wing of the ilium should be prepped to harvest the adipose tissue. This is usually done at the start of the procedure (see below).

The patient is then placed on the surgical table in a "sphinxlike" position (i.e. in sternal recumbency with limbs flexed alongside the body), with the head above the level of the thoracolumbar spine. The CCJ must be fully flexed for the first portion of the surgery, with the hard palate perpendicular to the cervical spine (i.e. nose perpendicular to the surgical table). This can be accomplished using commercially available positioning system or pegboard, or using a vacuum system such as the "Hug-U-Vac Surgical Positioning System" (www.vetorsolutions.com). Of note, a surgical assistant must be able to release CCJ from its flexed position at a later point in the surgery. To accomplish this, it is helpful to have a separately movable positioning device for the head, from that of the neck and body (e.g. Hug-U-Vac surgical head positioner, surgical tape across the bridge of the nose to the body/surgical table bilaterally). Regardless of the method of restraint used, care must be taken to avoid jugular vein pressure throughout the surgery; this will avoid the negative effects of jugular vein compression on intracranial pressure (i.e. Queckenstedt's maneuver) [19, 20]. Once desirable positioning is achieved, the area is aseptically prepped.

Surgical Technique

If a fat graft is to be used, this must be harvested first, using separate gloves and instruments [1]. The harvested tissue must be large enough to easily cover the surgery site, with accommodation for it shrinking by a third of its size during revascularization, and should be of a thickness of approximately 0.5–0.8 cm. The fat graft is wrapped in saline-soaked gauze post-harvesting and is set aside for later use. It is then rinsed again in saline prior to its use [21, 22].

An incision is made from a point 2 cm rostral to the underlying external occipital protuberance and is continued caudally to the caudal aspect of the third cervical vertebra. The underlying subcutaneous tissue and fat are sharply dissected along the midline to the level of the superficial cervical muscles. These and the underlying deep cervical muscles (see above) are separated along the median raphe. The use of electrocautery as a method of dissection here can improve hemostasis and efficiency at this point in the surgical approach, particularly during dissection of the superficial cervical muscles. Additionally, sharp tipped Gelpi retractors can be used throughout the dissection to optimize visibility and are moved down as the dissection continues. Right-angled Gelpi retractors are particularly helpful in retracting the cervical musculature as it is divided. Saline lavage is used throughout surgery to maintain hydration of the exposed tissues and aid in maintaining optimal visibility. Cooled saline may be used, instead, in patients where additional hemostasis is needed.

Once these muscles are dissected, periosteal elevators are used to expose the cervical musculature from the spinous process sees and lamina of the atlas and axis, bilaterally. These same instruments are used then to expose the super occipital bone, separating the overlying musculature bilaterally. As described above, vessels of the vertebral venous plexus and branches of the great auricular artery are encountered in this area. Bipolar cautery can be used to target these. Throughout this dissection, great care must be taken to identify bony edges, at the cranial and caudal aspects of the laminate of the cervical vertebrae, and at the atlantooccipital junction, to avoid inadvertent damage of the underlying neural structures. Additionally, as described above, the shape and size of the foramen magnum can vary substantially between individuals. Patients with occipital dysplasia may have larger-than-expected foramen magnum, with the enlarged area being covered by a thin periosteum membrane [16, 17]. This should be noted before surgery and considered in the dissection.

The area exposed will vary depending on the area to be targeted, extending through to the caudal aspect of the axis if decompression of the dorsal atlantoaxial junction is planned. In these cases, following muscle dissection, the spinous process of the axis is removed using double-action Lempert rongeurs, to allow access to the dorsal atlas and atlantoaxial junction.

Once all necessary structures are exposed, surgery is continued using a high-speed pneumatic drill. A craniectomy is performed first; the margins of this exposure include the area ventral to the nuchal crest and external occipital protuberance dorsally, and the FM ventrally, dorsal to the occipital condyles. Care must be taken when dissecting the muscles overlying the supraoccipital bone and foramen magnum, particularly in dogs diagnosed with occipital dysplasia on imaging. While occipital dysplasia is not a pathologic finding on its own, the larger foramen magnum created by this anatomic variation and/or the markedly thin areas of the supraoccipital bone that results, creates a larger area of exposure of underlying neural structures [16, 17]. Of note, the supraoccipital bone is typically irregular in its surface and thickness, which must be accounted for in the drilling process. There is also a central prominence overlying the vermis (i.e. the vermiform impression), over which the bone is typically thinner than in surrounding areas. In thinner and/or irregular areas. Lempert and Kerrison rongeurs can help safely complete the craniotomy to expose the underlying meninges (Figure 16.6). A dental sickle scaler, and or a nerve hook can be helpful in elevating thin bony remnants, so that these can most easily be removed using Lempert rongeurs. If drilling is inadvertently extended dorsally or laterally into the bone encasing the transverse

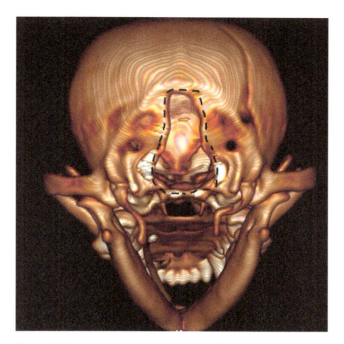

Figure 16.6 A craniectomy is performed first; the margins of this exposure include the area ventral to the nuchal crest and external occipital protuberance dorsally, and the FM ventrally, dorsal to the occipital condyles as outlined in this figure. After the initial opening of the occipital bone, Lempert and Kerrison rongeurs can help safely complete the craniotomy to expose the underlying meninges.

venous sinuses, hemostasis can be achieved using bone wax as a means of mechanical hemostasis [23].

A dorsal laminectomy of the atlas is then performed medial to the lateral vertebral foramina, using a pneumatic air drill, exposing the underlying dura along the length of this vertebra. This allows visualization of the AO atlantooccipital junction, identification, and resection of atlantooccipital fibrous bands. It is also important in patients diagnosed with atlantooccipital overlapping. Safe access to the cranial-most extent of the atlas is facilitated by full flexion of the CCJ; this can reduce the extent of cerebellar herniation and improve overlapping between the atlas and the foramen magnum [24, 25]. When preparing to perform the dorsal laminectomy, care must be taken to define the cranial and caudal-most extents of the lamina of the atlas prior to drilling, to help prevent inadvertent damage to neural tissue. Removal of the overlapping portion of the spinous process of the axis is needed to allow full access to the lamina of the atlas; this is accomplished using Lempert rongeurs. Lastly, during exposure for the dorsal laminectomies, maintaining the soft tissues overlying the dorsal atlantoaxial and atlantooccipital junctions intact (e.g. the dorsal atlantoaxial membrane and dura) can help protect underlying neural tissues during drilling, and will prevent the release of cerebrospinal fluid from the subarachnoid space, which may impair visibility during drilling. Cerebrospinal fluid is initially released as a large volume, then continues to emanate from durotomy/dural tear sites in a pulsatile manner.

The laminectomy must be extended to include the axis if atlantoaxial fibrous band-associated compression is present. This is done in the manner described for the atlas, above. Of note, once the lamina of the atlas and axis have been removed, if dural tissues remain intact, focal dilation of the subarachnoid space is notable immediately cranial (and, to a lesser extent caudal) to sites of atlantoaxial band-associated compression. Fibrous tissue is identified at this point and gently dissected from the underlying dura using Bishop Harman iris forceps to stabilize the tissue and a combination of the gross hook and spoon and a fresh number 11 blade to isolate and incise the band on midline, and gently dissect and excise it bilaterally. Bleeding may be encountered as it is resected and at the time of incision of the dorsal atlantoaxial membrane. This is controlled using bipolar cautery and Gelfoam®[1]. Following incision and resection of the fibrous band, resolution of the focal dilation of the subarachnoid space can be noted at this level, as the compressive band is removed. If present, compressive fibrous tissue overlying the atlantooccipital junction is also excised, in the same method described above.

A durotomy is then performed overlying the cerebellum, continuing caudally through the laminectomy area. To begin the durotomy, it is safest to elevate the portion of the dura that is to be excised, to separate it from the underlying cerebellum. This can be accomplished directly using a number 12 scalpel; alternatively, a dental scythe scaler or a 25-gauge needle with its tip bent upward into a 45° angle (held with a hemostat) can be used first to elevate the dura at the planned point of incision. The dura is then incised over the elevating object using a number 11 or number 12 surgical blade. The needle/scaler is then replaced with a nerve hook as a blunt means of continuing to elevate the dura, if desired. The durotomy may be continued along its full length with either a surgical blade, or Castroviejo, Potts, or angled iris scissors. The durotomy is extended mediolaterally at the atlantooccipital junction and at the caudal aspect of the laminectomy area, in an "I" formation. This allows the freed dura to be marsupialized to surrounding tissues at each cranial and caudal extent, using an absorbable 5–0 monofilament suture. Placement of these sutures through the four fixation points at one time and using these as stay sutures can

---

1 Gelfoam Sponges, Pharmacia and Upjohn Company, Kalamazoo, MI 49001.

help to plan marsupialization globally prior to tying each individual suture.

Hemostasis is maintained throughout using bipolar electrocautery, neurosurgery sponges/patties, Gelfoam[1], and thrombin topical agents (e.g. Recothrom[®2]), and as needed. Visualization can be aided using cellulose spears to gently clear the nervous system from blood clots that may remain following gentle lavage with saline.

At this point in the surgery, the head is released from its flexed position to one that resembles a normal standing posture. The cerebellum will frequently slide caudally as the head position is changed (i.e. will appear increasingly displaced through the foramen magnum). This variation in position of the cerebellar tonsils with variations in head position has been described previously [25]. Of note, if implants are to be placed, head release should be withheld until screw placement has been completed (see below).

The surgical site is then copiously lavaged, taking care to avoid having the exposed neural tissue in direct line of the saline's jet. The durotomy site is then covered using either biological or synthetic dural substitutes, taking care to cover the exposed area fully. The biological substitute most used is a porcine origin dural substitute (i.e. lyophilized swine submucosa) covered by an autologous fat graft harvested prior to the start of the main surgical procedure [1, 21, 22, 26, 27]. Synthetic agents include collagen matrix-based dural grafts (e.g. Duragen[®3]) with or without added PEG-based hydrogel sealants (e.g. DuraSeal[®4] spinal sealant) [28–30]. A recent study showed, however, that use of a hydrogel sealant can improve craniotomy outcomes in dogs when used in combination with duroplasty onlays [31]. However, there is little consensus as to which dural graft type is preferable to use in CCJ decompression surgeries among surgeons, partly due to a paucity of studies evaluating their superiority over one another in the veterinary literature. Factors to be considered in deciding the type to be used include cost, availability, potential for infection, and/or reaction to the material used (e.g. lipoid meningitis/necrosis vs. foreign body reaction potential) [26]. These agents are used to obtain a protective covering, to prevent meningoneural adhesions, create a scaffold for scar tissue formation, and to help prevent an excess of the latter from developing in the CCJ postoperatively [29].

Regardless of the material used, it must be cut to a size that will entirely cover the durotomy site and affixed to the underlying dura to maintain its postoperative position using 5–0 absorbable monofilament suture. The need for a

watertight seal when affixing this has not been demonstrated in veterinary patients in contrast to their human counterparts [1]. Closure is completed routinely. Close apposition of the muscular layers helps to prevent seroma formation postoperatively. The epaxial musculature is closed first, using an absorbable monofilament suture (e.g. polydioxanone) placed in a simple continuous suture pattern. The musculature overlying the cerebellum is then brought together using the same suture material and pattern. The subcutaneous tissues are similarly closed on midline, followed by the subcuticular and skin layers (routine closure).

An alternate surgical option described is the use of a surgical implant covering the exposed area of the neuraxis. If this is to be performed, care must be taken to avoid drilling the supraoccipital bone completely, to allow room for screw placement without needing to impinge upon the nuchal crest and its underlying transverse sinus. At this point 3–6, 1.5 mm, titanium self-drilling (a.k.a. drill-free) screws are inserted approximately into the edge of the supraoccipital bone, arranged in an arc surrounding the craniectomy site (larger screw size may be needed in large breed dogs). Titanium is chosen as the material of preference to allow for MR imaging to be performed, if needed, in the future. The use of self-drilling screws helps to limit the risk of iatrogenic damage to the underlying cerebellum during drilling and shorten overall surgical time and, if available, are preferable to self-tapping screws in their biomechanical properties [32, 33]. The length of the screws is chosen to accommodate a depth of placement of 2–3 mm, and an external presence of 3–4 mm (i.e. chosen to be longer than their depth of insertion to accommodate attachment to the overlying mesh-polymethylmethacrylate plate). The head position is then released, as described above. A titanium mesh implant is cut to cover the craniectomy site and screws, in a shape resembling a guitar pick, with its wider portion positioned dorsally and its narrower portion overlapping the atlantooccipital junction. The implant is molded to retain the decompression accomplished by the craniectomy, with its ventral margin partially bent caudodorsally so that compression of the underlying tissues can be prevented during awake movement of the head. Polymethylmethacrylate cement is then used to thinly cover both sides of the mesh and affix it to the underlying screws. The area is then copiously lavaged and closed routinely [34]. Postoperatively, either orthogonal radiographic images or CT imaging of the CCJ must be obtained to assess implant placement.

---

2 ZymoGenetics, Inc., 1201 Eastlake Avenue East, Seattle, WA 98102.
3 Duragen, IntegraLifeSciences Corporation, Princeton, NJ 08540.
4 DuraSeal Spinal Sealant System, IntegraLifeSciences Corporation, Princeton, NJ 08540.

Outcomes

Whether duroplasty or implant placement is performed, surgery must be coupled with long-term medical management. The use of adjunctive treatment modalities such as an Assisi loop and/or acupuncture can help to improve postoperative comfort and healing. Routine in hospital and at home care is employed. In the short term, substantial improvement in quality of life is reported, principally noticed in patient comfort and neurologic function, regardless of the surgery type employed (i.e.

titanium-PMMA implant placement vs. duroplasty). However, scratching is not substantially affected [5, 12, 27, 34, 35]. Recurrence of signs may be noted, however, longer term (i.e. greater than six months postoperatively), regardless of the surgical technique employed. This is typically the result of scar tissue formation accumulating at the surgery site, overlying the cervicomedullary junction. Of note, surgical reports are restricted to management of CLM alone [27, 28, 30, 34], AOO alone [36, 37], but do not describe outcome of surgery for globally managed CCJ disease.

References

1. Akin, E.Y. and Shores, A. (2017). Suboccipital craniectomy/foramen magnum decompression. In: *Current Techniques in Canine and Feline Neurosurgery* (ed. A. Shores and B. Brisson), 115–120. Hoboken NJ: Wiley.

2. Hechler, A.C. and Moore, S.A. (2018). Understanding and treating Chiari-like malformation and syringomyelia in dogs. *Top. Companion Anim. Med.* 33 (1): 1–11. https://doi.org/10.1053/j.tcam.2018.03.002. Epub 2018 Mar 15. PMID: 29793722.3.

3. Cerda-Gonzalez, S. and Dewey, C.W. (2010). Congenital diseases of the craniocervical junction in the dog. *Vet. Clin. North Am. Small Anim. Pract.* 40 (1): 121–141. https://doi.org/10.1016/j.cvsm.2009.10.001. PMID: 19942060.

4. Cerda-Gonzalez, S., Olby, N.J., and Griffith, E.H. (2015). Dorsal compressive atlantoaxial bands and the craniocervical junction syndrome: association with clinical signs and syringomyelia in mature cavalier king Charles spaniels. *J. Vet. Int. Med.* 29 (3): 887–892.

5. Loughin, C.A. and Marino, D.J. (2016). Atlantooccipital overlap and other Craniocervical junction abnormalities in dogs. *Vet. Clin. North Am. Small Anim. Pract.* 46 (2): 243–251. https://doi.org/10.1016/j.cvsm.2015.10.008. Epub 2015 Nov 27. PMID: 26631588.

6. Driver, C.J., Volk, H.A., Rusbridge, C., and Van Ham, L.M. (2013). An update on the pathogenesis of syringomyelia secondary to Chiari-like malformations in dogs. *Vet. J.* 198 (3): 551–559.

7. Lu, D., Lamb, C.R., Pfeiffer, D.U., and Targett, M.P. (2003). Neurological signs and results of magnetic resonance imaging in 40 cavalier king Charles spaniels with Chiari type 1-like malformations. *Vet. Rec.* 153: 260–263.

8. Freeman, A.C., Platt, S.R., Kent, M. et al. (2014). Chiari-like malformation and syringomyelia in

American Brussels griffon dogs. *J. Vet. Intern. Med.* 28 (5): 1551–1559. https://doi.org/10.1111/jvim.12421. Epub 2014 Aug 21. PMID: 25145262; PMCID: PMC4895564.

9. Kiviranta, A.M., Rusbridge, C., Laitinen-Vapaavuori, O. et al. (2017). Syringomyelia and Craniocervical junction abnormalities in chihuahuas. *J. Vet. Intern. Med.* 31 (6): 1771–1781. https://doi.org/10.1111/jvim.14826. Epub 2017 Sep 11. PMID: 28892202; PMCID: PMC5697179.

10. Korff, C.P. and Williamson, B.G. (2020). Clinical presentation of Chiari-like malformation in 2 Persian cats. *Top. Companion Anim. Med.* 41: 100460. https://doi.org/10.1016/j.tcam.2020.100460. Epub 2020 Jun 25. PMID: 32823159.

11. Minato, S. and Baroni, M. (2018). Chiari-like malformation in two cats. *J. Small Anim. Pract.* 59 (9): 578–582.

12. Cerda-Gonzalez, S., Olby, N.J., and Griffith, E.H. (2016). Longitudinal study of the relationship among Craniocervical morphology, clinical progression, and syringomyelia in a cohort of cavalier king Charles spaniels. *J. Vet. Intern. Med.* 30 (4): 1090–1098. https://doi.org/10.1111/jvim.14362. Epub 2016 Jun 17. PMID: 27311874; PMCID: PMC5094541.13.

13. Hechler, A.C. and Moore, S.A. (2018). Understanding and treating Chiari-like malformation and syringomyelia in dogs. *Top. Companion Anim. Med.* 33 (1): 1–11. https://doi.org/10.1053/j.tcam.2018.03.002. Epub 2018 Mar 15. PMID: 29793722.

14. Rusbridge, C. and Jeffery, N.D. (2008). Pathophysiology and treatment of neuropathic pain associated with syringomyelia. *Vet. J.* 175 (2): 164–172.

15. Evans, H.E. and deLahunta, A. (ed.) (2013). *Miller's Anatomy of the Dog*, 4e. St Louis: Elsevier / Sanders.

16. Rusbridge, C. and Knowler, S.P. (2006). Coexistence of occipital dysplasia and occipital hypoplasia/

syringomyelia in the cavalier king Charles spaniel. *J. Small Anim. Pract.* 47 (10): 603–606. https://doi.org/10.1111/j.1748-5827.2006.00048.x. PMID: 17004953.

17. Wright, J.A. (1979). A study of the radiographic anatomy of the foramen magnum in dogs. *J. Small Anim. Pract.* 20 (8): 501–508.

18. Janeczek, M. and Chrószcz. (2011). The occipital area in medieval dogs and the role of occipital dysplasia in dog breeding. *Turk. J. Vet. Anim. Sci.* 35 (6): 453–458. https://doi.org/10.3906/vet-1012-672.

19. Pearce, J.M. (2006). Queckenstedt's manoeuvre. *J. Neurol. Neurosurg. Psychiatry* 77 (6): 728.

20. Chi-Hsiang, C., Ming-Luen, D., Jong-Ling, F. et al. (2013). Queckenstedt's test affects more than jugular venous congestion in a rat. *PLoS One* 8 (3): e59409.

21. Akin, E.Y., Ortinau, N.H., Shores, A. et al. (October 2009). Foramen magnum decompression with free autogenous adipose tissue graft for treatment of caudal occipital malformation syndrome in dogs. Poster presented at the ACVS Symposium, Washington, DC.

22. Trevor, P.B., Martin, R.A., Saunders, G.K., and Trotter, E.J. (1991). Healing characteristics of free and pedicle fat grafts after dorsal laminectomy and durotomy in dogs. *Vet. Surg.* 5: 282–290.

23. Pluhar, G.E., Bagley, R.S., Keegan, R.D. et al. (1996). The effect of acute, unilateral transverse venous sinus occlusion on intracranial pressure in normal dogs. *Vet. Surg.* 25 (6): 480–486. https://doi.org/10.1111/j.1532-950x.1996.tb01447.x. PMID: 8923727.

24. Cerda-Gonzalez, S., Dewey, C.W., Scrivani, P.V., and Kline, K.L. (2009). Imaging features of atlanto-occipital overlapping in dogs. *Vet. Rad. Ultrasound* 50 (3): 264–268.

25. Upchurch, J.J., McGonnell, I.M., Driver, C.J. et al. (2011). Influence of head positinoing on the assessment of Chiari-like malformation in cavalier king Charles spaniels. *Vet. Rec.* 169 (11): 277.

26. Di Vitantonio, H., De Paulis, D., Del Maestro, M. et al. (2016). Dural repair using autologous fat: our experience and review of the literature. *Surg. Neurol. Int.* 7 (Suppl 16): S463–S468. https://doi.org/10.4103/2152-7806.185777. PMID: 27500007; PMCID: PMC4960926.

27. Ortinau, N., Vitale, S., Akin, E.Y. et al. (2015). Foramen magnum decompression surgery in 23 Chiari-like malformation patients 2007-2010: outcomes and owner survey results. *Can. Vet. J.* 56 (3): 288–291. PMID: 25750451; PMCID: PMC4327144.

28. Abla, A.A., Link, T., Fusco, D. et al. (2010). Comparison of dural grafts in Chiari decompression surgery: review of the literature. *J. Craniover. Jun. Spine* 1 (1): 29–37. https://doi.org/10.4103/0974-8237.65479. PMID: 20890412; PMCID: PMC2944852.

29. Calikoglu, C., Cakir, M., and Tuzun, Y. (2019). Histopathological investigation of the effectiveness of collagen matrix in the repair of experimental spinal dura mater defects. *Eur. J. Med.* 51 (2): 133–138. https://doi.org/10.5152/eurasianjmed.2018.17422. Epub 2018 Dec 3. PMID: 31258352; PMCID: PMC6592439.

30. Vermeersch, K., Ham, L.V., Caemaert, J. et al. (2004). Suboccipital craniectomy, dorsal laminectomy of C1, durotomy and dural graft placement as a treatment for syringohydromyelia with cerebellar tonsil herniation in cavalier king Charles spaniels. *Vet. Surg.* 33: 355–360.

31. Preul, M.C., Campbell, P.K., Bichard, W.D., and Spetzler, R.F. (2007). Application of a hydrogel sealant improves watertight closures of duraplasty onlay grafts in a canine craniotomy model. *J. Neurosurg.* 107 (3): 642–650. https://doi.org/10.3171/JNS-07/09/0642. PMID: 17886566.

32. Goelzer, J.G., Avelar, R.L., de Oliveira, R.B. et al. (2010). Self-drilling and self-tapping screws: an ultrastructural study. *J. Craniofac. Surg.* 21 (2): 513–515. https://doi.org/10.1097/SCS.0b013e3181d023bd. PMID: 20216445.

33. Kumar, V.K., Prasad, K., Sansgiri, T. et al. (2021). Self-drilling versus self-tapping screws: a 3D finite element analysis. *Craniomaxillofac. Trauma Reconstr.* 14 (1): 4–10. https://doi.org/10.1177/1943387520904212. Epub 2020 Apr 12. PMID: 33613829; PMCID: PMC7868515.

34. Dewey, C.W., Marino, D.J., Bailey, K.S. et al. (2007). Foramen magnum decompression with cranioplasty for treatment of caudal occipital malformation syndrome in dogs. *Vet. Surg.* 36 (5): 406–415. https://doi.org/10.1111/j.1532-950X.2007.00286.x. PMID: 1761492135.

35. Plessas, I.N., Rusbridge, C., Driver, C.J. et al. (2012). Long-term outcome of cavalier king Charles spaniel dogs with clinical signs associated with Chari-like malformation and syringomyelia. *Vet. Rec.* 171 (20): 501.

36. Dewey, C.W. and Cerda-Gonzalez, S. (2009). Case report – surgical stabilization of a craniocervical junction abnormality with atlantooccipital overlapping in a dog. *Compend. Contin. Educ. Vet.* 31 (19): E1–E6.

37. Takahashi, F., Hakozaki, T., Kouno, S. et al. (2018). Atlantoaxial overlapping and its effects on outcomes after ventral fixation in dogs with atlantoaxial instability. *J. Vet. Med. Sci.* 80 (3): 526–531.

17

Ventral Approach to the Cervicothoracic Spine

Isidro Mateo

Veterinary Hospital, Universidad Alfonso, Villanueva de la Cañada, Spain

Introduction

Several common pathological conditions affect the cervicothoracic spine including disk herniations (either extrusions or protrusions), cervical spondylomyelopathy, and vertebral fractures and luxations (Figure 17.1) [1–6]. Some of them can be managed with a conventional dorsal or lateral approach for laminectomy or hemilaminectomy (particularly when lateralized) [1–3, 6, 7]. However, if the lesion is midline located in the ventral spinal canal or implant placement in the vertebral bodies is desirable, an approach to the ventral aspect of C6–T2 vertebral bodies and corresponding intervertebral disk spaces is required [4, 5, 8–10]. The exposition of these structures is limited using the conventional ventral approach to the cervical spine as they are hindered by the manubrium and the depth of the access (Figure 17.1b). Resection of the manubrium and median manubriotomy are surgical techniques that can be performed to improve exposure of the ventral aspect of C6–T2 vertebral bodies and intervertebral disks [8, 10].

Surgical Anatomy [10–12]

Most neurosurgeons are familiar with the ventral anatomy of the neck but the complex anatomy and delicate neurovascular structures near the thoracic inlet and mediastinum may dissuade them from a deep cervicothoracic approach. A precise knowledge of the anatomy will allow a safe access to this region.

Muscles

After a superficial midline skin incision is made from the mid-cervical region to the cranial margin of the second sternebra, the sternocephalicus and superficial pectoral muscles are exposed (Figure 17.2A). Superficial pectoral muscles originate paramedially on the cranial end of the sternum and run laterally and distally covering the biceps brachii muscle to the humerus. The sternocephalicus muscle is a flat muscle arising on the manubrium and has two components: the mastoid and occipital part. The mastoid part is cranially directed to the mastoid part of the temporal bone, whereas the occipital part attaches to the dorsal nuchal line of the occipital bone. At their origin the muscles of the two sides are intimately joined, but they separate at the middle of the neck and each crosses under the external jugular vein of its own side. Because of this divergence, there is a space ventral to the trachea in which the bilateral sternohyoideus and sternohyoideus muscles appear. The sternohyoideus muscle arises from the deep surface of the manubrium and the cranial edge of the first costal cartilage and extends cranially as flat longitudinal fibers to be inserted on the basihyoid bone covering the ventral surface of the trachea. The sternothyroideus muscle lies deep to the sternohyoideus muscle and arises from the first costal cartilage to be inserted on the lateral surface of the thyroid lamina, adjacent to the lateral surface of the trachea on its course. Dorsal to the trachea, the deep fascia of the neck can be visualized covering the longus coli muscle, which is a long muscle composed of separate bundles that lies in the ventral aspect of the bodies of cervical and six first thoracic vertebrae. Bundles in the cervical portion arise on the

---

Advanced Techniques in Canine and Feline Neurosurgery, First Edition. Edited by Andy Shores and Brigitte A. Brisson.
© 2023 John Wiley & Sons, Inc. Published 2023 by John Wiley & Sons, Inc.
Companion site: www.wiley.com/go/shores/advanced

162 | *Advanced Techniques in Canine and Feline Neurosurgery*

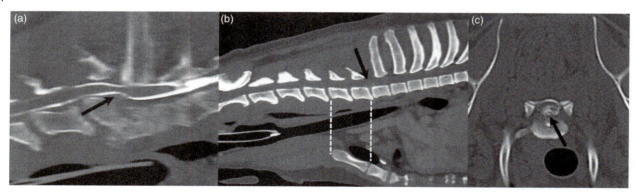

Figure 17.1 Sagittal CT myelogram (a) and CT (b) reconstruction and transverse CT myelogram at C7–T1 intervertebral disk space (c) showing C7–T1 vertebral subluxation associated with discospondylitis (a) and disk extrusions (b and c) causing severe spinal cord compression (arrows). Note the position of the manubrium relative to caudal cervical vertebrae (dashed lines in B) hindering its access.

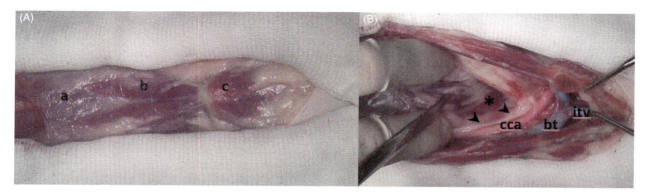

Figure 17.2 The cranial is to the left and caudal to the right in all of the images. (A) A ventral midline skin incision made from the mid-cervical area to the second sternebra exposes the sternohyoid (a), sternocephalicus (b), and pectoral muscles (c). (B) Deep ventral cervical spine with median manubriotomy. The trachea and esophagus have been retracted to the left (top of the image). The fingers pinpoint the transverse processes of C6, and the tip of the scissors pinpoints the C6–C7 intervertebral disk space. Note the V-shaped disposition of the longus coli muscle (asterisk). The vagosympathetic trunk (arrowheads), right common carotid artery (acc), right brachiocephalic trunk (bt), and internal thoracic vein (itv) are also depicted in the image.

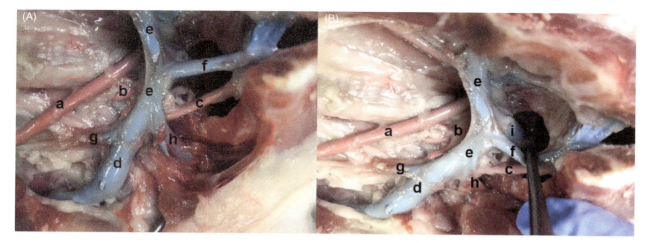

Figure 17.3 The cranial is to the left and caudal to the right in all of the images. (A) Vascular anatomy of the thoracic inlet. The right sternocephalicus muscle and the first right rib have been removed to allow visualization of deep vascular structures: (a) right common carotid artery; (b) right subclavian artery and ramifications; (c) internal thoracic artery; (d) external jugular vein; (e) right and left brachiocephalic veins; (f) internal thoracic vein; (g) internal jugular vein (not filled with colored latex); and (h) right subclavian vein. (B) Retraction of the internal thoracic vein allows visualization of cranial vena cava (i).

ventral border of the transverse process of the sixth to the third cervical vertebrae and end on the ventral spine of the next preceding vertebra, making a V shaped pattern running cranially (Figure 17.2B). The thoracic portion of the muscle arises on the ventral surface of the first six thoracic vertebrae to be inserted on the ventral border of the wing of the sixth cervical vertebra and on the transverse process of the seventh cervical vertebra.

Vessels

In the midline between the sternohyoideus muscles, the unpaired caudal thyroid vein can be observed with bilateral branches. This vein arises primarily from the deep surfaces of the sternothyrohyoideus muscles, but on one or both sides its most cranial tributary may arise in the thyroid lobe or lobes. It terminates in the cranial angle formed by the merging brachiocephalic veins which, cranial to the thoracic inlet, form the cranial vena cava (Figure 17.3). Brachiocephalic veins of both sides are formed by the confluence of caudally coursing external jugular and the medially coursing subclavian vein of each side (Figure 17.3). The external jugular vein receives the venous blood from the head. It crosses the lateral surface of the brachiocephalic muscle obliquely superficially under the skin. The internal jugular vein usually terminates in the caudal portion of the external jugular vein, but rarely terminates in the brachiocephalic vein (Figure 17.3).

The brachiocephalic trunk, the first branch of the aortic arch, passes obliquely to the right across the ventral surface of the trachea and gives rise to the left common carotid artery and terminates at the right common carotid artery and the right subclavian artery (Figure 17.3). Common carotid arteries are included in their respective carotid sheaths with the vasosympathetic trunk and internal jugular vein, which lie in the angle formed by the longus coli or longus capitis dorsally, the trachea ventromedially, and the brachiocephalicus and sternocephalicus muscles laterally (Figure 17.2B).

Nerves

The right recurrent laryngeal nerve, a branch that leaves the right vagus nerve at the level of the caudal side of the subclavian artery, is intimately associated with the lateral surface of the trachea until its end in the larynx. The left recurrent laryngeal nerve, a branch of the left vagus nerve, has similar disposition to the left but arches caudally around the aorta. Although care should be taken during manipulation, laryngeal dysfunction due to surgical trauma is extremely rare. Sympathetic innervation of the head is transmitted via the sympathetic trunk, which runs with the internal jugular vein, common carotid artery, and vagus nerve in the carotid sheath (Figure 17.2B). The vagus nerve contains parasympathetic preganglionic axons that course caudally down the neck to thoracic and abdominal organs.

Viscera

The trachea is immediately dorsal to the sternohyoideus muscle. It occupies a midline position under the longus coli muscle from the larynx to its bifurcation at the level of the fourth or fifth thoracic vertebra dorsal to the cranial part of the base of the heart.

The cervical portion of the esophagus traverses the neck closely related to the left longus coli and longus capitis muscles dorsally and to the trachea ventrally and to the right. At its origin, it starts to incline ventrally to the left, so that at the thoracic inlet it usually lies left ventrolateral to the trachea. This disposition should be considered during retraction of the trachea to expose the longus coli muscle near the thoracic inlet to avoid esophageal damage. The thoracic inlet is the oval opening of the thoracic cavity into the neck (Figure 17.3). The aperture is wider dorsally than ventrally and it is delimited by the longus coli muscle dorsally, the manubrium ventrally, and bilaterally by the first pair of ribs and costal cartilages. Through the thoracic inlet pass the trachea, esophagus vagosympathetic trunk, recurrent laryngeal nerve, phrenic nerve, first two thoracic nerves, left and right common carotid arteries, left subclavian artery, internal jugular veins, brachiocephalic veins and subclavian veins and lymphatic vessels. The rostral apices of the pleural cavities lie in the thoracic inlet.

Surgical Technique [10, 12]

The dog should be positioned in dorsal recumbency with the cervical spine extended over a sandbag or vacuum positioning pad with the thoracic limbs retracted caudally and attached to surgical table (Figure 17.4A). Access to the caudal cervical spine can be improved with the positioning pad placed as caudally as possible, near to thoracic spine, and with gentle traction of the neck using a weight on the maxilla. Tape should be used to immobilize the head and the thorax in a straight position for a perfect alignment of the neck. Clipping should extend midline from the mandible to the middle of the sternum. Proper positioning is mandatory before draping as incorrect positioning results in rotation of the cervical and thoracic spine, hindering the approach of the deep cervical and thoracic vertebral bodies. The surgeon is typically positioned to the right of the patient. Landmarks are the larynx and the manubrium and

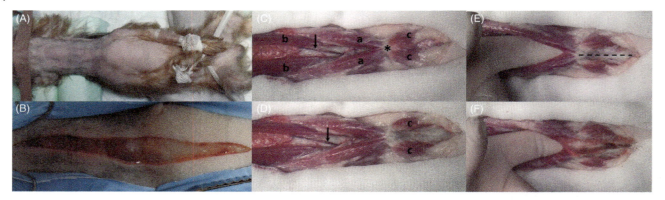

Figure 17.4 Positioning for manubriotomy and ventral access to the caudal cervical and cranial thoracic spine. The cranial is to the left and caudal is to the right in all images and the surgeon should be positioned on the right of the animal (bottom of the image). (A) The patient is positioned in dorsal recumbency with thoracic limbs drawn caudally, preferably crossed to improve stability. Observe the positioning pad under the neck and the tape to secure the maxilla. (B) Midline skin incision from the mid–cervical region to the second sternebra. (C) The sternocephalicus muscles (a) are divided to the cranial end of the manubrium (asterisk). The caudal thyroid vein can be observed (arrow) between the divided sternohyoideus muscles (b). (D) Pectoral muscles (c) are elevated from the manubrium. The index finger is dorsally positioned to the manubrium to facilitate median manubriotomy (broken line) and avoid pleural or vascular damage. (E) Image showing completed median manubriotomy.

a ventral midline skin incision is made from the mid-cervical region to the cranial margin of the second sternebra (Figure 17.4B). This incision exposes the sternocephalicus, sternohyoideus, and superficial pectoral muscles. The sternocephalicus muscles are divided to the manubrium and the superficial and deep pectoral muscles elevated (Figures 17.4C,D). Monopolar electrocautery and a periosteal elevator facilitate exposure of the manubrium.

Two approaches are described to improve access to the ventral cervical spine: the resection of the manubrium and median manubriotomy. In manubriotomy, the mastoid part of the sternocephalicus muscles are identified and elevated from the origin on the cranial aspect of the manubrium to a point immediately cranial to the articulation of the first rib. The sternohyoideus muscle should be elevated from its origin on the cranial aspect of the manubrium allowing full exposure of the manubrium that can be excised at a cranial point just cranial to the articulation of the first ribs. With this procedure the sternohyoideus and sternocephalicus muscles should be re-attached to the soft tissue of the remaining first sternebra in a locking loop pattern. In median manubriotomy the insertions of sternohyoideus and sternothyroideus muscles can be maintained. Median manubriotomy is performed with a sagittal saw. During the procedure the index finger should be dorsally positioned to the manubrium to avoid vascular and mediastinal damage (Figures 17.4E,F). External irrigation with saline to prevent heat necrosis should be used. Care should be taken to avoid penetration into the mediastinum and to respect the common carotid artery and the external jugular vein in its union with the brachiocephalic trunk. Gelpi retractors can be used to keep the manubrium split throughout the procedure. Then, the approach to the ventral aspect of the cervical and first thoracic spine can be continued in the standard manner. The sternohyoideus muscles are divided in the midline and the caudal thyroid vein is exposed with small branches on each side that may be cauterized. Blunt dissection with scissors and fingers will expose the trachea that should be retracted, with the recurrent laryngeal nerve (which should remain associated with the trachea) to the left. The esophagus is also retracted to the left, whereas the right carotid sheath is retracted to the right. A midline incision is made in the deep fascia of the neck between the recurrent laryngeal nerve and the carotid sheath to expose the longus coli muscle. The more caudal the position in the neck is, the deeper the structures are, and the more midline the position of the esophagus is, and care has to be taken to avoid damage to the esophagus during division of the longus coli muscle. Although blunt self-retaining retractors have been advocated to retract vital structures during division of the longus coli muscle in the midline over the region of interest, retraction with the index and middle fingers of the left hand is more efficient for this task, as Gooset or Balfour retractors are difficult to place in this caudal position.

The large transverse processes of C6 and first ribs can be used as anatomical landmarks (Figures 17.5a). Dissection of the longus coli muscle from the ventral tubercles should be performed with Metzenbaum scissors for a right-handed surgeon. It is important to stay in the midline during dissection and identify the ventral tubercles and left and right left and right transverse processes, particularly those from C6 which will be the main anatomical reference. Bipolar electrocautery may help to prevent bleeding when longus

17 Ventral Approach to the Cervicothoracic Spine | 165

inlet is recommended, but not mandatory, to enhance visibility of the T1–T2 intervertebral disk space and avoid trauma to the esophagus, carotid sheath, or brachiocephalic vein as they enter the thoracic inlet. This can be performed with Senn retractors or application of moistened sponges. If exposure of the ventral aspect of T3–T5 vertebral bodies is desirable, further sternotomy should be performed and the cranial mediastinum penetrated. In this situation, the mediastinum and brachycephalic trunk should be bluntly dissected and the heart gently retracted to expose the thoracic longus coli muscle. Retractors should be placed near the thoracic inlet and caudally along the brachycephalic trunk to increase visualization of the spine and prevent vital structures from being damaged. Cranial lung lobes must be packed off caudally using moist laparotomy sponges. Once the required vertebral bodies or intervertebral disk space are fully exposed, the decompression and/or stabilization can begin. The use of an angulated drill may be preferred for the ventral slot because it will allow drilling in a more comfortable position, limiting the possibilities of soft tissue damage. The technique for ventral slot and implant placement are described elsewhere [4, 5, 10, 12].

After completion of the procedure, a lavage is used to remove any debris and blood clots. Surgical closure begins with the apposition of the longus coli muscle in a simple continuous pattern. As longus coli muscles are frequently resected during exposure of the caudal cervical spine, apposition is often incomplete. Then, the segments of the manubrium should be brought into apposition with circumferential ligatures in small dogs or with sutures placed through pre-drilled transverse holes in the manubrium. The pectoralis, sternohyoideus, and sternocephalicus muscles are also opposed using simple continuous patterns. Subcutaneous tissues and skin are routinely closed.

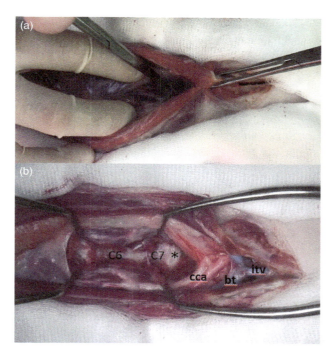

Figure 17.5 Deep ventral cervical spine with closed (a) and split (b) manubrium. Compare how improved the visualization of the deep caudal cervical spine is after manubriotomy (b). In (a) the fingers pinpoint the transverse processes of C6, and the tip of the scissors pinpoints the C7–T1 intervertebral disk space. Note the position of C7 – T1 intervertebral disk space (asterisk) and the right common carotid artery (acc), right brachiocephalic trunk (bt), and internal thoracic vein (itv). The trachea and esophagus have been retracted to the left (top of the image).

coli tendons are cut. Subperiostial elevation of the longus coli muscle with periosteal elevators cranial and caudal to the ventral tubercle and disk space should be performed. Retraction of the musculature is maintained with Gelpi retractors. For C6–C7 and C7–T1 intervertebral disk exposure, the tips of the left (rostral) Gelpi retractor should be positioned immediately caudal to the transverse processes of C6. The right (caudal) Gelpi retractor can be placed elsewhere caudal to this position. Although the use of moist sponges have been advocated to protect surrounding tissues for trauma with Gelpi retractors, their placement in this deep position can be difficult and obtrude visualization of the ventral aspect of vertebral bodies, and therefore may not be used. Particular care should be taken in this deep and caudal position to avoid damage to the esophagus and vasculature that is not usually identified with the conventional ventral approach. The external jugular, brachiocephalic, and internal thoracic veins can be visualized dorsal and lateral to the excised manubrium. With median manubriotomy, C5, C6, C7, T1, and T2 vertebral bodies are easily exposed and the cranial mediastinum should not be entered (Figure 17.5b). Caudal retraction of the thoracic

Clinical Results

To date, only a few reports describe ventral access to the caudal cervical and cranial thoracic spine [4, 5, 8–10]. Resection of the manubrium was performed in one case to facilitate access to the C7–T1 intervertebral space and ventral slot in a case of disk extrusion with successful outcome and without complications [8]. Median sternotomy has been described in two cases with traumatic fractures of cranial thoracic spine (T2–T3 luxation and comminute T5 vertebral fracture) also with successful outcome [4, 5]. In both cases median sternotomy allowed for satisfactory exposure of the ventral aspect of cranial thoracic vertebral bodies and safe application of the implants. Vital structures were adequately retracted and protected from iatrogenic injury.

The thoracic cavity and the pleural space were entered in both cases and therefore a thoracic drain and mechanical ventilation were required [4, 5]. However, when the lesion is restricted to the caudal cervical and first two thoracic vertebrae, a more restrictive approach by means of median manubriotomy can be performed avoiding the potential complications of entering the thoracic cavity. Median manubriotomy has been described in a case with T1–T2 disk extrusion [9]. Recently, the largest case series of dogs with lesions affecting the spinal cord at C6–T2 vertebral bodies has been published [10]. It included five dogs with disk extrusions, one dog with C7–T1 and T1–T2 disk protrusions, and three dogs with caudal cervical misalignment (one with C7–T1 vertebral subluxation due to discospondylitis, one with C6–C7 spondylomyelopathy and disk protrusion, and one with traumatic C6–C7 vertebral subluxation). Median manubriotomy was easily performed and substantially improved the visualization of C6, C7, T1, and T2 vertebral bodies, allowing a comfortable position for ventral slot in dogs with disk extrusions or protrusions and the placement of implants for vertebral fixation between C5 and T2 (Figure 17.6). In five dogs the brachiocephalic trunk was identified and exposed. Pneumomediastinum or significant blood loss was not observed in any case (Video 17.1). Neurological improvement was observed in seven cases. Five dogs (four dogs with disk extrusions and one dog with C6–C7 vertebral luxation) had excellent outcomes (without neurological deficits) and two dogs had good outcomes (one dog with C7–T1 and T1–T2 disk protrusion and the dog with C7–T1 subluxation due to discospondylitis). The poor outcome observed in two cases (one dog did not recovered in the first two postoperative weeks and was euthanatized at the owner's request; and one dog died from pulmonary thromboembolism five days after surgery) could not be attributed to the surgical technique [10].

Although caudal cervical or cranial thoracic disk extrusions can be addressed with hemilaminectomy via dorsolateral or lateral approaches, ventral access should be preferred, particularly if disk material is centered in the midline over the intervertebral disk and has not migrated. The ventral approach and ventral slot are less aggressive to the musculature, require less soft tissue dissection, and allow substantially less spinal cord and nerve root manipulation. It is the author's opinion that this combination of benefits results in less morbidity and mortality during the postoperative period. In cases when stabilization is required, exposure of the vertebral bodies is mandatory for implant placement and, therefore, ventral access is the only approach that should be considered.

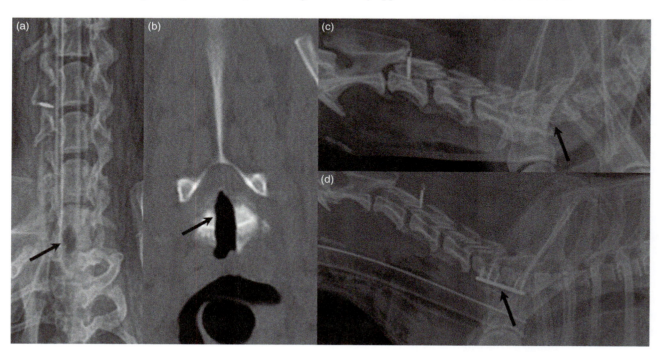

Figure 17.6 Ventrodorsal radiography of the cervical spine (a) and CT at C7–T1 intervertebral disk space (b) showing the position for C7–T1 ventral slot (arrows). Preoperative (c) and postoperative (d) lateral radiographies showing C6–C7 vertebral subluxation (arrow in c) realigned and stabilized with two locking plates (arrow in d). Locking plates are superimposed in image d.

Conclusion

Ventral approach to the cervicothoracic spine should be considered with lesions affecting the spinal cord at the level C6–T2 vertebral bodies, particularly when ventral slot or implant placement are required. Median manubriotomy is a simple method that facilitates visualization of the ventral aspect of the caudal cervical and cranial thoracic vertebral bodies and corresponding intervertebral disk spaces, particularly C7–T1 and T1–T2. This technique can help to reduce surgical time and allows the neurosurgeon to work in a comfortable position. Care must be taken to avoid injury to vascular (external jugular and brachiocephalic veins and common carotid artery) and cranial mediastinum structures at the thoracic inlet, but the procedure does not seem to be associated with increased morbidity or mortality. When exposure of more caudal vertebral bodies is needed, a complete median sternotomy should be performed. Although multiple risks can be associated with the procedure, they can be addressed by having a thorough knowledge of the regional anatomy.

Video clips to accompany this book can be found on the companion website at:
www.wiley.com/go/shores/advanced

References

1. Gilmore, D.R. (1983). Cranial thoracic intervertebral disk extrusion in a dog. *J. Am. Vet. Med. Assoc.* 182: 620–621.
2. Liptak, J.M., Watt, P.R., Thomson, M.J. et al. (1999). Hansen type I disk disease at T1-2 in a dachshund. *Aust. Vet. J.* 77: 156–159.
3. Mateo, I., Paniagua, R., Cloquell, A., and Vazquez, F. (2019). Intervertebral T3-T4 disc extrusions in two german shepherd dogs. *J. Am. Anim. Hosp. Assoc.* 55 (3): e553–e503. https://doi.org/10.5326/JAAHA-MS-6883.
4. Guiot, L.P. and Allman, D.A. (2011). Median sternotomy and ventral stabilisation using pins and polymethylmethacrylate for a comminuted T5 vertebral fracture in a Miniature Schnauzer. *Vet. Comp. Orthop. Traumatol.* 24: 76–83.
5. Klatzkow, S., Johnson, M.D., James, M., and Carrera-Justiz, S. (2018). Ventral stabilization of a T2-T3 vertebral luxation via median sternotomy in a dog. *Case Rep. Vet. Med.* 10 (2018): 9152394. https://doi.org/10.1155/2018/9152394.
6. De Risio, L., Muñana, K., Murray, M. et al. (2002). Dorsal laminectomy for caudal cervical spondylomyelopathy: postoperative recovery and long-term follow-up in 20 dogs. *Vet. Surg.* 31: 418–427.
7. Rossmeisl, J.H. Jr., Lanz, O.I., Inzana, K.D., and Bergman, R.L. (2005). A modified lateral approach to the canine cervical spine: procedural description and clinical application in 16 dogs with lateralized compressive myelopathy or radiculopathy. *Vet. Surg.* 34: 436–444.
8. Bush, M.A. and Owen, M.R. (2009). Modification of the ventral approach to the caudal cervical spine by resection of the manubrium in a dog. *Vet. Comp. Orthop. Traumatol.* 22: 514–516.
9. Cappelle, K.K. and Reaugh, H.F. (2018). Sternotomy and ventral slot decompression for treatment of T1-2 intervertebral disk disease in a Dachshund. *J. Am. Vet. Med. Assoc.* 253: 215–218.
10. Mateo, I. (2020). Median manubriotomy for ventral access to the caudal cervical and cranial thoracic spine. *Vet. Surg.* 49: 923–929.
11. Evans, H.E. (1993). *Miller's Anatomy of the Dog*, 3e. Philadelphia: WB Saunders.
12. Sharp, N.J.H. and Wheeler, S.J. (2005). Cervical disc disease. Approach to the ventral neck. In: *Small Animal Spinal Disorders. Diagnosis and Surgery*, 2e (ed. N.J.H. Sharp and S.J. Wheeler), 106–120. Elsevier Mosby. ISBN: 0723432090.

Part II

Intracranial Procedures

18

Intraoperative Ultrasound in Intracranial Surgery

Alison M. Lee, Chris Tollefson and Andy Shores

Mississippi State University, Mississippi State, MS, USA

Introduction

Primary and secondary brain tumors are often treated with a combination of maximal surgical resection followed by radiation and/or chemotherapy [1]. The ability to completely remove an intraparenchymal tumor depends on many factors, including lesion location, the surgeon's ability to recognize the tumor, the ability to define tumor margins, and the ability to detect residual tumor following excision [1–4]. In addition, these factors must be identified quickly in order to minimize surgery and anesthesia time. In order to ensure best patient outcomes, real-time and accurate assessment of brain parenchyma and parenchymal lesions intraoperatively is essential. Real-time diagnostic imaging is used in concert with neurosurgery in order to accomplish this.

Diagnostic imaging has been used to help guide neurosurgery for many years. The first stereotactic frame designed for human use was built in 1918; however, the stereotactic system using three-dimensional Cartesian coordinates was not developed until 1947 [5]. Intraoperative computed tomography (CT) and magnetic resonance imaging (MRI) scans are available in some facilities and are highly accurate; however, the expense of such systems limits their availability in veterinary settings [1]. In addition, the use of these machines requires that stereotactic equipment be attached to the patient at all times prior to and during the procedure, which can interfere with the surgical approach. Any movement of the equipment results in inaccurate imaging results. Additionally, there can be significant shifting of lesions and normal brain structures during the surgical procedure as a result of resolving mass effect or intraoperative hemorrhage, which can result in significant errors when comparing the pre-surgical imaging.

In contrast, intraoperative ultrasound is a reliable, non-invasive, real-time tool that can be used to accurately assess tumor volume and residual tumor, without the need for stereotactic equipment attached to the patient and without the confounding effects of changing mass effect during the surgical procedure [1–4, 6]. Human studies have shown that intraoperative brain ultrasound images are comparable, and in some cases superior, to MRI images of tumors and normal anatomic landmarks (Figure 18.1) [7]. Although there are some concerns about the application of transducer pressure on the brain parenchyma during the procedure, to date there is no identified risk of mechanical injury to the brain parenchyma resulting from intraoperative ultrasound use. Because the exam is real-time, intraoperative complications such as hemorrhage can be immediately appreciated using this imaging modality. A standard ultrasound machine can be used for this purpose and, in addition, the ultrasound machine is portable, so there is no need to purchase a separate machine solely for the intraoperative suite.

Ultrasound is a real-time imaging modality, so the operator can account for changes to the intraparenchymal structures during the surgical procedure. Ultrasound, however, is highly operator dependent with a somewhat steep learning curve. It has been reported that operators who are familiar with MRI and CT images of the brain but who have not been trained on ultrasound struggle to identify anatomy and lesions during the procedure when comparing to preoperative cross-sectional images (Figure 18.2) [8, 9]. In cases where an experienced sonographer is not available to assist, a stereotactic approach may be preferred. In addition, ultrasound cannot be used preoperatively to help guide the approach; thus, a multimodality approach is preferred when planning and performing surgical removal of intracranial lesions.

Advanced Techniques in Canine and Feline Neurosurgery, First Edition. Edited by Andy Shores and Brigitte A. Brisson.
© 2023 John Wiley & Sons, Inc. Published 2023 by John Wiley & Sons, Inc.
Companion site: www.wiley.com/go/shores/advanced

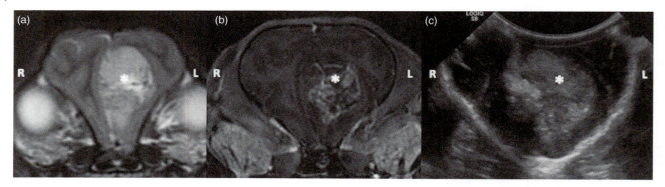

Figure 18.1 Transverse (a) T2, (b) T1 FSGR with Doteram, and (c) ultrasound images of a low-grade oligodendroglioma in the left frontal lobe (asterisk). (a) The hyperintense region that extends beyond the contrast enhancing border on image (b) is perilesional vasogenic edema. Notice (c) ultrasound also identifies the edema as abnormal tissue, thus care should be taken as to avoid removing too much tissue or biopsy of a non-representative area.

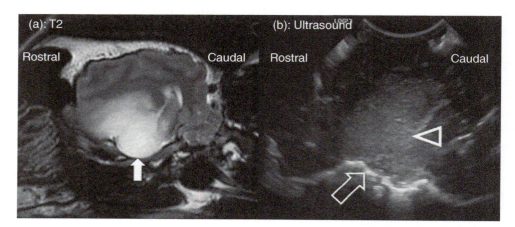

Figure 18.2 Sagittal (a) T2 MRI and (b) ultrasound images of a patient with a high-grade astrocytoma effacing the left amygdala, hippocampus, and piriform lobe. (a) This mass is ill defined and hyperintense on the T2 image (white arrow). (b) Notice the slight hyperechogenic region of the left amygdala on the ultrasound image (open white arrowhead). The base of the calvarium is a sharply marginated hyperechoic curvilinear line with distal acoustic shadowing (open arrow).

Artifacts in Imaging

Unfortunately, ultrasound is prone to many artifacts which can affect image quality and confuse inexperienced sonographers. Generally, these artifacts result from limitations to the width of the ultrasound beam or differences in the attenuation coefficients of intracranial structures [10]. The most common sources of error in intraoperative ultrasound are brightness errors. These errors result from the inclusion of air bubbles, coagulated blood, or hemostatic agents included in the surgical field, and result in the underlying tissues appearing more hyperechoic (Figure 18.3) [10, 11]. Interestingly, even the temperature of the saline infused into the surgical site has the potential to change the echogenicity of the underlying tissues [11].

The best way for sonographers to limit the introduction of artifact into the intraoperative exam is to choose a transducer which best fits the shape and size of the surgical craniotomy. Doing so will reduce the potential to include unwanted air bubbles into the site, and will limit the amount of sterile saline needed to infuse the surgical site. The sonographer should additionally keep the ultrasound probe as close to horizontal as possible. This minimizes air trapping within the surgical site. An additional strategy to reduce brightness artifact is to continually use time-gain compensation. This will keep the tissues the same echogenicity regardless of depth and will minimize the potential for overinterpreting artificially hyperechoic normal tissues as neoplastic [11].

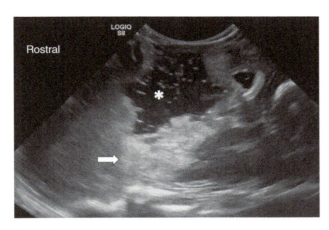

Figure 18.3 Following partial debulking of a mass. A common complication is intraventricular hemorrhage (asterisk). This can be identified as hyperechoic foci suspended and potentially swirling within the previously anechoic cerebrospinal fluid of the ventricles (asterisk). Notice the increased echogenicity of the mass distal (white arrow). This is likely due to a combination of distal acoustic enhancement, intraparenchymal hemorrhage, and edema. Avoid removing too much tissue or biopsy of a non-representative area.

Accuracy of Intraoperative Ultrasound

Although considered highly accurate, ultrasound is subject to registration errors as with any other non-frame-based imaging modality. Studies have shown that ultrasound is accurate up to 1.4 ± 0.45 mm [12]. Accuracy is mostly affected by probe calibration and can be improved significantly by the addition of Doppler images with B-mode images. In fact, when Doppler imaging is added to traditional B-mode imaging, accuracy had been shown to increase by over 10% [13]. An additional study showed that with the addition of Doppler imaging, misregistration errors that occurred with intraoperative ultrasound were less than 2.5 mm in more than 90% of cases (Figure 18.4) [14].

Although misregistration errors do occur with intraoperative ultrasound, the level of accuracy of this system is widely accepted in standard clinical practice as acceptable for neurosurgical guidance. With that in mind, the accuracy of the overall procedure can still be improved, largely by using a multimodal approach to the surgical procedure. This includes the use of preoperative cross-sectional imaging of the lesion (typically with MRI), as well as the use of intraoperative fluorescent dyes or Raman spectroscopy [11, 15].

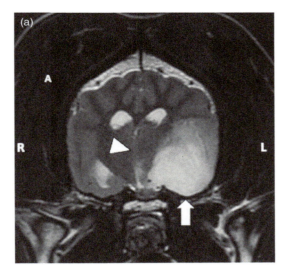

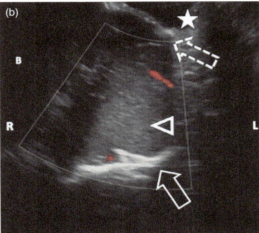

Figure 18.4 (Same patient as in Figure 18.2.) Transverse (a) T2 MRI and (b) ultrasound color Doppler images of a patient with a high-grade astrocytoma effacing the left amygdala, hippocampus, and piriform lobe. (a) This mass is ill defined and hyperintense on the T2 image (white arrow) with a mild rightward midline shift (white arrowhead). (b) Notice the slight hyperechogenic region of the left amygdala on the ultrasound image (open white arrowhead). At the top of the image, there is anechoic flush that aids with conduction of the ultrasound beam (star) and the hyperechoic meninges (dashed arrow). The base of the calvarium is a sharply marginated hyperechoic curvilinear line with distal acoustic shadowing (open arrow).

Scanning Procedure and Equipment

Typically, calvarial bone prevents a sonographer from being able to interrogate the brain. Therefore, brain ultrasound is usually accomplished by scanning through a defect in the calvarial bone. This can be done in animals with open or persistent fontanelles, but in most intraoperative procedures,

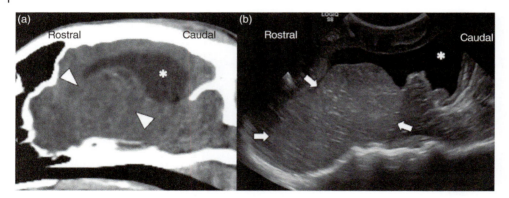

Figure 18.5 A. sagittal computed tomography, brain window W:150 L:50 and B. sagittal ultrasound images of a primitive glioma (white arrowheads) causing obstruction at the region of the foramen of Monro. The lateral ventricles were bilaterally enlarged with anechoic fluid (asterisk) and the third ventricle was near completely attenuated (not imaged). Notice the increased size of the mass on the ultrasound image compared to the computed tomographic image.

scanning is accomplished by creating windows in the calvarial bone via craniectomy or craniotomy through which to interrogate the underlying brain parenchyma. Probe selection is important when considering intraoperative ultrasound. Although both linear and microconvex probe geometries can be used successfully in brain scanning, microconvex probes tend to fit the geometry of the surgical field and osteotomy better and are thus preferred. There is a potential for gas to enter the site during sonography, so the sonographer should select the probe geometry which best fits the surgical osteotomy site. Generally, brain ultrasound is best performed with probes scanning from 7.5 to 12 MHz, depending on the size of the patient and the depth of the lesion. During scanning, gauze, cottonoid sponges, and other blotting equipment are removed from the field. Retractors and other surgical instruments are kept out of the field, and any blood overlying the site is washed with saline and suctioned in order to minimize artifacts and provide the best possible image quality.

It is vitally important to maintain sterility at all times when using the ultrasound equipment in an intraoperative setting. When the appropriate osteotomies have been made to allow for ultrasound interrogation, the probe should be draped in a sterile manner. This can be

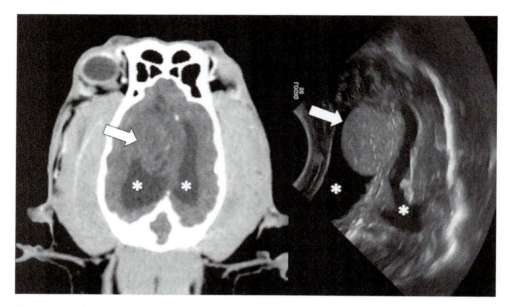

Figure 18.6 (a) Dorsal computed tomographic image of the same dog in Figure 18.5 after administration of Omniscan in a bone window (W:150 L:50) and (b) a right dorsolateral to left ventrolateral ultrasound image of same dog. The bilateral lateral ventriculomegaly is present on both images (asterisk). The primitive glioma is again in both images, but the ultrasound image is easier to delineate normal from abnormal tissue (white arrows).

18 Intraoperative Ultrasound in Intracranial Surgery | 175

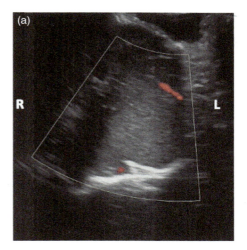

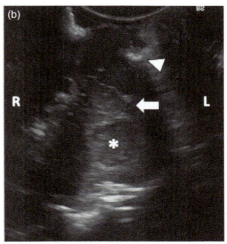

Figure 18.7 (a) Preoperative and (b), postoperative images of a high-grade glioma. The slightly hyperechoic region in (a) is now filled with echogenic fluid with distal acoustic enhancement, and a hyperechoic rim (asterisk) in the postoperative image. The postoperative region is a cavitated region with focal hemorrhage after biopsy and debridement of the mass. Additionally, the cerebrum is mildly collapsed with retraction of the hyperechoic meninges (white arrow) from the calvarium (white arrowhead).

accomplished by inserting the probe into a sterile surgical sleeve or palpation glove. Sterile lubricant must be placed into the end of the sleeve to eliminate any air at the probe-sleeve interface. The sleeve can then be clamped to the drape to prevent accidental dropping of the probe during the procedure. Probe–patient contact is maintained by infusing the surgical field with sterile saline. The probe must be handled at all times by a surgeon scrubbed in to the procedure and cannot be handed off to non-sterile assistants until the imaging portion of the procedure has been completed. As it is not possible to sterilize the console and viewing screen of the machine, a non-sterile assistant may manipulate the console and alter the image on the screen for the surgeon.

Scanning is accomplished by fanning the probe in a rostral–caudal and lateral–lateral manner in both the sagittal and transverse probe orientation. Anatomic landmarks that are typically used to assist in lesion localization with brain scanning include the lateral ventricles and choroid plexus, septum pellucidum, falx cerebri, and calvarial bone [8]. When the lesion is identified, an approximate size should be recorded in three planes (Figures 18.5 and 18.6). The overall echotexture and echogenicity of the lesion should also be recorded, as well as how well-defined the lesion margins are. Color or power Doppler interrogation is also recommended to identify any major blood vessels surrounding or entering the lesion prior to surgical removal. Ultrasound interrogation is recommended both prior to and following surgical removal (Figure 18.7). The sonographer should be aware that following removal of lesion material, there will likely be midline and tentorial shifts of the brain parenchyma, and thus the appearance and location of the lesion may change between scans during the procedure. The degree of change will depend on the initial size of the lesion, the lesion location, and the amount of lesion removed between scans. Ultrasound can also be used to guide surgical procedures, including biopsy instrument placement and location of bleeding vessels.

Appearance of Tumor on Ultrasound

The vast majority of tumors within brain parenchyma are hyperechoic; in one review in people, 100% of brain lesions (including high- and low-grade gliomas, neuronal tumors, and inflammatory lesions) identified were hyperechoic (Figure 18.2) [1]. Areas of hemorrhage within the lesion are more intensely hyperechoic in the acute phase, although chronic hemorrhage is hypo- to anechoic (Figure 18.8). In general, higher-grade tumors tend to be more heterogeneous in echotexture, while low-grade and benign lesions tend to be more homogeneous in echotexture [1]. This is probably related to the elevated water content with low-grade lesions, as opposed to a rich capillary network typically found in higher grade tumors. Most reports describe the transition between normal brain and lesion as sharp, with some reports describing either a hyperechoic or hypoechoic halo between the two tissues. This halo is likely a reflection of perilesional vessels, compressive edema, or active growth of the tumor [8]. In a study that analyzed the appearance of the borders of high-grade gliomas, all biopsy samples considered unequivocal by the surgeon based on their visual and tactile impressions were hyperechoic on ultrasound.

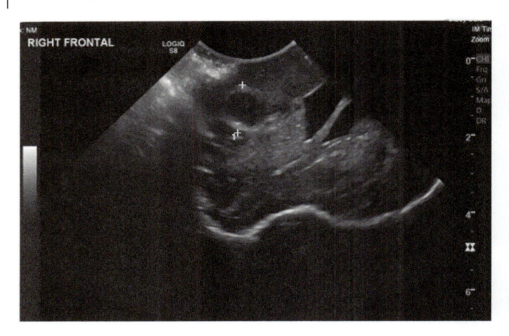

Figure 18.8 Ultrasound image of a chronic, intraparenchymal hematoma in an English Bulldog exhibiting intracranial signs. Note the hypoechoic appearance of this chronic hematoma.

Samples taken from the proposed edge of the lesion varied more. Seventeen samples came from hyperechoic tissues and showed tumor, inflammatory cells, and normal cells on biopsy. Eight samples were hypoechoic on ultrasound, and only one of these samples (12.5%) had any evidence of tumor tissue on biopsy [16]. Studies tend to agree that most lesions in the brain, and the majority of tumors, are hyperechoic on ultrasound, but ultrasound cannot reliably distinguish borders of tumors. Nevertheless, hypoechoic areas on ultrasound rarely contain tumor (Figure 18.9).

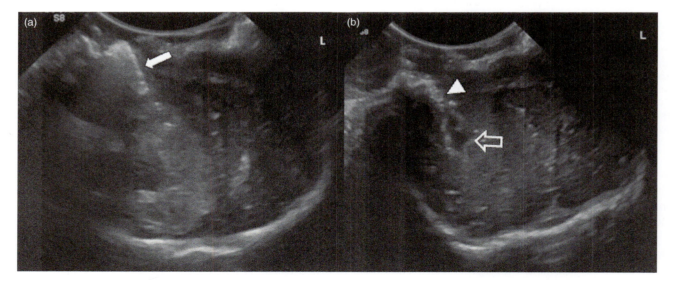

Figure 18.9 Transverse ultrasound images (a) with the placement of a Cavitron ultrasonic surgical aspirator (CUSA) and (b) post-procedure of a grade III astrocytoma within the right frontal lobe. (a) The hyperechoic linear structure (white arrow) with distal acoustic shadowing is the CUSA device. (b) a hyperechoic linear track which is likely due to hemorrhage (white arrow head) and a small anechoic cavitation with a hyperechoic rim (open arrow) are present.

Ultrasound Guided Procedures

An additional advantage of ultrasound is that it can be used intraoperatively to guide instrument placement for tissue sampling or tissue ablation. The probe selection is similar to intraoperative imaging applications, with the only exception being that the area must be big enough to allow for both probe contact and the introduction of the instrument into the surgical field. Sterile procedure is again vital, so the preparation of the probe is identical to imaging applications in the surgical suite.

The probe should be held such that the intended target (generally, the center of the lesion) is centered on the ultrasound monitor. Positioning a lesion off-center will result in inaccurate placement of the instrument and potentially erroneous tissue sampling or ablation. The focal zone of the ultrasound should be set at the deep portion of the lesion for optimal visualization. The instrument should be introduced into the surgical field on the side of the probe with the orientation marker, and should be aligned parallel to the marker. Ideally, the instrument or needle should be introduced into the tissue a few centimeters from the probe at an approximately 45° angle to the probe. The introduced object will appear ultrasonographically as a thin, sharply marginated, hyperechoic line with a distinct edge (Figure 18.10). The instrument should be advanced until the tip is seen within the desired location. If the instrument is not seen when introduced into the tissue, the sonographer should stop the advancement and should reposition the probe until the instrument is seen. This can be accomplished either by slowly scanning through the field in a sagittal orientation with a sweeping motion looking for the instrument, or by visually inspecting the alignment of the instrument with the orientation marker on the probe. If the instrument is not aligned with the orientation marker, the probe should be rotated into alignment and the screen reexamined. Once seen on the ultrasound, the instrument can then be repositioned or withdrawn as required.

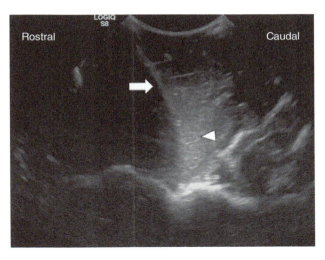

Figure 18.10 Sagittal ultrasound image. The sharply marginated linear line that casts distal acoustic shadowing (white arrow) is the biopsy device. The device is directed toward a hyperechoic region within the piriform lobe (white arrowhead).

Conclusion

Intraoperative ultrasound is a cost-effective and portable way to use real-time imaging in the intraoperative setting, while eliminating the need for bulky stereotactic equipment. Although operator dependent and prone to some artifacts and errors, ultrasound is highly accurate and is widely accepted as a reasonable imaging modality for intraoperative use. The best clinical results occur when intraoperative ultrasound is used in a multimodal approach with pre- and postoperative cross-sectional imaging.

 Video clips to accompany this book can be found on the companion website at:
www.wiley.com/go/shores/advanced

References

1. Chacko, A.G., Kumar, N.K., Chacko, G. et al. (2003). Intraoperative ultrasound in determining the extent of resection of parenchymal brain tumours – a comparative study with computed tomography and histopathology. *Acta Neurochir.* 145 (9): 743–748; discussion 748.
2. Maarouf, A.H., Ligon, B.L., Rabih, E. et al. (1996). Use of intraoperative ultrasound for localizing tumors and determining the extent of resection: a comparative study with magnetic resonance imaging. *J. Neurosurg.* 84 (5): 737–741.
3. Quencer, R.M. and Montalvo, B.M. (1986). Intraoperative cranial sonography. *Neuroradiology* 28 (5): 528–550.
4. Peter, D.L., Mitchel, S.B., George, A.O. et al. (1989). Correlation of intraoperative ultrasound tumor volumes and margins with preoperative computerized tomography scans. *J. Neurosurg.* 71 (5): 691–698.

5. Comeau, R.M., Sadikot, A.F., Fenster, A., and Peters, T.M. (2000). Intraoperative ultrasound for guidance and tissue shift correction in image-guided neurosurgery. *Med. Phys.* 27 (4): 787–800.

6. Shores, A., Lee, A.M., Kornberg, S.T. et al. (2021). Intraoperative ultrasound applications in intracranial surgery. *Front. Vet. Sci.* https://doi.org/10.3389/fvets.2021.725867.

7. Unsgaard, G., Ommedal, S., Muller, T. et al. (2002). Neuronavigation by intraoperative three-dimensional ultrasound: initial experience during brain tumor resection. *Neurosurgery* 50 (4): 804–812.

8. Elmesallamy, W.A.E.A. (2019). Demonstrative study of brain anatomical landmarks by intraoperative ultrasound imaging. *Egypt. J. Neurosurg* 34 (1): 30.

9. Prada, F., Del Bene, M., Mattei, L. et al. (2015). Preoperative magnetic resonance and intraoperative ultrasound fusion imaging for real-time neuronavigation in brain tumor surgery. *Ultraschall Med.* 36 (2): 174–186.

10. Selbekk, T., Jakola, A.S., Solheim, O. et al. (2013). Ultrasound imaging in neurosurgery: approaches to minimize surgically induced image artefacts for improved resection control. *Acta Neurochir.* 155 (6): 973–980.

11. Ganau, M., Ligarotti, G.K., and Apostolopoulos, V. (2019). Real-time intraoperative ultrasound in brain surgery: neuronavigation and use of contrast-enhanced image fusion. *Quant. Imaging Med. Surg.* 9 (3): 350–358.

12. Lindseth, F., Langø, T., Bang, J., and Nagelhus Hemes, T.A. (2002). Accuracy evaluation of a 3D ultrasound-based neuronavigation system. *Comput. Aided Surg.* 7 (4): 197–222.

13. Morin, F., Courtecuisse, H., Reinertsen, I. et al. (2017). Brain-shift compensation using intraoperative ultrasound and constraint-based biomechanical simulation. *Med. Image Anal.* 40: 133–153.

14. Chen, S.J.-S., Reinertsen, I., Coupé, P. et al. (2012). Validation of a hybrid doppler ultrasound vessel-based registration algorithm for neurosurgery. *Int. J. Comput. Assist. Radiol. Surg.* 7 (5): 667–685.

15. Doran, C.E., Frank, C.B., McGrath, S., and Packer, R.A. (2022). Use of handheld raman spectroscopy for intraoperative differentiation of normal brain tissue from intracranial neoplasms in dogs. *Front. Vet. Sci.* 8: 819200. https://doi.org/10.3389/fvets.2021.819200.

16. Mursch, K., Scholz, M., Brück, W., and Behnke-Mursch, J. (2017). The value of intraoperative ultrasonography during the resection of relapsed irradiated malignant gliomas in the brain. *Ultrasonography* 36 (1): 60–65.

19

Brain Biopsy Techniques

John Rossmeisl[1] and Annie Chen[2]

[1] *Virginia Tech, Blacksburg, VA, USA*
[2] *Washington State University, Pullman, WA, USA*

Introduction

Brain biopsy is a diagnostic surgical procedure that involves the removal of pieces of tissue from the brain which are then subjected to neuropathological, molecular, genetic, or microbiological analyses in order to establish a definitive etiologic diagnosis for the observed lesion [1]. Brain biopsy can be performed using open or closed techniques, and excisional or incisional biopsies performed during open craniotomy are currently the most frequently employed brain biopsy techniques in veterinary medicine [2]. In cases where open surgical approaches to a brain lesion may not be a possible or an optimal approach to case management, closed stereotactic brain biopsy (SBB) techniques are often a viable alternative method for sampling brain tissue [3–5].

This chapter will review closed SBB procedures, in which a stereotactic headframe – or in the case of frameless procedures, other types of fiducial markers – is affixed to the animal's head prior to the performance of a diagnostic imaging scan such that the target lesion can be precisely localized and referenced to the external headframe or fiducials [3–7]. The neurosurgeon then performs the biopsy procedure using a minimally invasive approach to the skull and burr-hole craniectomy technique.

Indications and Contraindications

While computed tomography (CT) and magnetic resonance (MR) imaging techniques are sensitive for the characterization of brain lesions, both of these modalities have limited specificity with the imaging features of neoplastic, vascular, and inflammatory brain diseases demonstrating significant overlap [8, 9]. Since CT and MR imaging

provide only a broad list of differential diagnoses for the observed lesions, brain biopsy allows for a definitive histologic diagnosis of the observed lesions which can subsequently guide specific and optimal treatment strategies.

The most common diseases diagnosed by brain biopsy in veterinary medicine are tumors and immune-mediated and infectious encephalitides, although theoretically any lesion that can be accurately targeted with imaging can be sampled [3–5, 9, 10]. A common clinical indication for brain biopsy is to establish a definitive diagnosis in a canine patient that presents with a focal intra-axial lesion with MR imaging characteristics that are consistent with a granuloma, neuroepithelial neoplasm, or infarction [8, 9]. Brain biopsy can be used to identify brain pathologies that do not require surgical treatment via open craniotomy, or to establish diagnoses in patients who are poor surgical candidates.

Closed brain biopsy is contraindicated in patients with underlying coagulopathies, and should be approached with caution in animals with clinical signs or MR imaging features consistent with increased intracranial pressure (ICP), animals with caudoventral lesions, or systemic medical disorders that result in increased anesthetic risk [3–5, 11].

Frame-based Stereotactic Brain Biopsy (SBBfb)

SBBfb is the most commonly described type of closed-brain biopsy procedure performed in animals with clinical signs of intracranial disease [3–7, 11]. SBBfb procedures require rigidly affixing the animal to an external reference system (i.e. headframe) and subsequently acquiring a set of diagnostic imaging data with the patient in the headframe such that the location of the target intracranial lesion can be transformed

---

Advanced Techniques in Canine and Feline Neurosurgery, First Edition. Edited by Andy Shores and Brigitte A. Brisson.
© 2023 John Wiley & Sons, Inc. Published 2023 by John Wiley & Sons, Inc.
Companion site: www.wiley.com/go/shores/advanced

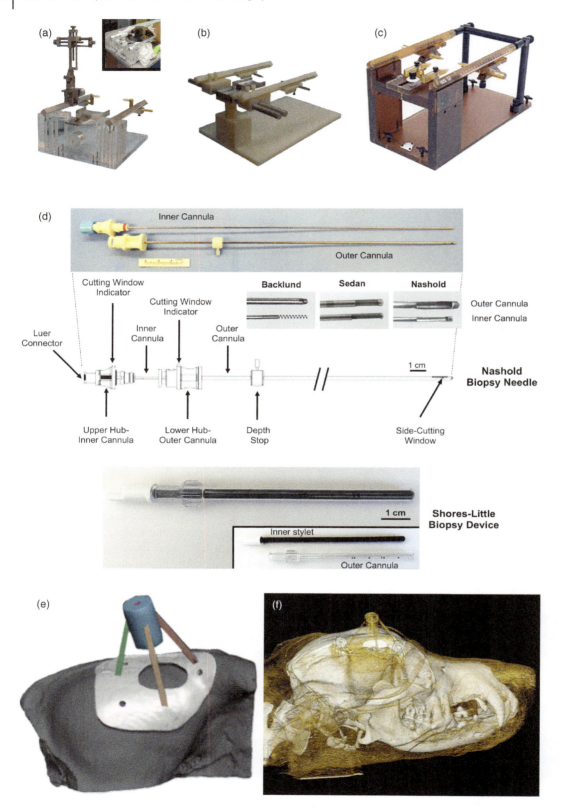

Figure 19.1 Instrumentation used for frame-based stereotactic brain biopsy. Dynatech with attached micromanipulator arm (a), Virginia tech custom (b), and Kopf 1530M (c) MRI compatible stereotactic headframes. A dog instrumented in the Dynatech headframe is illustrated in the inset of panel (a). (d) Schematic of design components of commonly used brain biopsy instruments. Computer rendering of a 3D printed, skull contoured patient-specific brain biopsy guide (e), and 3D reconstructed CT scan (f) demonstrating the surgically implanted biopsy guide *in situ*.

from the two-dimensional imaging data into three-dimensional stereotactic coordinates. Numerous types of stereotactic headframes (Figure 19.1) have been developed and modified for veterinary applications, and contemporary frames are constructed from non-ferromagnetic materials, such as titanium, thermoplastics, or aluminum, such that they can be used safely in CT or MR imaging environments [3, 12–14]. Additive manufacturing techniques are also being increasingly utilized in veterinary neurosurgery, and several SBBfb approaches using patient-specific 3D printed brain biopsy guides have been recently described [12–14] (Figure 19.1).

SBBfb Technique

Preoperative Evaluation

Prior to SBBfb, animals should have a complete blood count, serum biochemic profile, urinalysis, coagulation profile (i.e. PT/aPTT), and indirect blood pressure performed to screen for the animal's underlying risk factors for anesthetic or post-biopsy complications [3, 11]. Ideally, the initial diagnostic MR imaging that identified the lesion that is intended to be biopsied should have been performed within two weeks of the planned SBBfb procedure to avoid registration errors that can be associated with lesion evolution or resolution [3, 4].

Headframe Placement and Acquisition of Stereotactic Images

The target lesion is typically identified on an MR imaging scan of the animal's brain that was performed for diagnostic purposes. Following induction of general anesthesia and clipping of the head as required for the desired surgical approach, the animal is placed in sternal recumbency upon a rigid backboard. The neurosurgeon then affixes the head of the animal to the headframe. The majority of external stereotactic headframes described in veterinary medicine utilize a three-point immobilization system, which involve a patient-specific bite block and ear bars [3] (Figure 19.1). A dental impression of the patient's maxillary arcade is created using vinylpolysiloxane dental putty and molded into the bite block of the headframe. The patient is then placed into the bite block of the headframe, and the ear bars of the headframe placed into the horizontal ear canals. Memory foam or cloth pads can also be placed beneath the mandible to further support the head. Rigid patient immobilization can be further achieved by bolting the headframe baseplate to the rigid backboard using threaded nylon nuts and bolts placed through predrilled holes in the backboard

or plastic C-clamps [3]. Once the patient is immobilized, they are transported to the radiology suite for acquisition of diagnostic images while instrumented in the headframe.

If an MR imaging-compatible headframe is being used, CT or MR images can be used for stereotactic imaging [3, 6, 12]. Care should be exercised when transferring the patient onto and off the CT or MR imaging gantry, as this is a common potential source of patient movement and subsequent frame registration error. Regardless of the imaging modality used, the field of view (FOV) must include the headframe apparatus, and this can significantly limit the types of coils that can be used for MR imaging. The accuracy of the target coordinates on the imaging will be correlated to the resolution of the imaging matrix. The precision of the Z coordinate is directly related to the slice thickness, and the magnitude of error for the X and Y coordinates will be related to the pixel size [1]. When performing stereotactic MR imaging, the authors minimally acquire T2W sequences in three planes and pre- and post-contrast 3DT1W (isotropic $\leq 1\,mm$ slice thickness with no gap). If using CT stereotactic imaging, pre- and post-contrast images should also be obtained using $\leq 1\,mm$ slice thickness, with no gap [1, 3].

SBBfb Planning

DICOM formatted images of the diagnostic MR and stereotactic imaging dataset(s) are imported into an image analysis software package, and the diagnostic and stereotactic images are co-registered using the automated mutual information co-registration software feature. The neurosurgeon then uses the multiplanar reformatted image software interface to determine and visualize the desired stereotactic coordinates and trajectories for lesion biopsy [1, 3] (Figure 19.2). When planning the target location, it is optimal to choose a target location that is associated with both clinical and diagnostic imaging; evidence of pathology, areas of hemorrhage, and necrosis should be avoided, and the contrast-enhancing lesion burden should be sampled whenever possible [3–5, 15]. In general, the biopsy needle entry point and trajectory are planned to traverse the shortest distance of normal brain between the skull and the target, and simultaneously avoid sulci, major vasculature, and ventricular structures. However, depending on the lesion location, geometry, and position relative to critical structures, the shortest path to the target is not always optimal. Rostrocaudal (Z) coordinates are measured from the internal linear (ear bar) reference markers (Figure 19.2). Mediolateral (X) and dorsoventral (Y) coordinates and/or angular trajectories are measured directly from DICOM images using osseous anatomic landmarks, including the external sagittal crest and external surface of

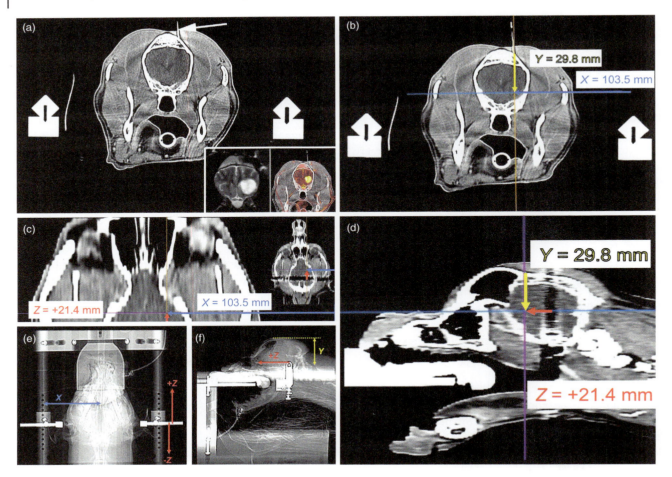

Figure 19.2 Frame-based stereotactic brain biopsy planning procedure with simulated biopsy needle placement (a, arrow). CT images are obtained with the patient instrumented in the headframe (a–e), and the diagnostic MRI images co-registered and fused with the stereotactic CT dataset (inset, a). The neurosurgeon imports stereotactic images into multiplanar reformatting software, plans the biopsy trajectory and target depth (intersection of colored crosshairs in b–d), and determines the X, Y, and Z stereotactic coordinates. Panels e and f illustrate the headframe and patient references from which the stereotactic coordinates are measured.

the skull, referenced to the rostrocaudal bars of the headframe. The target depth is measured from the external surface of the intended craniectomy defect to the intended distal most position of the biopsy needle within the lesion. The final stereotactic (X, Y, and Z) coordinates are verified and stored in the planning software and registered to the headframe [1, 3].

The neurosurgeon then chooses the type of instrument that will be used to harvest the biopsy. Multiple biopsy instruments are available for SBB, but they operate using three basic principles: side-cutting needles, suction coring devices, or microforceps (Figure 19.1). Side-cutting needles, such as the Nashold, Sedan, Latinen, and Backlund spiral, are the most frequently described instruments used in veterinary SBB applications [3–5, 10–14]. These needles produce a sample size of 2×8–10 mm. When microforceps are used they are introduced through a biopsy cannula and typically retrieve a biopsy sample in the 1–2 mm^3 range. Advantages of side-cutting needles compared to microforceps include larger sample size and superior preservation of cellular cytoarchitecture. In humans, side-cutting needles are associated with a higher incidence of symptomatic hemorrhage, which may be related to their sample size or the tissue tearing that occurs as the needle is turned within the brain [16]. The Shores–Little biopsy device (Figure 19.1) is an example of a suction coring instrument that is manufactured specifically for veterinary brain biopsy applications, although it was designed for use in open, ultrasound-guided biopsy procedures. A disadvantage of the Shores–Little biopsy device is its relatively short working length, which can limit its utility for use in closed SBB applications. Head-to-head comparisons of the diagnostic yield, tissue quality, and adverse effect profiles resulting from the use of different biopsy instruments have yet to be performed in veterinary patients with intracranial disease.

After the biopsy is planned, the neurosurgeon can elect to perform a phantom simulation to further verify the plan [17]. The phantom simulation involves attaching the micromanipulator arm to the stereotactic headframe and simulating the biopsy using a needle blank that is seated in position at the desired needle entry point into the calvarium [3, 17] (Figure 19.2). A CT or MR imaging scan is then repeated to include the headframe and attached needle phantom using the identical image acquisition parameters as the initial stereotactic scan for each patient.

SBBfb Procedure

Following stereotactic planning, SBBfb can be performed in the operating room without image guidance, or with image guidance in the CT suite [3–5, 15] (Figure 19.3). The surgical techniques are similar in both cases. The animal's clipped head is aseptically prepared for surgery, and the animal is transported to the location where the SBBfb procedure will be performed while being maintained under anesthesia and immobilized in the headframe, and the patient draped routinely. The stereotactic coordinates are transferred from the planning station and then re-registered onto the frame and verified. A routine approach to the skull ipsilateral to the location of the mass is performed, with the specific approach used dictated by the target location. Following completion of the surgical approach, a perforated drape is applied over the standard surgical drapes. The perforated drape assists coupling of the sterile micromanipulator arm to the non-sterile headframe. The micromanipulator arm and guide tube assembly are then mounted to the headframe, the final stereotactic coordinates verified and recorded, and the micromanipulator arm rotated out of the field to allow creation of a 3–5 mm diameter burr-hole craniectomy defect at the intended entry point in the skull using a high-speed pneumatic or manual twist drill [5]. The exposed dura is cauterized using bipolar cautery, and then the dura sharply perforated. After creation of the burr-hole and dural defects, the biopsy instrument is advanced down the guide tube mounted to the micromanipulator to confirm that no impediments to the intended trajectory are encountered.

Next, the depth to target is then verified and a depth stop applied to the proximal portion of the biopsy instrument. If a biopsy needle is being used, a saline-filled syringe is attached to the needle, and the assembly flushed and the needle port confirmed to be in the closed position. The biopsy instrument is then passed through the guide tube and gradually advanced to the planned target depth using the micromanipulator arm controls [3, 17]. If an image-guided

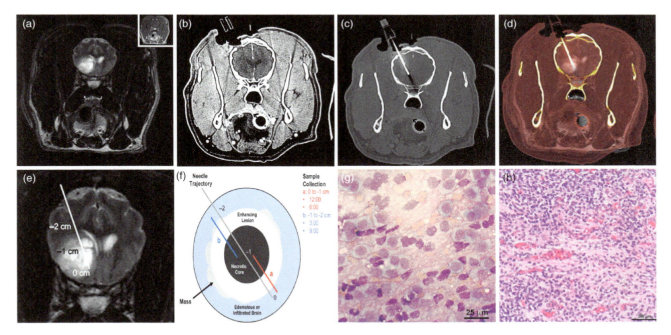

Figure 19.3 CT-guided stereotactic brain biopsy of an oligodendroglioma in the right frontal lobe of a dog. (a) The tumor appears as a heterogeneously T2-hyperintense, ring-enhancing (inset) mass on the diagnostic MRI. (b) The minimally invasive rostrotentorial approach, burr-hole craniectomy, and biopsy guide cannula. The biopsy needle is evident in situ within the target at the −2 cm needle position on the intraoperative CT (c) and fused CT-MR images (d). Stylized representations (e and f) of the geographic core biopsy technique utilized to harvest four biopsy samples along a single needle trajectory. Intraoperative, Giemsa-stained cytologic (g) specimens are used to confirm the quality of the biopsy samples and obtain a preliminary diagnosis of glial neoplasia, which was subsequently histopathologically confirmed to be a low-grade oligodendroglioma (f).

procedure is being performed, it is at this point the animal is advanced into the bore of the CT scanner and images obtained with the biopsy instrument in situ to confirm the desired placement within the target (Figure 19.3). Once the biopsy needle is at the desired location in the target depth, the biopsy is harvested. If a side-cutting needle is being used, the side-cutting port is opened by rotating the inner cannula hub 180°, and slight negative pressure applied by pulling back the plunger on the attached saline-filled syringe to pull a tissue core into the needle. The side-cutting port is then closed and the inner needle cannula withdrawn.

Biopsy specimens can be retrieved by flushing saline through the inner cannula to eject the specimen into a sterile tissue cassette, or in the case of microforceps, a 25- or 27-gauge needle used to remove the biopsy from the jaws of the microforceps into the cassette. To obtain multiple specimens along a singular needle trajectory, a geographic core technique can be used [15] (Figure 19.3). This involves collecting multiple specimens from the same target depth by rotating the biopsy needle aperture to different positions of the clockface for each collection, and repeating this technique at different target depths as the needle is withdrawn.

At the conclusion of the biopsy procedure, the needle is incrementally withdrawn from the brain to assess for hemorrhage. In the event hemorrhage is observed, blood should be permitted to flow from the needle until the bleeding ceases. Following completion of the biopsy, the operative field is lavaged copiously and the surgical wound closed routinely.

Postoperative Care and Adverse Events

In the absence of the development of complications, most animals require analgesic therapy for 24–48 hours after the procedure, and can be discharged from the hospital the following day. Adverse events reportedly occur in 15–27% of dogs following SBBfb, and most will manifest clinically within 24 hours of the biopsy [3–5, 11]. Approximately 5% of cases undergoing SBBfb experience fatal adverse events [3, 4, 11]. The development of de novo neurologic deficits or exacerbation of pre-existing neurologic deficits are the most common adverse event associated with SBBfb, and these deficits resolve within one week in the majority of cases [3, 11]. Seizures, surgical site infections, and tumor seeding along the biopsy tract are other reported complications of SBBfb [3–5]. Intracranial hemorrhage is the most frequent and importantly implicated cause of postoperative adverse events [3–5, 11]. In one study of dogs with brain tumors diagnosed with SBBfb, the presence of T2W heterogenous tumors and platelet counts lower than 185 000 mm^3 were identified as risk factors for the development of postoperative adverse events [11].

Some neurosurgeons perform a CT scan of the brain immediately after completion of the procedure to evaluate for the presence of intracranial hemorrhage [3, 4, 11]. While post-biopsy CT is valuable for the identification of intracranial hemorrhage, it is not predictive of the subsequent development of adverse events as asymptomatic intracranial hemorrhage was observed in over 50% of dogs that recovered uneventfully following SBBfb [11].

The other major complication of brain biopsy is a failed procedure, which occurs when biopsy specimens are unable to be collected, are non-diagnostic, or not representative of the primary underlaying pathology present in the patient. The performance of intraoperative cytology (Figure 19.3) and the collection of multiple brain biopsy specimens are techniques that can reduce the likelihood of failed brain biopsy [3–5, 15, 18].

Processing of Brain Biopsy Specimens

A primary intraoperative objective should be to confirm whether brain tissue satisfactory for an eventual definitive diagnosis has been obtained, and this can be facilitated by performing intraoperative touch or smear cytologic preparations [3, 18]. Tissue preparations intended for cytological evaluation are wet fixed with 95% alcohol and can be stained with Giemsa, hematoxylin and eosin (H&E), or toluidine blue. Although intraoperative specimens provide excellent cytologic detail and can generally determine if the biopsy is of sufficient quality, definitive and specific diagnosis of brain tumors and encephalitides often requires histopathologic examination of formalin fixation, paraffin embedded biopsy tissue (Figure 19.3) [15, 18]. In cases in which multiple biopsies are obtained, the authors sharply divide one biopsy specimen perpendicular to the axis of the needle trajectory immediately after harvesting and preserve it for ancillary diagnostic investigations [3]. Consultation with a pathologist is recommended prior to performance of the biopsy such that tissues can be adequately prepared and preserved for ancillary diagnostic tests appropriate for the patient's differential diagnoses [18].

Contemporary SBBfb techniques are associated with an overall diagnostic yield of $\geq$90% [3, 4]. Generally, diagnostic yields tend to be higher in dogs with intracranial tumors compared to inflammatory brain lesions [3, 4, 10]. The diagnostic accuracy of SBBfb is also higher in dogs with meningiomas compared to other types of brain tumors, with glioma grade being a frequent source of diagnostic discordance [4, 15].

Frameless Stereotactic Brain Biopsy (SBBfl)

With the advent of modern neuronavigation technology, SBBfl has become more available in veterinary medicine [6, 7, 19]. The frameless neuronavigation system utilizes typically a pointer system along with fiducials. This stereotactic technique allows for mapping of the brain onto a three-dimensional (3D) coordinate system by utilizing preoperative imaging, typically MR imaging or CT, in conjunction with fiducials. The fiducials are attached to the patient's head and used as reference to allow for the definition and calibration of the surgical space relative to the patient's head on the images. Targets are then chosen based on the reference system to guide the biopsy needle through a small burr-hole toward the intended lesion in real time. One major advantage of a frameless system is that preoperative imaging can be done without a frame with fiducials attached to the patient instead. This then allows the flexibility of performing the biopsy procedure on a separate day outside of the imaging gantry [6, 7, 19, 20].

Currently, there are two described SBBfl systems in the veterinary literature [6, 7]. Both of these systems utilize neuronavigation. The MR imaging-guided modified Brainsight™ stereotactic system (Rogue Research, Montreal, Quebec) was able to target the caudate nucleus, thalamus, and midbrain of canine cadaver brains with a mean needle placement error of 1.79 +/− 0.87 mm with an upper bound of error at 3.31 mm [6]. The CT-guided Radionics Omnisight™ Excel system (Integra Radionics, Burlington, MA) was able to target various brain lesions in canine cadaver brain with a mean application accuracy of 2–3.9 mm [7]. Both systems supported the use of this system for canine brain lesions > 3.31 mm [6] and 3.9 mm [7], respectively. The main difference between the two systems was the attachment of the fiducials. The MR imaging-guided system had fiducials attached to the patient via a dental bite block while the CT-guided system had the fiducials attached to the position device rather than a separate dental mold. Both systems have been used successfully in live dogs with naturally occurring intracranial diseases [7, 21].

SBBfl Technique

The modified Brainsight™ frameless stereotactic system will be described (Video 19.1) [6, 21]. This system was modified to accommodate the variable sizes of the canine skull. Components of this stereotactic system include a standard computer with Brainsight™ neuronavigation software, Polaris® Vicra optical position sensor, surgical headclamp, articulated arm with digital ruler guide and needle, subject tracker, and neuronavigation pointer (Figure 19.4).

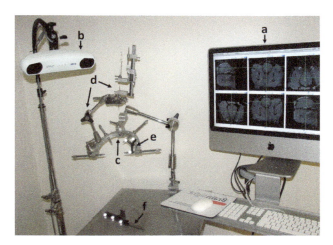

Figure 19.4 Components of the Brainsight™ stereotactic system include a standard computer with Brainsight™ neuronavigation software (a), Polaris® Vicra optical position sensor (b), surgical headclamp (c), articulated arm with digital ruler guide and needle (d), subject tracker (e), and neuronavigation pointer (f).

Attachment of the Fiducial Markers

Fiducial markers are constructed of material visible to MR imaging or CT. They create a disk-shaped hyperintense landmark on the MR images that can be easily identified with the neuronavigation software. Fiducials are generally made from MR-safe plastics and co-labeled with copper sulfate and iodinated contrast [19]. Fiducials need to be firmly attached to the patient because any movement in the fiducials relative to the head can cause registration and sampling error. The closer the fiducials are to the target lesion, the higher the accuracy. Fiducials can be attached to the patient through dental bite blocks or be skull implanted [6, 19, 22]. The placement of the fiducials is strategic so that they are easily visible to the optical position sensor and nonobstructive to the potential entry point of the biopsy needle.

For the dental bite block, thermoplastic dental material is softened in hot water and placed on the custom-made mouthpiece to make a maxillary dental impression (Figure 19.5). Once the dental mold is hardened, the mouthpiece is then secured to the dorsal aspect of the maxilla using a velcro strap and white tape. An adjustable sidebar that extends along the lateral aspect of the maxilla is attached to both sides of the mouthpiece with a starburst articulated joint. This articulated joint can be easily adjusted so that the fiducials can be placed in the best position. Three to four fiducial markers are attached to each sidebar. A small divot is located in the center of each fiducial marker, which is important for the registration procedure (Figure 19.5). This dental mold technique allows positioning reproducibility so that the SBB procedure can be performed under a separate anesthetic event [6].

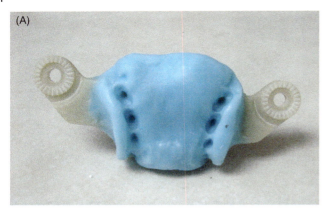

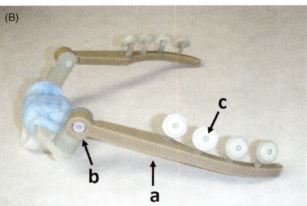

Figure 19.5 Dental bite block. (A) Thermoplastic dental material is softened in hot water and placed on the custom-made mouthpiece to make a maxillary dental impression. (B) Once the dental mold is hardened, the sidebar arms (a) are attached to each side of the mouthpiece via a starburst articulated joint (b). Four fiducial markers are attached to each of the sidebars. The small divot (c) located in the center of each fiducial marker is used for the registration process.

Acquisition of Magnetic Resonance Images

The head with the fiducials attached is positioned in the MR imaging gantry in dorsal recumbency using the appropriately sized imaging coil. Careful attention is needed to make sure no pressure is placed on the fiducials while imaging. It is crucial that the fiducials are in the same position for the biopsy procedure as they were during the acquisition of the MR images in order to minimize error. The smallest volume isotropic voxels should be selected without compromising signal-to noise ratio [6, 19]. Signal averaging can also be increased for higher resolution, but this will require longer anesthesia time. A T1W post-contrast 3D sequence is typically acquired with set parameters such as the following on a 1.0 Tesla MR imaging system: TR = 34 ms, TE = 9 ms, flip angle = 45°, FOV = 260 mm, 0.9×0.9×0.9 mm³ voxels, 256×256 matrix, 2 signal averages [6]. FLAIR images can also be obtained and overlaid on top of the T1W post-contrast images to identify the perilesional edema if present. MR images are then uploaded and saved to the Brainsight™ neuronavigation software. The dental bite block with the fiducials can be removed and saved for later use. Careful attention is needed to keep the fiducials undisturbed and in the same position.

Registration Procedure

On the day of the biopsy procedure, the dental bite block with fiducials is reattached to the patient. In the surgical suite, the head is placed in ventral recumbency in the surgical headclamp using skull screws. Typically, two screws are placed just ventral to the temporal line on either side, and two screws are placed just ventral to the nuchal crest on either side (Figure 19.6). The skull screws are specifically designed to be rigidly fixed to the skull without penetrating through. It is important for the head to be stable and secured so that it remains in the same position relative to the headclamp for the entire procedure. The subject tracker with three reflective spheres is then attached to the surgical headclamp to act as the reference coordinate system. The Polaris® optical position sensor is placed in a position so that it can visualize the reflective spheres on the subject tracker and the neuronavigation pointer. The tip of the neuronavigation pointer will be placed in the divot of each fiducial marker on the cadaver's head in succession, corresponding to the homologous markers on the MR image which is displayed on the neuronavigation computer screen (video). Once all the fiducial markers are registered, the neuronavigation software applies a least square fit to map the surgical space to the image space. The neuronavigation pointer can be

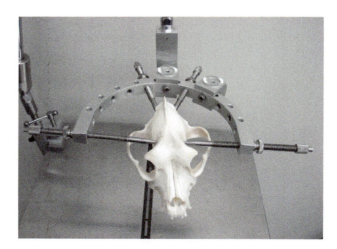

Figure 19.6 The skull is attached to the surgical C-shaped headclamp using four specifically engineered skull screws. Two screws are placed ventral to the nuchal crest on either side while the other two screws are placed just ventral to the temporal like on either side.

moved to various locations on the scalp surface and its corresponding location is displayed in real-time on the computer screen (video). It is important to note that there are other systems that utilize a patient position device for the head; therefore, not utilizing a surgical head frame [7].

Trajectory Planning

The neuronavigation pointer will be placed in the instrument sleeve of the articulated arm to determine a favorable path to the brain lesion (target) using the Brainsight^{TM} software. The shortest trajectory to the target will be chosen to minimize tissue trauma while also avoiding critical brain structures such major vasculatures and the ventricular system. Once the favorable path is determined, the articulated arm is locked in position. With the feedback capability of the neuronavigation system, the trajectory path chosen can be checked by looking at the corresponding 3D MR images to assure the surgeon that critical areas of the brain are missed (video). The target approach can also be altered easily to accommodate a different entry point during the biopsy procedure without having to reimage the patient. Once the fiducials are registered, the patient's head attached to the headclamp can be rotated as a unit in different positions to allow for best access to a specific entry point on the skull.

Brain Biopsy

With the articulated arm locked in place, the neuronavigation pointer is lowered down to the zeroing platform and the distance from the platform to target is measured by the neuronavigation software. A twist drill is then inserted in the instrument sleeve and a 5 mm craniectomy hole is made in the skull (Video 19.1). The twist drill can be set to only drill a specific depth based on the skull thickness at the entry point. If the drill is slipping due to the irregular skull contour, the locked articulated arm can be temporarily removed as a unit to allow drilling of the skull with a pneumatic drill. The articulated arm can easily be placed back on the headclamp in the same position. Minor adjustments can be made with the pointer in the instrument sleeve to make sure needle tip is still on target.

A 16- or 14-gauge (approximately 1.6–2 mm diameter) side-cutting biopsy needle with a lateral window of 5–10 mm is typically used for the brain biopsy procedure. The side-cutting needle has both an inner and outer cannula and the window can be closed or open. The digital ruler guide with the biopsy needle attached is inserted in the instrument sleeve. The needle in the closed position is lowered manually to the zeroing platform, and the digital ruler guide is then set to zero. With the platform removed,

the closed needle is manually lowered to the previously determined depth to reach target, utilizing the digital ruler guide. Once at target, the window of the needle is opened, and a 3-cc syringe system is attached to the needle. Gentle negative pressure is applied by aspirating up to 2-cc, and the window is closed by twisting the inner cannula 180° against the outer cannula [23]. The inner canula is then removed with the syringe system attached and the biopsy sample can be visualized in the window (video). Once the biopsy sample is removed, the inner cannula is flushed with saline and reinserted in the outer cannula to obtain more samples. This procedure can be repeated multiple times, and the window of the outer cannula can be rotated to sample various parts of the brain lesion. Once the biopsy is completed, the needle is removed slowly from the brain. If hemorrhage is flowing out of the needle, it is best to allow that to cease before pulling the needle. The surgical site is then lavaged, and a piece of gel foam can be placed in the burr-hole. The surgical site is closed in routine fashion.

Biopsy Sample Processing

Biopsy samples can be used to make touch or smear impressions for cytology and placed in formalin for histopathology and immunohistochemistry analysis [3, 18]. Frozen sections (FS) can also be used if immediate diagnosis is needed for therapeutic purposes. In human medicine, FS is routinely performed for suspect brain tumors to assess the adequacy of the submitted tissue particularly in the setting of stereotactic brain biopsies [24, 25]. This is not commonly done in veterinary medicine because it requires an onsite pathologist experienced in FS who understands the common challenges and limitations that can be faced with FS in the diagnosis of CNS lesions. Obtaining multiple SBB samples has been shown to increase the diagnostic yield [25]. Three to four biopsy samples are ideally taken, assuming the patient is stable under anesthesia and excessive hemorrhage is not encountered.

Conclusion

Both SBBfb and SBBfl are considered safe and effective for biopsy of intracranial lesions [7, 21]. More clinical studies are needed on the diagnostic accuracy of SBBfl in veterinary medicine. In human medicine, the diagnostic accuracy of both systems is comparable [20]. In a recent meta-analysis, there was no significant difference in either biopsy diagnostic yield or the presence of negative clinical outcomes between techniques [20]. In the absence of any objective evidence to suggest one technique is better than the other, the system used should be based on the neurosurgeon's experience and the system that is readily available.

There are definite advantages to having neuronavigation technology in real-time. With this feedback capability and the ability to register a variety of tools in the virtual space, this technology can be utilized to optimize electrode placement, margin definition for surgical approaches, and image-guided tumor resection. It is important to note that brain shift is inevitable and can occur when the skull or dura is opened. In humans, brain shift up to 5.6 mm can happen from durotomy alone and up to 2 cm during full craniotomy [26–28]. If brain shift happens, the initial image space created is no longer accurate until repeat imaging and registration occur. Having intraoperative imaging capability in the neurosurgical suite can help combat this limitation, but is costly and likely not readily feasible in veterinary medicine.

 Video clips to accompany this book can be found on the companion website at: www.wiley.com/go/shores/advanced

References

1. Gildenberg, P.L. (1990). The history of stereotactic neurosurgery. *Neurosurg. Clin. N. Am.* 1: 765–780.
2. Miller, A.D., Miler, A.C., and Rossmeisl, J.H. (2019). Canine primary intracranial cancer: a clinicopathologic review of glioma, meningioma, and choroid plexus tumors. *Front. Oncol.* 9: 1151.
3. Rossmeisl, J.H., Andriani, R.T., Cecere, T.E. et al. (2015). Frame-based stereotactic biopsy of canine brain masses: technique and clinical results in 26 cases. *Front. Vet. Sci.* 2: 20.
4. Koblik, P.D., LeCouteur, R.J., Higgins, R.J. et al. (1999). CT-guided brain biopsy using a modified Pelorus Mark III stereotactic system: experience with 50 dogs. *Vet. Radiol. Ultrasound* 40: 434–440.
5. Moissonnier, P., Blot, S., Devauchelle, P. et al. (2002). Stereotactic CT-guided brain biopsy in the dog. *J. Small Anim. Pract.* 43: 115–123.
6. Chen, A.V., Wininger, F.A., Frey, S. et al. (2012). Description and validation of a magnetic resonance imaging-guided stereotactic brain biopsy device in the dog. *Vet. Radiol. Ultrasound* 53: 150–156.
7. Taylor, A.R., Cohen, N.D., Fletcher, S. et al. (2013). Application and machine accuracy of a new frameless computed-tomography-guided stereotactic system in dogs. *Vet. Radiol. Ultrasound* 54: 332–342.
8. Young, B.D., Fosgate, G.T., Holmes, S.P. et al. (2014). Evaluation of standard magnetic resonance characteristics used to differentiate neoplastic, inflammatory, and vascular brain lesions in dogs. *Vet. Radiol. Ultrasound* 55: 399–406.
9. Diangelo, L., Cohen-Gadol, A., Heng, H.G. et al. (2019). Glioma mimics: magnetic resonance imaging characteristics of granulomas in dogs. *Front. Vet. Sci.* 6: 286.
10. Flegel, T., Oevermann, A., Oechtering, G., and Matiasek, K. (2012). Diagnostic yield and adverse effects of MRI-guided free-hand brain biopsies through a mini-burr hole in dogs with encephalitis. *J. Vet. Intern. Med.* 23: 969–976.
11. Shinn, R.L., Kani, Y., Hsu, F.C. et al. (2020). Risk factors for adverse events occurring after recovery from stereotactic brain biopsy in dogs with primary intracranial neoplasia. *J. Vet. Intern. Med.* 34: 2021–2028.
12. James, M.D., Bova, F.J., Rajon, D.A. et al. (2017). Novel MRI and CT compatible stereotactic brain biopsy system in dogs using patient-specific facemasks. *J. Sm. Anim. Pract.* 58: 615–621.
13. Gutmann, S., Winkler, D., Muller, M. et al. (2020). Accuracy of a magnetic resonance imaging-based 3D printed stereotactic brain biopsy device in dogs. *J. Vet. Intern. Med.* 34: 844–851.
14. Shinn, R.L., Park, C., DeBose, K. et al. (2021). Feasibility and accuracy of 3D printed patient specific skull contoured brain biopsy guides. *Vet. Surg.*; e-pub 5/11/2021 ahead of print https://doi.org/10.1111/vsu.13641.
15. Kani, Y., Cecere, T., Lahmers, K. et al. (2019). Diagnostic accuracy of stereotactic brain biopsy for intracranial neoplasia in dogs: comparison of biopsy, surgical resection, and necropsy specimens. *J. Vet. Intern. Med.* 33: 1384–1391.
16. Riche, M., Amelot, A., Peyre, M. et al. (2021). Complications after frame-based stereotactic brain biopsy: a systematic review. *Neurosurg. Rev.* 44: 301–307.
17. Sidhu, D.S., Ruth, J.D., Lambert, G. et al. (2017). An easy to produce and economical three-dimensional brain phantom for stereotactic computed tomographic-guided brain biopsy training in the dog. *Vet. Surg.* 46: 621–630.
18. Vernau, K.M., Higgins, R.J., Bollen, A.W. et al. (2001). Primary canine and feline nervous system tumors: intraoperative diagnosis using the smear technique. *Vet. Pathol.* 38: 47–57.
19. Wininger, F. (2014). Neuronavigation in small animals: development, techniques and applications. *Vet. Clin. North Am. Samll Anim. Pract.* 44 (6): 1235–1248.
20. Kesserwan, M.A., Ahakil, H., Lannon, M. et al. (2021). Frame-based versus frameless stereotactic brain

biopsies: a systematic review and meta-analysis. *Surg. Neurol. Int.* 12 (52): 1–8.

21. Chen, A.V., Tucker, R.L., Haldorson, G.J. et al. (2011). Clinical evaluation of a magnetic resonance imaging guided frameless stereotactic brain biopsy system in the dog. *J. Vet. Intern. Med.* 25: 751–752.

22. Long, S., Frey, S., Freestone, D.R. et al. (2014). Placement of deep brain electrodes in the dog using the Brainsight frameless stereotactic system: a pilot feasibility study. *J. Vet. Intern. Med.* 28: 189–197.

23. Schneider, A.R., Chen, A.V., and Haldorson, G.J. (2010). Evaluation of a 14 and 16 gauge side-cutting biopsy needle and four different aspiration pressures used to obtain brain tissues from dogs. *J. Vet. Intern. Med.* 24: 743.

24. Obeidat, F.N., Awad, H.A., Mansour, A.T. et al. (2019). Accuracy of frozen section diagnosis of brain tumors: an 11 year experience from a tertiary care center. *Turk. Neurosurg.* 29 (2): 242–246.

25. Brainard, J.A., Prayson, R.A., and Barnett, G.H. (1997). Frozen section evaluation of stereotactic brain biopsies: diagnostic yield at the stereotactic target position in 188 cases. *Arch. Pathol. Lab. Med.* 121 (5): 481–484.

26. Kuhnt, D., Bauer, M.H., and Nimsky, C. (2012). Brain shift compensation and neurosurgical image fusion using intraoperative MRI: current status and future challenges. *Crit. Rev. Biomed. Eng.* 40: 175–185.

27. Harkens, T., Hill, D.L., Castellano-Smith, A.D. et al. (2003). Measurement and analysis of brain deformation during neurosurgery. *ILEE Trans. Med. Imaging* 22: 82–89.

28. Roberts, D.W., Hartov, A., Kennedy, F.E. et al. (1998). Intraoperative brain shift and deformation: a quantitative analysis of cortical displacement in 28 cases. *Neurosurgery* 43: 749–758.

20

Surgical Management of Sellar Masses

Tina Owen, Annie Chen-Allen and Linda Martin

Washington State University, Pullman, WA, USA

Introduction

Hypophysectomy is the removal of the pituitary gland. Transsphenoidal hypophysectomy (TSH) is the removal of the pituitary gland via the sphenoid bone. Victor Horsley, a human neurosurgeon, experimentally approached the pituitary gland in two dogs through a temporal approach in 1886. He performed surgery on two animals that survived five and six months after removal of the pituitary gland. Horsley went on to become the first to expose and remove a pituitary adenoma with a successful outcome in a human case in 1889 [1].

In veterinary medicine in 1968, Rijnberk et al. performed hypophysectomy for pituitary dependent hyperadrenocorticism (PDH) in four dogs. All four dogs improved after hypophysectomy; they had hair regrowth, resolution of their pendulous abdomen, and became stronger in their gait [2]. Aleida Lubberink in her thesis entitled: 'Diagnosis and Treatment of Canine Cushing's Syndrome', in 1977, compared the results of treatment of hyperadrenocorticism in the dog by surgical hypophysectomy and by chemotherapy with o,p'-DDD. In this case series of 28 dogs with PDH treated by hypophysectomy, 12 of 28 patients made a complete recovery, 6/28 improved but without complete recovery or with considerably delayed recovery, 4/28 had no improvement, 1 was lost to follow up and 5/28 died within one week after surgery [3].

Between 1970 and 1997, with the exception of Lubberink's thesis, there were no clinical studies reported on hypophysectomy in dogs [4]. A transoral approach to hypophysectomy via mandibular symphysiotomy in the dog was described [5]. Niebauer described a new localization technique using metallic bone markers and venous sinus angiography in a terminal setting in an attempt to improve localization of the pituitary gland [6]. Niebauer

and Lantz both published on hypophysectomy in clinically normal dogs, assessing the surgical technique, hormonal abnormalities, and completeness of resection [7, 8]. The surgical approach in these studies was followed as described by Markowitz et al. in 1964 [9]. The patient was placed in dorsal recumbency with the maxilla parallel with the table and the mandible pulled back over a metal bar. There were several studies done in clinically normal dogs assessing this surgical technique, survival, and the ability to remove the pituitary gland in its entirety; however, there were no case series on the treatment of PDH using hypophysectomy [4, 6–8]. Studies began again in earnest in 1993 at Utrecht University on TSH in the dog. Meij, through several publications, concluded that the surgical approach was better carried out in sternal recumbency with the maxilla held open over a bar [10, 11]. Sternal recumbency improved anatomic visualization, reduced intracranial pressure, and allowed easier suctioning of fluid, blood, and bone debris, reducing potential postoperative dyspnea. Meij also preferred the extraction technique for removal of the pituitary gland rather than the suction technique. The extraction technique utilizes a small ball-tipped probe and neurosurgical graspers to remove the pituitary gland. Meij reported the results of TSH in 52 dogs with PDH in 1998 [11]. The one- and two-year survival rate was 84% and 80% respectively [11]. This paper and subsequent papers out of Utrecht University initiated a resurgence of TSH for PDH [11–13]. These studies laid the groundwork for other groups to perform TSH for not only PDH in dogs but for PDH in cats, hypersomatotropism (HST) in cats, and for non-functional or silent pituitary tumors [14–18].

Currently, indications for TSH in veterinary medicine are PDH in dogs and cats, HST in cats, and clinical, non-functional sellar tumors in dogs and cats.

Advanced Techniques in Canine and Feline Neurosurgery, First Edition. Edited by Andy Shores and Brigitte A. Brisson.
© 2023 John Wiley & Sons, Inc. Published 2023 by John Wiley & Sons, Inc.
Companion site: www.wiley.com/go/shores/advanced

Treatment options other than surgery for clinical pituitary masses include medical management and radiation therapy. Medical management for dogs with PDH includes the following drugs: trilostane, mitotane, selegiline, ketoconazole, pasireotide, and cabergoline with varying degrees of success [19–24]. Trilostane has also been used to treat cats with PDH [25]. HST in cats is medically treated using increasing insulin doses, with little success, but pasireotide has had some minimally positive effect for HST in cats [26]. Non-functional sellar masses in the dog and cat have been treated medically with a corticosteroid to control brain edema.

As with medical management, radiation therapy has been used with varying degrees of success to treat pituitary tumors in dogs and cats. Throughout the literature there are an array of protocols that have been proposed in an attempt to shrink the pituitary tumor and control the clinical signs, be they endocrine or neurologic [27–33]. Neither radiation therapy nor medical management offer a cure for patients with pituitary tumors. They may ameliorate clinical signs and/or shrink the pituitary tumor, but either treatment option is rarely curative. Surgical treatment for clinical pituitary tumors is the only treatment modality that offers a cure, can provide decompression and a rapid resolution of clinical signs, and provide a definitive diagnosis.

An extensive discussion on medial and radiation treatment of pituitary tumors in the dog and cat is beyond the scope of this book chapter.

Case Selection

Case selection for hypophysectomy in veterinary medicine is dependent on clinical signs, endocrine testing, tumor size, and concurrent co-morbidities in a given patient. Dogs diagnosed with PDH, showing endocrine signs (polyuria (PU)/polydipsia (PD), truncal alopecia, polyphagia, panting etc.), and with or without a definable pituitary mass based on brain imaging, are candidates for TSH. Clinical signs may be controlled with medical management but rarely is the pituitary tumor quiescent. If the pituitary gland is not enlarged, then based on counseling, owners may choose to treat medically and monitor pituitary growth with serial imaging. Some dogs diagnosed with PDH fail medical therapy and, therefore, owners may pursue treatment with surgery.

Cats diagnosed with HST without significant co-morbidities are excellent candidates for TSH. Cats with HST typically suffer from severe insulin resistant diabetes mellitus (DM), and the hallmark of successful treatment is hypophysectomy [16, 18].

Dogs and cats with pituitary or sellar tumors may present with only neurologic signs without evidence of endocrine dysfunction. These silent tumors without the clinical manifestation of endocrine disease are considered non-functional sellar masses. Non-functional pituitary tumors do not secrete a sufficient concentration of hormones for detection in the blood nor result in endocrine symptoms [34–36]. Pituitary adenoma is the most common non-functional tumor in dogs and cats. Other tumors of the sellar region are meningioma, craniopharyngioma, pituitary carcinoma, and leptomeningeal oligodendrogliomatosis [17, 37].

Currently, dogs considered for TSH are those [38]:

- diagnosed with PDH with a normal size pituitary gland;
- diagnosed with PDH who have failed medical management and have either a normal-sized or enlarged pituitary gland;
- diagnosed with PDH who have an enlarged pituitary tumor with or without neurologic signs;
- diagnosed with a non-functional sellar mass causing neurologic signs or otherwise documentation of tumor growth.

Currently cats considered for TSH are those [38]:

- diagnosed with PDH or HST and a normal or enlarged pituitary gland;
- diagnosed with DM exhibiting insulin resistance secondary to HST;
- diagnosed with a non-functional sellar mass causing neurologic signs or otherwise documentation of tumor growth.

Patients being considered for TSH must have a complete work up with their veterinarian and consultation with either an internal medicine specialist, neurologist, or both. Owners need to be fully informed of the treatment options for pituitary tumors to include medical management, radiation therapy, and surgery. Owners must understand the limitations and complications of each treatment modality in order to make a fully informed decision as to how to proceed.

Tumor size does play a role in the successful outcome after surgery and potential long-term complications [13, 39, 40]. The bigger the tumor, the higher the mortality rate, the shorter the disease-free interval and survival time, the higher the recurrence rate, and the longer a patient may require desmopressin acetate (DDAVP) post-surgery to effectively treat central diabetes insipidus (CDI) [13, 40]. Sato et al. developed and published on a tumor classification system to aide in preoperative prognostic evaluation of dogs with PDH with respect to stage and tumor size [39]. Five stages were established according to extent of tumor growth: Grade 1, no tumor extension beyond the dorsum sellae; Grade 2, tumor extension beyond the dorsum sellae up to the third ventricle but no contact with the optic chiasm and mamillary body; Grade 3, tumor extension beyond the dorsum sellae up to the third ventricle and contact with the optic chiasm and/or mamillary body but not the interthalamic adhesion; Grade 4, tumor extension beyond the dorsum sellae and contact with the optic chiasm, mammillary body, and interthalamic adhesion; and Grade 5, tumor occupation of the third ventricle. Tumors were further classified as either Type A or Type B, without or with involvement of the arterial circle or the cavernous sinus, respectively. Sato concluded that dogs with type A, Grades 1, 2, and 3 had a good prognosis following TSH. Grade 3B, 4, and 5 classifications may not be suitable for this surgery as incomplete resection and recurrence rate may be higher with these grades [39]. However, debulking and adjunctive therapy such as radiation and/or chemotherapy may be beneficial when considering surgery for larger masses. Initial debulking to decrease tumor size and decompress, followed by radiation, is an option [39, 41].

Each patient must be screened for current co-morbidities. Routine blood work and urinalysis, coagulation panel, thromboelastography (TEG), appropriate endocrine testing, thoracic radiographs, echocardiogram, abdominal ultrasound, and brain imaging should be performed in all prospective patients. Hypercortisolemia can result in co-morbidities such as diabetes mellitus, recurrent urinary tract or skin infections, hypertension, gallbladder mucoceles, poor wound healing, and hypercoagulability or thromboembolic events [42–46].

Preoperative Work up

Neurologic Exam

A thorough neurologic exam is crucial to the success of TSH. Determining this baseline will help clinicians identify nuances that are important to monitor both pre- and postoperatively. Animals with sellar masses are typically older. With that comes more potential neurologic deficits that may or may not be related to the sellar mass. The art of the neurologic exam is to help decipher what abnormalities are important and pertinent to the sellar mass.

Animals with sellar masses can present with normal neurologic exams [47–52]. Although larger sellar masses can lead to more neurologic deficits, the size of the sellar mass does not always correlate with the severity of neurologic deficits [47, 50, 52]. One published study in dogs with PDH found that the sensitivity of CNS-specific neurologic signs used to predict whether a dog had a pituitary macrotumor (tumor > 10 mm) was low [52]. However, non-specific neurologic signs such as lethargy, mental dullness, and inappetence were found to be highly specific for the

detection of a pituitary macrotumor in dogs with PDH. Sellar masses are typically slow growing in nature allowing the brain to compensate for some time, leading to minimal neurologic deficits. The degree of neurologic dysfunction is often correlated more to tumor type and less to tumor size. Aggressive tumors with rapid growth rate will enlarge quickly, not allowing the surrounding brain to compensate, causing neurologic signs to develop sooner and more severely [52]. These sellar masses can also acutely bleed causing sudden secondary mass effect which can lead to acute neurologic deterioration.

Most animals with functional pituitary masses are neurologically sound at initial presentation [48, 52]. This is because these animals are presenting to the hospital earlier in the course of disease due to clinical signs associated with the hormonal imbalance. Animals with non-functional pituitary masses tend to present with more profound neurologic deficits associated with a larger mass [17, 53]. These animals are usually presenting to the hospital later in the course of disease for a primary neurologic problem since there are no hormonal imbalances of note. In a study evaluating detectable functional and non-functional pituitary masses on magnetic resonance (MR) imaging, neurologic signs were found to be positively associated with increased pituitary/brain (P/B) ratio and MR imaging signs of brain compression (mass effect) [54]. Due to the retrospective nature of this study, not all dogs in this study had endocrine testing and most did not have histopathologic confirmation that the mass was of pituitary origin. Overall, the most common complaint noticed by the owners is usually associated with mentation changes [47, 50–52, 54–56]. Dogs with altered mental status had significantly higher odds of brain compression than other dogs [54]. The onset of these signs is usually non-specific and somewhat insidious, such as subtle lethargy and inappetence. This can progress to more obvious disorientation, dullness, obtundation, and stupor [47, 50–52, 54–56]. One important thing to note is that the degree of mental dullness can vary throughout the exam dependent on the amount of environmental stimulation. Other behavioral changes such as excessive pacing, circling, head pressing, or aggression can also be seen [47, 50–52, 54–56].

Cranial nerve deficits can also be seen, although this is less common [50, 52, 54, 55, 57–59]. Decreased to absent menace response leading to blindness is the most common cranial nerve finding in dogs showing brain compression on MR imaging [54]. This can be associated with the pituitary mass causing forebrain dysfunction or compression of the optic chiasm, optic nerves, and post-chiasmal tracts leading also to decreased to absent pupillary light reflex [50, 52, 54, 58, 59]. Overall, visual deficits are uncommon in dogs with sellar masses because the pituitary fossa of the dog is covered by an incomplete diaphragma sellae, facilitating dorsal growth of the tumor rather than involving the optic chiasm rostrally [60, 61]. Other cranial nerves can be affected secondary to significant cerebral edema or mass effect that can lead to caudal transtentorial herniation and brainstem compression, particularly at the level of the oculomotor nerve [50, 52, 55, 57].

Gait alterations such as paraparesis, tetraparesis, and ataxia have also been reported [47, 52, 54–57]. These animals can have concurrent proprioceptive deficits. Spinal reflexes are normal to increased indicative of an upper motor neuron dysfunction. Because of the supratentorial location of these masses, these animals will usually remain ambulatory even if the gait is altered. Head and cervical spinal pain can be palpated in 25–50% of dogs with a detectable pituitary mass, likely secondary to brain compression leading to increased intracranial pressure [54, 56].

Seizures are an uncommon manifestation of sellar masses but are reported [50, 52, 55, 56] In fact, it has been suggested that dogs with PDH that have seizures or blindness should not be assumed to have large pituitary masses and other causes should be ruled out first [52]. In even rarer cases, signs related to hypothalamic disturbance, such as adipsia and hyperthermia, are possible [57, 62]. A pituitary macroadenoma causing narcolepsy-cataplexy has also been reported in a dog [63]. It is speculated that the mass caused disruptions in the downstream signaling of hypocretin secondary to the mass effect. Acute neurologic decompensation due to sudden increased intracranial pressure can lead to severe obtundation, pupillary changes, and hypertension with bradycardia (Cushing Reflex).

Preoperative Testing and Diagnostics

In addition to a thorough physical and neurologic examination, the following diagnostics are recommended to establish base-line values for anesthesia and surgery and to identify co-morbidities that may preclude surgery.

- Complete blood count (CBC), serum chemistry panel, and urinalysis.
- Urine culture and susceptibility.
- Coagulation screening – prothrombin time (PT), activated partial thromboplastin time (PTT), TEG, and D-dimer.
- Blood type and cross match.
- Three-view thoracic radiographs.
- Abdominal ultrasound.
- Echocardiogram and electrocardiogram (ECG) – these are specifically important for diabetic cats with HST.

- Serial blood pressures.
- Schirmer tear test (STT).
- Total T4 or full thyroid panel, if indicated.
- Feline Leukemia Virus (FeLV) antigen/Feline Immunodeficiency Virus (FIV) antibody test.

Endocrine Testing

To confirm the presence of a functional sellar mass, endocrine testing will be needed. In brief, low-dose dexamethasone test, high-dose dexamethasone test, endogenous adrenocorticotropic hormone (ACTH), urine cortisol and creatine ratio (UCCR), along with evaluating the adrenal glands on abdominal ultrasound can be used to confirm PDH [51]. HST can be confirmed with an elevation in serum insulin-like growth factor-1 (IGF-1) or growth hormone (GH) [64, 65]. This is especially important in the diabetic and/or acromegalic cat. Measuring IGF-1 is most commonly performed because GH has an extremely short half-life, secretions are pulsatile, and assays are also not widely available in the United States [65, 66]. Endocrine testing is not the focus of this chapter, and it is recommended that readers consult other sources for details. Confirmation of PDH or HST is crucial prior to considering surgery as a treatment option.

Brain Imaging

Magnetic resonance imaging and computed tomography (CT) are the primary modalities used for diagnosing sellar masses in dogs and cats [48, 51, 52, 67]. Brain imaging provides valuable information regarding probable diagnosis and is essential prior to implementing treatment options. With both imaging modalities becoming increasingly available to clinicians, early diagnosis of sellar masses is now possible, which can lead to better prognosis with treatment [13, 38, 51].

Magnetic resonance imaging is the modality of choice for evaluation of sellar masses in humans [68]. MR imaging gives better intracranial anatomic resolution and soft tissue contrast than CT [55, 57]. Intravenous (IV) injection of paramagnetic contrast agent further increases the sensitivity and specificity of MR imaging by better delineating the extent of tumor expansion into the parasellar tissues [55, 69, 70]. Use of CT for evaluation of the brain is more limited due to poor soft tissue contrast and potential artifacts from bone [57]. However, CT can be helpful for surgical planning by providing the exact location of the sellar mass relative to important boney surgical landmarks [15]. CT is also less expensive and does not require anesthesia, making it a convenient modality used for initial screening of sellar masses in dogs and cats [52].

A retrospective study of skull base neoplasia in dogs found pituitary adenomas to be the most common sellar masses, followed by meningiomas. Less common sellar masses included craniopharyngioma, oligodendroglioma, and pituitary adenocarcinoma [37]. Pituitary metastases are rare but have also been reported in dogs with a solitary sellar mass [71, 72].

Imaging of Pituitary Masses

The pituitary gland lies outside of the blood–brain barrier allowing contrast medium in the vascular space to diffuse freely in. Following IV contrast administration, the pituitary gland will enhance on both CT and MR images [48, 73]. The normal pituitary gland is 6–10mm in length, 5–9mm in width, and 4–6mm in height in dogs [74, 75]. These values are highly variable amongst breeds and individual dogs of the same breed and do not account for the size of animal [61, 73]. In cats, the normal pituitary gland measurements are based on whether the cat is brachycephalic or mesocephalic [76]. For brachycephalic cats, the mean pituitary gland sagittal length is 3.14+/−0.30mm, the mean transverse width is 4.44+/−0.27mm, the mean transverse height is 2.42+/−0.21mm. and the mean sagittal height is 2.15+/−0.15mm. For mesocephalic cats, the pituitary gland dimensions are 4.88+/−0.30mm, 4.73+/−0.31mm, 3.09+/−0.26mm, and 2.94+/−0.16mm for mean pituitary gland sagittal length, transverse width, transverse height, and sagittal height, respectively.

Historically, pituitary adenomas were classified into microadenomas (≤10mm) and macroadenomas (>10mm) based on the height of the mass [48, 51, 77]. This is not very applicable in veterinary medicine because pituitary adenomas in the dog that are between 6 and 10mm in height enlarge the gland and, therefore, cannot be classified technically as microadenomas [75]. Instead, some have defined macroadenomas as anything that extends beyond the sella turcica [78, 79].

Pituitary height to brain area ratio is used to standardize the size of the pituitary gland relative to the patient size. P/B ratio is the height of the pituitary in mm/area of the brain in cm^2. The pituitary gland is considered enlarged when the ratio is >0.31 and non-enlarged when the ratio is ≤0.31 in dogs [79]. In cats, the pituitary gland is considered enlarged when the ratio is >0.4. P/B ratio allows for detection of even the smallest increase in height of the pituitary gland and, therefore, it seems appropriate to adjust the definition of microadenomas to adenomas that do not affect the size or shape of pituitary gland [79, 80].

Pituitary tumors can be classified as an adenoma, invasive adenoma, or adenocarcinoma. Adenomas are more likely to be round instead of oval or irregular. Invasive adenoma should be suspected if a dog with a pituitary tumor is <7.7years of age and has a mass >1.9cm in vertical height. Mineralization of the pituitary mass may also indicate an invasive adenoma. The tumor functionality does not predict the tumor type [81].

A five-point MR imaging classification system based on tumor extension in dorsal and cranio-caudal directions has been developed in evaluating pituitary tumors, with grade 1 having no extension and grade 5 having the most extension [39]. Cases were classified as Type A if there was no arterial circle of Willis or cavernous sinus involvement and Type B if these blood vessels were involved. This study concluded that dogs with grade 1–3, Type A classification had better prognosis following TSH. The authors advocated utilizing this classification system in determining whether TSH should be performed [39]. It is important to note that dogs with grades 3–5B have been treated successfully with TSH despite larger tumors having more surgical morbidity and mortality [13, 15, 82].

Dorsal extension of the macroadenoma can cause compression of the hypothalamus and interthalamic adhesion, dorsal displacement of the third ventricle, and dilation of lateral and third ventricles secondary to obstructive hydrocephalus [48, 49, 55, 57]. Cranial extension of the macroadenoma can result in displacement of the optic chiasm and optic tracts [39, 55, 58].

Typical MR imaging features for pituitary tumors are iso- to hyperintense on T2-weighted (T2W) images, iso- to hypointense on T1-weighted (T1W) images and avid homogenous contrast enhancement on T1W post-contrast images (Figure 20.1) [48, 49, 52, 67, 83]. Adenomas are typically round with smooth delineated borders. Hemorrhage within the mass may be seen on the gradient echo T2*W images. MR imaging has been reported to detect pituitary tumors as small as 3mm at the greatest height [48]. Typical CT imaging features for a pituitary tumor are an enlarged isodense mass that enhances homogeneously after contrast administration [73, 80].

Non-enlarged pituitary masses can be difficult to delineate, particularly with CT [49, 84]. With conventional CT, 40% of dogs with microadenomas have a normal size and shape of the pituitary gland [79]. Non-enlarged pituitary masses often cannot be localized on routine contrast enhanced CT images because of isoattenuation and because the enhancement usually represents the secondary capillary phase, which is weaker and less visible [80, 85, 86]. Dynamic contrast enhanced CT can be used identify a so-called pituitary flush [73, 80]. This represents the arterial blood supply of the neurohypophysis (posterior pituitary) that is slightly earlier than the enhancement of the adenohypophysis (anterior pituitary) through the portal blood supply. The displacement, distortion, reduction,

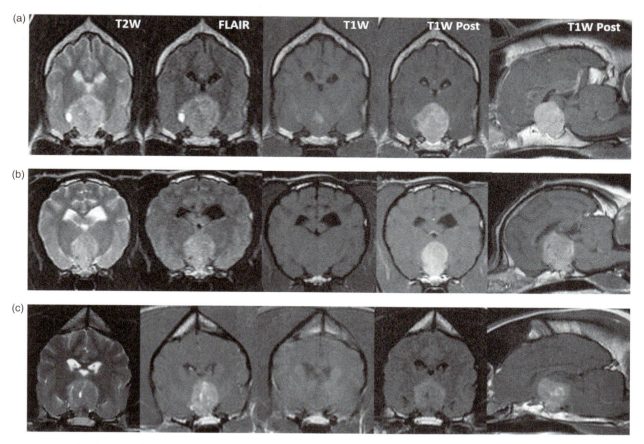

Figure 20.1 MR images of a dog with a pituitary adenoma (a), a meningioma (b), and a craniopharyngioma (c). The MR imaging features are very similar between the three diagnoses. The masses are predominately hyperintense on T2W and FLAIR images, isointense on T1W images, and contrast enhance avidly delineating a discrete, well-marginated circular mass in the area of the sella with dorsal extension into the thalamus causing mass effect.

or disappearance of the pituitary "flush sign" in the early phase of dynamic CT can be used to identify non-enlarged pituitary tumors [80].

The diagnosis of smaller pituitary tumors on MR imaging is influenced by slice thickness [87]. Thicker slices (> 3 mm) may result in false negative finding in dogs with small pituitary tumors [87]. Also, microadenomas may have delayed enhancement, appearing hypointense to the normal pituitary immediately after contrast administration; whereas macroadenomas often show rapid enhancement after contrast administration, possibly due to their increased vascularity, making visualization easier [70, 88]. The posterior lobe (neurohypophysis) can have a high signal intensity on non-contrast T1W images. The high signal intensity represents the density of secretory granules containing arginine vasopressin. Anatomically, the posterior lobe is located slightly to the dorsal side of the center of the pituitary. Displacement of this high signal intensity of the posterior lobe may suggest the presence of an adenoma [89]. The absence of this high signal intensity is not indicative of a pituitary tumor because this hyperintensity is not seen in all pituitary glands of healthy dogs [84, 89]. Overall, a normal pituitary appearance does not exclude the presence of microadenomas because these tumors may not change the size or shape of the pituitary [75].

In acromegalic cats with confirmed pituitary tumors, increased frontal bone thickness and evidence of soft tissue accumulation in the nasal cavity, sinuses, and pharynx have been reported with MR imaging and CT [90]. These findings may be helpful in affected cats with no clinical signs of facial enlargement or upper respiratory disease and may provide further support for the diagnosis of HST.

Imaging of Non-Pituitary Sellar Masses

Non-pituitary origin tumors, such as meningiomas, ependymomas, craniopharyngiomas, oligodendrogliomas, lymphoma, and metastatic neoplasia, can involve the sella [17, 37, 83]. These tumors often have MR imaging characteristics indistinguishable from pituitary tumors

(Figure 20.1) [83]. Associated hemorrhage can also be seen within the tumor similar to pituitary tumors. Because these tumors are non-functional, the P/B ratio is often increased since these animals are presenting later in the disease course after neurologic signs become apparent.

Expansion of the sella along with compression of the parasellar tissues in the cranial, caudal, and dorsal directions are often noted. This can lead to obstructive hydrocephalus and cause dilatation of the lateral and third ventricles [83]. Some of these tumors can grow rapidly and cause rapid neurologic deterioration secondary to acute mass effect. Acute mass effect can then result in perilesional edema and vasogenic edema depicted as T2W and fluid attenuated inversion recovery (FLAIR) hyperintensity in the surrounding brain parenchyma or white matter tracts on MR imaging. Herniation can also be seen on MR imaging secondary to the mass effect, particularly in the area of the tentorium. Overall, imaging diagnosis is presumptive and often much more difficult with non-functional sellar masses. Although the majority of non-functional sellar masses are of pituitary origin [83], definitive diagnosis can only be made with tissue histopathology, not with imaging alone.

Surgery

Anatomy

The pituitary gland is attached to the ventral midline of the brain. The size varies greatly with breed and even among dogs within the same breed [91]. The pituitary gland sits in a boney fossa of the basisphenoid bone at the base of the skull. On the dorsal side of the bone, the rostral extent of the fossa is a minimally elevated boney prominence, the tuberculum sellae. The caudal extent of the pituitary fossa, which tends to be more prominent than the tuberculum sellae, is the dorsum sellae. On the ventral aspect of the skull, the basisphenoid bone where the fossa is located is bounded by the pterygoid bone. There are two projections off the caudal aspect of the pterygoid bone named the hamular process. The center of the pituitary fossa is approximately located between the base of the hamular process and the caudal extent of the tip of the hamular process. In the cat, there is a sphenoid sinus at the rostral extent of the pituitary fossa that can be used as a landmark for localization. The ventral aspect of the basisphenoid bone is covered by mucoperiosteum. At the base of the hamular process there are two slits in the mucoperiosteum which are the entry into the eustachian canal.

The pituitary gland is covered by dura mater which divides into two layers laterally and contains the paired cavernous sinus in which the internal carotid artery passes. The cavernous sinus is lateral to the pituitary gland and is connected caudal to the dorsum sellae by the caudal intercavernous sinus and rostral to the dorsum sellae by the rostral intercavernous sinus. There is on occasion a third fragile sinus connecting the cavernous sinus rostral to the hypophysis [91].

The internal carotid artery enters the skull via the tympanooccipital fissure, transverses the carotid canal, as it passes rostrally it passes ventrally through the foramen lacerum, forms a loop, and reenters the cranial cavity through the same foramen. Upon reentering the cranial cavity, the internal carotid artery perforates a layer of dura to enter the cavernous sinus that is contained within the dura and courses rostrally within the cavernous sinus, at first obliquely toward the dorsum sellae, then directly rostral to the level of the optic chiasm. Here the artery again perforates the cavernous sinus and the adjacent dura and arachnoid and comes to lie in the subarachnoid space. It then branches into the rostral cerebral, middle cerebral, and caudal communicating arteries [92].

The arterial blood supply to the hypophysis is from the arterial circle. The arterial circle, on the ventral surface of the brain, is formed by the right and left rostral cerebral arteries and their rostral communicating arteries, the caudal communicating arteries from the internal carotid arteries and the basilar artery. Several rostral hypophyseal arteries leave the caudal communicating artery to supply the stalk of the hypophysis. These vessels supply the major portion of the gland. The pars nervosa is supplied by the caudal hypophyseal artery, a branch of the caudal intercarotid artery [92].

The oculomotor, trochlear, and abducent nerves and the ophthalmic branch of the trigeminal nerve pass in close proximity to the hypophysis [4]. The oculomotor nerve lies caudal lateral to the hypophysis and the optic chiasm lies immediately rostral to the hypophysis. These two nerves are typically those nerves in the vicinity of the hypophysis that may be damaged during TSH.

Localization

Localization of the pituitary fossa has been described and is dependent on proximity to equipment and comfort level with the chosen system [15, 93, 94]. Unfortunately, the pituitary fossa can vary in location and is significantly dependent on breed, skull anatomy, and size of the patient. CT imaging and localization of landmarks with respect to the location of the pituitary fossa has been described [93]. Given the angle of the head and angle of drilling, navigation to the exact location of the pituitary fossa can be challenging. Drilling two pilot holes through the outer cortex of the basisphenoid bone at the approximate location of the pituitary fossa followed by a CT imaging for surgical planning and measurement is very helpful in locating the exact position of the pituitary fossa and accounts for the drilling angle [15]. The eustachian slits and the point at which the hamular process of the pterygoid bone enters the base of the skull can be used as a rough estimation of the location of the pituitary fossa. The latter being an anatomic location visible on the CT imaging. Drilling two pilot holes allows for precise measurement and location of the bone window using the location of the pilot holes on the CT [15]. A neuronavigational system, Brainsight™, can also be used for localization of the pituitary fossa [94].

Positioning

The patient is positioned in sternal recumbency with the canine teeth suspended over a metal bar encircled by rubber. The maxilla is taped to the bar for security so the head will not move for the duration of the surgery. The surgery table is tilted to approximately 40° to allow in-line observation of the hard palate and basisphenoid bone [15]. A roll gauze is secured to one side of the front of the surgery table, passed over the mandible, behind the canines, and secured to the opposite side of the surgery table. The roll gauze is not tightened until surgery commences and once tightened, is released and the mandible is put through a range of motion for 1 minute every 30 minutes (every 20 minutes in cats). The patient's rear legs are placed into a harness which is secured to the front of the table to prevent slipping and relieve pressure on the head and neck when the table is tilted. The chest and neck of the dog are supported with either towels or a surgical positioning vacuum pad, and a heating blanket is placed over the patient. Ophthalmic ointment is liberally applied to both eyes and the eyelids are taped shut. The oral cavity is wiped out with dilute chlorhexidine solution. The oropharynx is packed with moistened radiopaque sponges. The head is draped, maintaining an opening to the mouth.

Approach

The surgical approach to the pituitary gland is a transsphenoidal approach and was initially described by Meij et al. [93]. It is an open mouth procedure, through the soft palate to the base of the skull. The surgery is performed using the VITOM system, a high-definition (HD) exoscope, for better magnification and visualization (Karl Storz-Endoskope, Tuttlingen, Germany) (Figure 20.2). The surgeon operates looking at the HD screen during the remainder of the surgery (Figure 20.3).

Palpation of the hamular process of the pterygoid bone facilitates approximation of the location of the incision into the soft palate. A midline incision in the soft palate, using either a CO^2 LASER or scalpel blade, is centered over the location of the hamular process and held open by stay sutures, small gelpi retractors, or a ring retractor. The mucoperiosteum is incised on midline and elevated off the basisphenoid bone to expose the sutures of the basisphenoid bone. Identification of the sutures allows drilling to proceed on midline. It is very important to keep the boney window on midline to avoid inadvertent injury to the surrounding vasculature. Using either measurements from CT imaging, correlating measurements associated with the pilot holes and the CT image, or neuronavigation, the rostrocaudal and lateral extents of the sella are marked with the drill. Drilling of the basisphenoid bone is performed with a high-speed drill with an elongated and angled tip with a 2 mm diamond burr. The table is tilted at 40°, to allow for perpendicular drilling of the basisphenoid bone. It is necessary to direct the drill in a rostral trajectory to prevent inadvertent drilling in the caudal direction which can be catastrophic. Drilling progresses, through the outer cortex, through the medullary bone to the inner cortical bone, until there is a thin layer of the inner cortical bone present. Dependent on tumor size the bluish hue of the cavernous sinus can generally be seen at the lateral edges of the bone window and is avoided. Once the boney window is drilled to the desired dimensions, the remaining cortical bone over the pituitary dura is removed with a ball-tipped probe, cup curettes, and Kerrison rongeurs [15].

The dura is opened in a cruciate fashion using a microblade. The normal to mildly enlarged pituitary gland is gently teased around the edges using a ball-point probe to detach it from the fossa and typically removed in its entirety using grasping forceps. For larger tumors that cannot be removed en bloc, initial debulking is carried out using ring curettes, ball-point probes, and teasers (Tew Dissectors, KLS Martin, Jacksonville, FL) (Figure 20.4) to bring the tumor to the center of the fossa and detach it from the surrounding tissues for removal with grasping forceps. Suction can be used to bring the tumor to the boney opening for removal. Aspiration devices (e.g. Myriad; Nico Corp., Indianapolis, IN) with side ports are also useful for drawing tissues toward midline. Hemostasis is obtained by packing the site with gelfoam and surgical patties for several minutes and then removed. This is repeated as necessary to control bleeding. Bovine thrombin-soaked gelfoam may be used in situations where it is difficult to gain adequate hemostasis. The thrombin-soaked gelfoam is removed once hemostasis is achieved. Identification of the opening to the third ventricle and lateral walls of the hypothalamus are important landmarks to indicate extensive

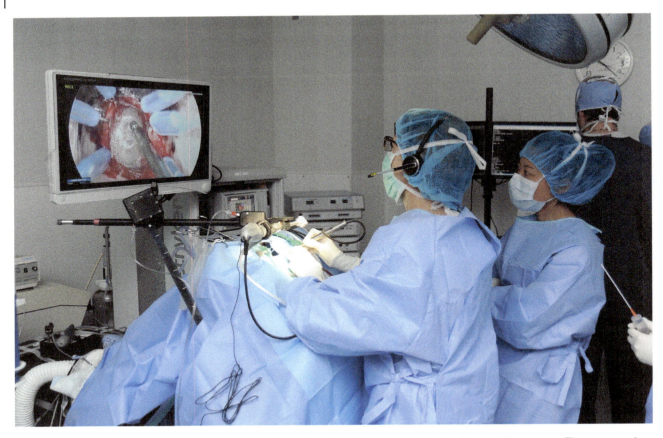

Figure 20.2 With the 90° VITOM exoscope in place, the patient is on the surgery table head toward the surgeon. The exoscope is held in front of the open mouth using a pneumatic scope holder (Wingman Stryker, San Jose, CA). *Source:* Courtesy of Henry Moore Jr, College of Veterinary Medicine/Biomedical Communications Unit, Washington State University, Pullman, WA.

tumor removal. Palpation of the dorsum sella is useful to determine the caudal extent of tumor removal. Probing of the rostral aspect of the boney defect will often yield additional tumor tissue and, therefore, the boney window is opened further rostral to assess for complete tumor removal. When satisfied with complete tumor removal and hemostasis, the surgical site is copiously lavaged. A gelatin hemostatic sponge is placed in the boney defect and covered by a single layer of porcine submucosa as an overlay graft. The soft palate is debrided and closed in two layers.

Surgical Outcome

Dogs with PDH have a remission rate of 86–95% following TSH with a recurrence rate of 25% and a mortality rate of 10–12% [13, 15]. The mortality rate for TSH is defined as death by any cause within four weeks of surgery [11]. Long-term estimated survival rates for dogs with PDH following TSH at one, two, three, and four years were 86%, 79%, 74%, and 72%, respectively [13]. In this same study by van Rijn et al., of 306 dogs with PDH undergoing TSH, the median survival time of 300 dogs for whom follow-up information was available was 781 days, and the median disease-free remission interval was 951 days for 257 dogs with confirmed remission of hypercortisolism after surgery [13]. Over time, 69 of 257 (27%) of the dog with confirmed remission developed recurrence of hypercortisolism after a median period of 555 days [13].

The larger the pituitary mass, the worse the prognosis [13]. A normal P/B ratio is ≤ 0.31. A pituitary tumor is considered enlarged when P/B ratio is > 0.31 [79]. Dogs undergoing TSH with a presurgical P/B ratio > 0.3 had a significantly shorter survival time and a shorter disease-free interval than those with a P/B ratio of ≤ 0.31 [13]. Dogs that died within four weeks of surgery had a significantly higher P/B ratio [13].

The outcome for cats with HST treated with hypophysectomy is reported by Fenn and van Bokhorst [16, 18]. Fenn reported on a group of 68 cats with HST and DM treated by TSH: 85% of cats were alive four weeks postoperative with 10 postoperative deaths; 95% of the 58 surviving cats had improved control of diabetes. Diabetic remission occurred in 41/58 surviving cats with insulin administration discontinued after median of nine days (range 2–120).

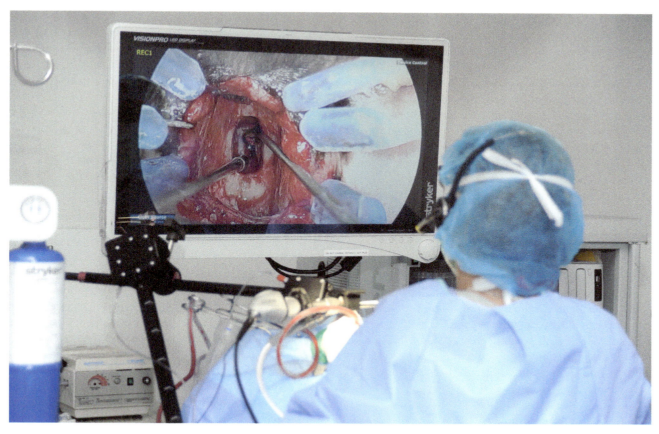

Figure 20.3 The VITOM exoscope (STORZ, Karl Storz-Endoskope, Tuttlingen, Germany) shows how the surgeon views the HD screen positioned over the head of the animal to perform surgery. *Source:* Courtesy of Henry Moore Jr, College of Veterinary Medicine/Biomedical Communications Unit, Washington State University, Pullman, WA.

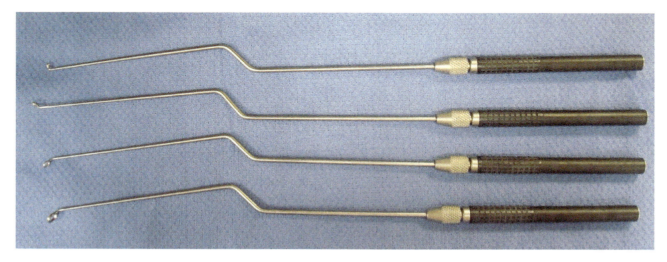

Figure 20.4 Tew (KLS Martin, Jacksonville, FL) neurosurgical instruments are elongated and bayonetted to facilitate use around the exoscope.

Postoperative four-weeks serum IGF-1 concentration nadir was significantly lower in cats achieving diabetic remission. Recurrence of DM occurred in 5 of 41 cats (12%) after a median of 248 days (range 84–1232). Median survival time of all cats was 853 days (range, 1–1740) [16].

van Bokhorst reported on a group of 25 client-owned cats that underwent TSH. One cat died. Normalization of plasma IGF-1 concentration occurred in 23/24 cats, and 22/24 cats entered diabetic remission. Median survival time was 1347 days and the overall one-, two-, and three-year all-cause survival rates were 76%, 76%, and 52% respectively [18].

The outcome for non-functional pituitary tumors in dogs is good to excellent [17, 53]. A study currently in progress reveals the median survival time for 15 dogs with a non-functional sellar mass post TSH is 232 day (range 0–1658 days). For those dogs that survived four weeks postoperatively, the median survival time is 708 days; 73% of the dogs had a non-functional pituitary adenoma; the rest had one of each of the following tumor types: meningioma, ependymoma, craniopharyngioma, and one primitive neuroectodermal tumor. Post TSH, three dogs received chemotherapy, four dogs underwent radiation therapy. and one dog underwent a second TSH surgery [53].

In Hospital Care

Postoperative Management and Monitoring

Following surgery, patients are recovered in an intensive care unit and extubated when they are breathing spontaneously and can protect their airways [11, 15]. Postoperative management of these patients includes monitoring of vital signs, neurological status, fluid intake and output, serum electrolyte concentrations, palate incision site, and tear production. Fluid balance can be assessed by measuring fluid intake, urine output, urine specific gravity, body weight, packed cell volume, total solids, lactate, and central venous pressure. For patients with co-morbidities such as DM, chronic renal failure, or cardiac disease, these conditions are also closely monitored. In the immediate postoperative period, patients are administered glucocorticoids, DDAVP, antibiotics, analgesia, artificial tears, and IV fluid therapy. (See below for specific details.) The administration of IV fluid therapy type, volume, and rate are generally guided by serum electrolyte concentrations, fluid intake, urine output, urine specific gravity, packed cell volume, total solids, lactate, central venous pressure, and acute changes in body weight. Eating and drinking are encouraged following surgery and when the patient can tolerate oral medications, thyroid hormone supplementation is started, and injectable formulations of glucocorticoids, DDAVP, antibiotics, and analgesics are converted to oral medications. Neurological status, visual capabilities, and tear production are also assessed and monitored at regular intervals following surgery.

Postoperative Complications

Endocrine and Metabolic Complications

Central Diabetes Insipidus (CDI). CDI is a polyuric syndrome that results from insufficient production of anti-diuretic hormone (ADH) which results in the inability to concentrate urine for water conservation. Selective resection of pituitary and sellar masses is difficult in animals undergoing TSH and, therefore, the entire pituitary gland including normal tissue is frequently resected [40]. Following complete TSH, there is a sudden cessation of ADH secretion from the neurohypophysis which results in the development of CDI. In the authors' experience, CDI can be transient or permanent, and also partial or complete. This has also been noted in pediatric and adult human patients following surgery to remove pituitary or suprasellar tumors [95]. The development of CDI following TSH may also reflect the sensitivity of the hypothalamic-neurohypophysis to surgical alterations in blood flow, edema, and manipulation of the pituitary stalk when there is incomplete resection of the pituitary gland and/or pituitary mass [11]. Most, if not all, animals will develop CDI following TSH. It can be a transient condition since ADH produced in the hypothalamus can still be secreted into the systemic circulation via the portal capillaries in the median eminence [11, 12] and CDI can resolve within days to months following TSH [11, 12, 15, 40, 96]. There are also reports that CDI can persist for longer time periods (months to years) following TSH [12]. Permanent disturbance of ADH secretion has additionally been documented following TSH in dogs [11, 12, 40], can be due to direct damage to the neurohypophysis or hypothalamic nuclei, and can depend on the size and location of the tumor and extent of the surgical resection [11, 12, 40]. Pituitary tumor extension that occurs in the dorsal direction and results in a prolonged mass effect of the tumor on the hypothalamic nuclei may result in damage to the ADH producing nuclei, such as the paraventricular and supraoptic nuclei [12]. Efforts to completely remove dorsally located tumor tissue in animals with large pituitary tumors may also lead to damage to the pituitary stalk and cell bodies in the hypothalamic nuclei, leading to the development of permanent CDI [12, 97, 98]. The incidence of permanent CDI appears to be higher in dogs with a P/B ratio > 0.31 than in dogs with a P/B ratio ≤ 0.31 [12, 40]. Endogenous and exogenous glucocorticoids can also inhibit ADH release by a direct effect on the hypothalamus and/or neurohypophysis. This inhibition of ADH release is characterized by both an increase in osmotic threshold and a decrease in the sensitivity to increasing osmolality [99, 100]. Additionally, glucocorticoids can cause resistance to the effects of ADH on the kidney, possibly by interfering with the action of ADH at the level of the renal collecting tubules or by decreasing renal tubular permeability to water [40]. These factors may also affect ADH release in the early postoperative period.

The preferred agent for treating postoperative CDI is DDAVP, a synthetic vasopressin analogue. Compared to the natural hormone, DDAVP has a greater anti-diuretic activity, longer duration of action, fewer pressor actions and adverse effects, and a greater capacity to cause platelet aggregation and the release of hemostatic factors [101, 102]. DDAVP is a highly selective agonist for vasopressin V2 receptors, making it an effective treatment for CDI [103]. When given IV or (subcutaneously) SQ to human patients with CDI, DDAVP induces anti-diuresis that lasts from 8 to 24 hours [104]. The duration of action is similar in dogs and cats [105–107]. DDAVP is available for clinical use via nasal or conjunctival sac administration as well as per os (PO), SQ, and IV administration [103, 108]. Although administration of medication to dogs and cats via the intranasal route is possible, it is not well tolerated in some cases. Therefore, the intranasal drops placed in the conjunctival sac are generally a more suitable alternative. Poor or erratic response in some dogs and cats can be due to incomplete absorption caused by conditions that alter the absorptive capacity of the nasal mucosa or from atresia or blockage of the nasolacrimal duct [103] as well as concurrent administration of ophthalmic artificial tear ointment for the treatment of keratoconjunctivitis sicca (KCS) that can occur following TSH. Because of individual differences in absorption and metabolism, the dose required to achieve complete, around-the-clock control varies from animal to animal. Usually 1–4 drops of the intranasal solution (0.01%) administered two to three times daily in the conjunctival sac is sufficient to control the signs of CDI [103]. The maximal effect of the drug is evident 6–10 hours after the administration and the duration of effect of DDAVP varies from 8 to 24 hours [105–107, 109, 110]. The oral preparation of DDAVP is available as 0.1 and 0.2 mg tablets. Each 0.1 mg tablet of DDAVP is comparable to 5 µg (1 large drop) of the intranasal DDAVP preparation and it is generally dosed at 0.1−0.2 mg PO q 8–12 hours [103]. The parenteral dose of DDAVP for CDI is 0.5–2 µg SQ or IV q 12–24 hours [103]. The dose ranges given can be used as a starting point for the treatment of CDI following TSH. The dose is then adjusted based on changes in urine output, urine specific gravity, body weight, packed cell volume, total solids, and sodium concentrations. DDAVP therapy is titrated over time to the lowest dose that controls the patient's clinic signs and is continued until the PU is resolved, the patient can concentrate urine, and serum sodium concentrations remain in the normal reference range.

DDAVP is generally safe for dogs and cats with CDI. The main complications of administration are the development of water intoxication and hyponatremia. These complications can result from overzealous administration of DDAVP in conjunction with failure to reduce IV fluid administration. Serum sodium concentrations should be monitored after the initiation of DDAVP therapy. If hyponatremia develops, treatment with DDAVP should be delayed or temporarily stopped [103].

Hypernatremia can occur following TSH due to ADH deficiency and results from hypotonic or pure water loss via PU. In the immediate postoperative period, rising serum sodium concentrations can reflect the presence of CDI and the development of hypernatremia can be prevented by the administration of DDAVP and appropriate fluid therapy. Prompt diagnosis and treatment of CDI are essential to prevent the extreme alterations in sodium and water balance that accompany this disorder. CDI is easily recognized by the PU that develops early in the postoperative period, commonly occurring within the first 24 hours after TSH [96]. The authors have noted that the development of CDI can occur rapidly following TSH, within one to four hours after surgery. Urine output can be dramatic (> 10 ml/kg/h) and urine specific gravity quickly becomes hyposthenuric (frequently < 1.005) and in addition serum sodium concentrations can rapidly rise (> 160 mEq/l) [40, 96]. Basic requirements of successful management of CDI include meticulous assessment of fluid intake and output, measurement of body weight and of serum electrolyte concentrations. A urinary catheter with a closed collection system is placed preoperatively to monitor urine output intra- and postoperatively. Initially in the postoperative period, fluid intake, urine output, urine specific gravity, body weight, packed cell volume, total solids, central venous pressure, and serum electrolyte concentrations are monitored every three to four hours. Once CDI develops, the volume and/or rate of IV fluid therapy generally needs to be increased to keep up with urinary losses. Intravenous replacement of fluid losses is typically done with lactated Ringer's solution, 0.45% NaCl, 5% dextrose in water, or a combination of these fluid solutions. Patients that can take oral fluids should be allowed to regulate their own intake and water balance. This will help to normalize fluid and sodium imbalances [11, 15, 40]. Serum sodium concentrations should initially be checked every three to four hours until a consistent trend of change has been established, and then sodium monitoring can be adjusted accordingly.

Cerebral Salt Wasting Syndrome (CSWS). CSWS is a disorder of sodium and water handling that occurs as a result of cerebral disease in the setting of normal kidney function. It is characterized by hyponatremia, hypochloremia, and metabolic alkalemia in association with PU and hypovolemia [111]. As the name implies, it is caused by natriuresis and chloruresis. In humans, CSWS is uncommon and can be seen following subarachnoid hemorrhage, cerebral infarction, head injury, neurosurgery, and expansion of intracranial neoplasia [112–114]. In the authors' experience, CSWS has been noted in a few veterinary patients (both cats and dogs) following TSH. The mechanisms underlying CSWS are unclear, but are likely multifactorial and may involve increased concentrations of circulating natriuretic peptides and decreased sympathetic input to the kidney [111, 112, 115]. In humans, CSWS is generally a temporary condition that develops within two to three days of the cerebral insult and usually resolves within a few to several weeks [112]. CSWS and CDI can develop concurrently in human patients, making clinical diagnosis and management extremely challenging [95, 111, 112, 114]. In the authors' experience, we have noted a similar timeline and transient condition in our veterinary patients that developed CSWS following TSH. All cases that developed CSWS, concurrently had CDI.

Differentiating CSWS from other causes of hyponatremia (overzealous administration of DDAVP, over administration of hypotonic or isotonic IV fluid solutions, or the development of the syndrome of inappropriate ADH secretion) is important in postoperative TSH patients [115]. Extracellular volume assessment may be the key factor to distinguish CSWS from the other causes of hyponatremia during recovery from TSH. Overzealous administration of DDAVP, over administration of hypotonic or isotonic IV fluid solutions, and the syndrome of inappropriate ADH secretion generally result in a positive fluid balance whereas CSWS results in fluid volume depletion [115]. Serum bicarbonate concentrations are also increased in CSWS due to large volumes of sodium-rich, chloride-rich, and bicarbonate-poor fluid loss by the kidneys, and many of these cases subsequently develop metabolic alkalemia.

The mainstay of treatment for CSWS is the replacement of sodium, chloride, and water that is lost as a result of pathologic natriuresis, chloruresis, and diuresis. In patients that are hypovolemic, the initial management is the administration of 0.9% NaCl to restore intravascular volume. Once euvolemia is achieved, attention is directed at correcting the hyponatremia by administering IV hypertonic saline solutions. The use of 1.5% sodium chloride solutions can be administered through a peripheral IV catheter, and can safely and effectively restore and maintain intravascular volume and serum sodium concentrations when administered at rates that are titrated to achieve a normal fluid balance [111]. The use of 3% sodium chloride should be reserved for those patients with CSWS who have severe hyponatremia because it must be administered through a central venous catheter and generally cannot be given at rates high enough to restore or maintain intravascular volume [111]. Salt tablets or salt solutions (if the patient will drink them) can also be given orally or they can be given through a feeding tube. Serum sodium concentrations and intravascular volume can also be augmented by administering fludrocortisone at a dose of 0.1–0.2 mg/patient PO q 12 hours [111, 115]. Fludrocortisone can be started once the diagnosis of CSWS is made and continued until serum sodium concentrations and intravascular volume are stable and then weaned off over a period of several days [111]. Fludrocortisone administration can lead to the development of hypokalemia; therefore, serum potassium concentrations should also be monitored closely [111].

Hypoadrenocorticism. Total resection of the pituitary gland which occurs with TSH, not only induces CDI, but also hypoadrenocorticism which requires careful postoperative management by hormone supplementation therapy [116]. Treatment consists of hydrocortisone sodium succinate (Solu-Medrol) at a dose of 1 mg/kg IV prior to the start of surgery and is continued at the same dose every six hours for the first 48–72 hours. Equivalent doses of dexamethasone sodium phosphate can also be used. When the patient can tolerate oral medications, it is then switched to cortisone acetate at a dose of 0.5–1 mg/kg PO q 12–24 hours. Over the next four weeks the dose of cortisone acetate is gradually tapered to 0.25 mg/kg PO q 12–24 hours. Long term, the dose can generally be further reduced to 0.10–0.2 mg/kg PO q 24 hours. Equivalent doses of hydrocortisone, prednisone, or prednisolone (cats) can also be used. Dose adjustments are based on endocrine monitoring and clinical status. Therapy will likely be lifelong unless there is regrowth of the functional pituitary adenoma.

Hypothyroidism. Complete resection of the pituitary gland also results in hypothyroidism and requires postoperative management and monitoring. Treatment consists of starting levothyroxine at a dose of 0.02 mg/kg PO q 12–24 hours once the patient can tolerate oral medications. The dose of levothyroxine is titrated based on thyroid function testing and typically this is a lifelong therapy for the patient.

Hypoglycemia. Following successful TSH, cats with HST can develop hypoglycemia even after the discontinuation of exogenous insulin [16, 18]. van Bokhorst and colleagues reported that 4/25 (16%) cats developed clinical signs of hypoglycemia after discontinuation of exogenous insulin and 5/25 (20%) cats developed hypoglycemia without clinical signs. In three of the hypoglycemic cats, an inappropriately elevated or normal endogenous insulin concentration was noted [18]. Fenn et al. found that 9/68 (13%) cats with HST experienced hypoglycemia following TSH. In 4/9 cats, the hypoglycemia occurred during tapering of the exogenous insulin dosage; however, in the remaining cats their hypoglycemia developed after insulin therapy had been discontinued [16]. In 4/9 cats the hypoglycemia was suspected to be due to sepsis, whereas in another 4 cats the hypoglycemia resolved or responded to appropriate therapy. In one cat, the hypoglycemia was unresponsive to treatment and the cat was subsequently euthanized 17 days after surgery [16]. Some of these hypoglycemic events have been interpreted as the direct consequence of surgical intervention and the rapid remission of HST leading to hyperinsulinemia. It is hypothesized that the hyperinsulinemia is secondary to hyperplasia of the pancreatic beta cells as a compensatory mechanism during the insulin resistance phase of HST [18]. In some patients following TSH, HST may resolve more rapidly than beta cell hyperplasia. Postoperative plasma IGF-1 concentrations can decrease rapidly and normalize within seven days or less [18].

Treatment for hypoglycemia can include reducing the dose and frequency of exogenous insulin or discontinuing insulin therapy if still being administered to the cat, IV dextrose supplementation, and frequent feedings. The dose of glucocorticoid supplementation can be temporarily increased to stimulate hepatic gluconeogenesis [18]. If this is insufficient, diazoxide at a dose of 5 mg/kg PO q 12 hours can be administered to help inhibit pancreatic insulin secretion, stimulate hepatic gluconeogenesis and glycogenolysis, and inhibit tissue use of glucose [18, 117]. Diazoxide can result in anorexia, vomiting, and diarrhea. These side effects may be reduced by giving the medication with food [117].

Respiratory Complications

Aspiration Pneumonia. Aspiration pneumonia has been documented in patients following TSH [11, 12, 82], and this complication can potentially be life threatening. It is unknown why this complication occurs; however, it is possible that the etiology is multifactorial. Possible etiologies include immunosuppression of PDH dogs, medications given to the patient that predispose to vomiting and/or regurgitation, copious lavage of the oral cavity during surgery, and prolonged length of surgery and time under anesthesia. If aspiration pneumonia develops postoperatively, broad spectrum antibiotic therapy should be instituted and supplemental oxygen therapy should be started if the patient is hypoxemic. Nebulization, coupage, and recumbency care can also be considered as additional therapies.

Pulmonary Thromboembolism and Hypercoagulability. Hyperadrenocorticism is associated with multisystemic complications, of which the coagulation system is not spared. Hypercoagulability associated with human hyperadrenocorticism appears to be due to increases in procoagulant parameters (Factor (F) II, FV, FVIII, von Willebrand factor, FIX, FXII, and fibrinogen), decreased fibrinolysis, platelet dysfunction, and endothelial dysfunction [118–121]. Hypercoagulability accompanying canine hyperadrenocorticism appears to be associated with increases in FII, FV, FVII, FIX, FX, FXII, and fibrinogen, and in some cases decreases in antithrombin [43, 122–125]. Some dogs also have ongoing thrombin generation, decreased fibrinolysis, and platelet dysfunction [122, 125]. In humans with hyperadrenocorticism, arterial and venous thrombosis can cause significant morbidity and mortality and the postoperative time period can be a critical time where significant thromboembolic events can occur [118]. Almost 50% of all thromboembolic events occur within two months following a surgical intervention [118]. Thrombotic events can be arterial (coronary, cerebral, aortic) and venous (pulmonary, cerebral, jugular, caval, portal, splenic, mesenteric) in both humans and canines [43, 118, 126–130]. The authors have experienced arterial and venous thromboembolic events in dogs with PDH following TSH, some occurring within 36 hours of surgery and others occurring several days following surgery.

In humans, the risk of thrombotic events appears to be proportional to the degree of hypercortisolism [118]. In dogs, duration of hyperadrenocorticism may not predict hypercoagulability and hemostatic abnormalities can persist in dogs despite appropriate treatment and normalization of cortisol concentrations [42, 122, 125]. Clinical evaluation of thromboembolic risk in human and veterinary patients with PDH is complex. Although hemostasis is altered, the use of coagulation parameters alone to determine risk has not been firmly established [42, 118, 122, 125].

Canine PDH patients may benefit from thromboprophylaxis following TSH. Use of low molecular weight heparin, unfractionated heparin, rivaroxaban, or clopidogrel can be considered to reduce the risk or treat the presence of thromboembolism based on thrombus location (arterial vs. venous). The timing of thromboprophylaxis should always be a concerted decision among the surgical team and individualized for each patient. For most cases, thromboprophylaxis can be considered after the first 24 hours of an uncomplicated surgical course [118]. Non-pharmacological therapies such as passive range of motion and early mobilization may also be beneficial in preventing thromboembolic events.

Fluid Overload. Cardiac abnormalities such as left ventricular concentric hypertrophy, left atrial enlargement, and diastolic dysfunction have been noted in cats with HST [131, 132].Therefore, these cats are at risk for the development of fluid overload and subsequent pulmonary edema and/or pleural effusion. Kenny et al. reported that 4/19 (21%) cats developed congestive heart failure post hypophysectomy. All four cases occurred prior to the reduction of postoperative IV fluid volume [133]. Subsequently, Fenn and colleagues described the development of transient congestive heart failure that occurred after surgery in 5/65 (7%) cats, which was presumed to be due to volume overload. Only one case occurred in 57 (2%) cats after instituting a reduction in postoperative IV fluid administration [16]. To prevent the development of fluid overload, fluid intake and output, urine specific gravity, body weight, packed cell volume, total solids, central venous pressure, respiratory rate and effort, and auscultation of the lungs should be closely monitored and assessed. If fluid overload develops, appropriate therapies can include reducing or discontinuing IV fluid therapy, furosemide administration, and supplemental oxygen therapy.

Neurologic Complications

Increased Intracranial Pressure. Postoperatively, each patient is monitored for signs of increased intracranial pressure. Initially, repeat assessments of mental status, cranial nerve status, pupil size, pupillary light reflexes, and signs of the Cushing Reflex are monitored every 3–6 hours until neurologic status is deemed stable for 24 hours. Serial neurologic exams are crucial to a successful outcome because neurologic status can change rapidly and dramatically in the first 24 hours post surgery which may require medical intervention. If there are concerns that increased intracranial pressure is present, mannitol is given at a dose of 1 gm/kg IV over 15–30 minutes and/or hypertonic saline (7.5% solution) can be given at a dose of 3–5 ml/kg IV over 5–10 minutes. Due to the likelihood that CDI and subsequent hypernatremia could develop, mannitol is generally the preferred treatment in this situation to avoid the development or worsening of hypernatremia.

In the authors' experience, most patients recover neurologically relatively rapidly assuming there are no secondary complications. Patients are usually ambulatory shortly after surgery but may have worsening of proprioception and paresis. These deficits are usually transient, and patients are often back to their initial presentation status within the first week after surgery.

Blindness. The optic chiasm and optic nerves are parasellar structures that can be damaged while performing TSH and lead to blindness. Blindness can result from direct damage, neuropraxia, or secondary damage via postoperative hemorrhage or cerebral edema causing compression of the optic chiasm or nerves. If the optic chiasm or optic nerves have not been directly damaged, the condition is typically transient and resolves within a few days [14, 15].

Procedural Related Complications

Keratoconjunctivitis Sicca (KCS). KCS is a complication that can occur following TSH. Its development has been attributed to direct (traumatic) or indirect (ischemic) neuropraxia of the major petrosal nerves, resulting in decreased tear production from the lacrimal glands [10]. In most cases, the decrease in tear production is transient following TSH. Hanson and colleagues reported that in 47/150 (31%) dogs that developed KCS after TSH, ophthalmologic treatment was required for 3–547 days (median: 70 days) for the patient's left eye and for 3–717 days (median: 58 days) for the patient's right eye [12]. In addition, Meij et al. reported that following TSH, 18/52 (35%) dogs developed KCS and treatment was needed for 3–20 weeks (median: 10 weeks) until the condition resolved [11]. Currently there does not appear to be a relationship between the frequency of KCS development and size of the pituitary mass [12].

Decreased tear production has also been noted in cats with HST following TSH [16, 18]. van Bokhorst et al. reported decreased tear production as a major complication following surgery. Eleven of twenty-five (44%) cats had decreased tear production; however, this complication was temporary in all cats and eye lubricant treatment could be discontinued in the weeks following surgery as tear production normalized [18]. In another report of 68 cats with HST treated with TSH, reduced tear production was also noted in 2/65 (3%) of cats [16]. The authors did not indicate if or when this complication resolved in these cats.

Routine pre- and postoperative monitoring of STT values should be performed on each patient. Tear production can be monitored on the first day following TSH and then every two days while the patient is hospitalized. The STT can also be rechecked during subsequent follow-up visits, if appropriate. Ophthalmologic treatment with artificial tears is started postoperatively and continued until tear production has normalized. Initially, artificial tears are instilled into each eye every six hours and the frequency of administration is reduced as tear production improves.

Soft Palate Dehiscence. Complete dehiscence of the soft palate or development of an oronasal fistula is another potential complication of TSH [134, 135]. Complete dehiscence can be seen on the second to fourth day following surgery [135] and oronasal fistulas typically reveal themselves several days postoperatively. The soft palate incision is monitored daily until the patient is discharged from the hospital to assess for dehiscence of the surgical site. Clinical signs that may indicate the presence of soft palate dehiscence include nasal discharge, sneezing, and food or water coming from the nose after eating or drinking. If untreated, the patient may develop rhinitis, middle ear infections, or aspiration pneumonia [134, 135]. The incidence of dehiscence can be minimized by not placing undue traction on the soft palate edges when the retractor is inserted during surgery. In small dogs, the use of retention sutures instead of instrument retractors is recommended [135]. Debridement of the edges of the soft palate prior to closure is important to decrease the incidence of dehiscence as well as a two-layer closure. If soft palate dehiscence occurs, debridement and resuturing is done as soon as possible.

This complication can also occur in cats following TSH. van Bokhorst et al. reported dehiscence of palate wounds in cats with HST following TSH [18]. After electrocautery incision was replaced by scalpel incision of the soft palate, no other cases of major palate dehiscence were noted. All dehisced palate wounds were reoperated successfully. Additionally, there were 2/25 cats (8%) that had minor palate wound dehiscence which healed without specific treatment [18].

Surgical Site Infection. Patients are typically placed on antibiotic therapy following TSH due to the surgical location (mouth/soft palate) being contaminated with bacteria. Antibiotics with a spectrum appropriate for oral flora should be used. The authors utilize ampicillin and sulbactam at a dose of 30 mg/kg IV q 8 hours or clindamycin at a dose of 5–10 mg/kg IV q 12 hours for 48–72 hours following TSH. When the patient can tolerate oral medication, amoxicillin, and clavulanic acid at a dose of 13.75 mg/kg PO q 12 hours or clindamycin at a dose of 5–10 mg/kg PO q 12 hours is given for 10 days.

Long term Follow Up

Long-term follow up is necessary for optimal success post-TSH. Because TSH causes diabetes insipidus, hypothyroidism, and hypoadrenocorticism, specific parameters will need to be monitored regularly post surgery. Additionally, patients with functional sellar masses will need endocrine testing regularly to adjust medical management as needed.

For all postoperative TSH patients, the following is recommended at 1 week and at 1, 3, 6, 9, and 12 months postoperatively and yearly thereafter.

- physical and neurologic examinations;
- CBC, serum chemistry, urinalysis;
- STT until tear production has normalized;
- total T4 +/− full thyroid panel if indicated.

For patients with PDH, endogenous ACTH and UCCR are recommended at the above time points. For patients with HST, monitoring IGF-1 is recommended at the above time points. The diabetic cat will also need regular glucose checks for insulin dose adjustments.

Serial brain imaging, ideally MR imaging, is recommended at 3 months postoperatively to reevaluate residual disease and at 6, 9, 12 months postoperatively, and yearly thereafter, for regrowth. This becomes important if adjunctive therapy such as radiation therapy or chemotherapy is being considered. If residual tissue is highly suspected postoperatively, MR imaging is typically performed sooner at four to six weeks postoperatively in preparation for radiation therapy. The type of adjunctive therapy to consider depends on histologic tumor type. Pituitary adenomas and meningiomas are reported to respond to radiation therapy [50, 136–140]. Radiation is effective and complications are lower with smaller tumor sizes [50, 136]. If the tumor is not surgically removed in its entirety, it is still advantageous to decrease tumor size for better radiation outcome. Larger pituitary tumors and more severe preoperative neurologic signs have been shown to adversely affect radiation prognosis [50, 136, 140].

The overall reported recurrence rate for PDH following TSH is 27% in dogs [13] and 20% in cats [134]. The recurrence rate in cats with HST-induced diabetes mellitus following TSH is reported to be up to 12% [16, 18]. The recurrence rate following TSH for non-functional sellar masses has not been reported in the literature. When recurrence occurs, repeat brain imaging is important in identifying regrowth and to determine what type of adjunctive therapy is warranted. The best adjunctive therapy for each tumor type is not the focus of this chapter, and it is recommended that readers consult other sources for details. Repeat surgery is also a potential option, but many factors play a part in this decision.

 Video clips to accompany this book can be found on the companion website at: www.wiley.com/go/shores/advanced

References

1. Laws, E.R. Jr. (1980). Functional pituitary tumors. The neurosurgeon and neuroendocrinology. *Clin. Neurosurg.* 27: 3–18.
2. Rijnberk, A., der Kinderen, P.J., and Thijssen, J.H. (1968). Spontaneous hyperadrenocorticism in the dog. *J. Endocrinol.* 41: 397–406.
3. Lubberink, A.A. (1977). *Diagnosis and Treatment of Canine Cushing's Syndrome*, 44–74. Utrecht University.
4. Meij, B.P. (1998). Transsphenoidal hypophysectomy for the treatment of pituitary-dependent hyperadrenocorticism in dogs. *Vet. Q.* 20 (Suppl 1): S98–S100.
5. Henry, R.W., Hulse, D.A., Archbald, L.F. et al. (1982). Transoral hypophysectomy with mandibular symphysiotomy in the dog. *Am. J. Vet. Res.* 43: 1825–1829.
6. Niebauer, G.W. and Evans, S.M. (1988). Transsphenoidal hypophysectomy in the dog. A new technique. *Vet. Surg.* 17: 296–303.
7. Lantz, G.C., Ihle, S.L., Nelson, R.W. et al. (1988). Transsphenoidal hypophysectomy in the clinically normal dog. *Am. J. Vet. Res.* 49: 1134–1142.
8. Niebauer, G.W., Eigenmann, J.E., and Van Winkle, T.J. (1990). Study of long-term survival after transsphenoidal hypophysectomy in clinically normal dogs. *Am. J. Vet. Res.* 51: 677–681.
9. Markowitz, J., Archibald, J., and Downie, H.G. (1964). Hypophysectomy in Dogs. *Exp. Surg.* 630–643.
10. Meij, B.P., Voorhout, G., Van den Ingh, T.S. et al. (1997). Transsphenoidal hypophysectomy in beagle dogs: evaluation of a microsurgical technique. *Vet. Surg.* 26: 295–309.
11. Meij, B.P., Voorhout, G., van den Ingh, T.S. et al. (1998). Results of transsphenoidal hypophysectomy in 52 dogs with pituitary-dependent hyperadrenocorticism. *Vet. Surg.* 27: 246–261.
12. Hanson, J.M., van 't Hoofd Martine, M., Voorhout, G. et al. (2005). Efficacy of transsphenoidal hypophysectomy in treatment of dogs with pituitary-dependent hyperadrenocorticism. *J. Vet. Intern. Med.* 19: 687–694.
13. van Rijn, S.J., Galac, S., Tryfonidou, M.A. et al. (2016). The influence of pituitary size on outcome after transsphenoidal hypophysectomy in a large cohort of dogs with pituitary-dependent hypercortisolism. *J. Vet. Intern. Med.* 30: 989–995.
14. Hara, Y., Tagawa, M., Masuda, H. et al. (2003). Transsphenoidal hypophysectomy for four dogs with pituitary ACTH-producing adenoma. *J. Vet. Med. Sci.* 65: 801–804.
15. Mamelak, A.N., Owen, T.J., and Bruyette, D. (2014). Transsphenoidal surgery using a high definition video telescope for pituitary adenomas in dogs with pituitary dependent hypercortisolism: methods and results. *Vet. Surg.* 43: 369–379.
16. Fenn, J., Kenny, P.J., Scudder, C.J. et al. (2021). Efficacy of hypophysectomy for the treatment of hypersomatotropism-induced diabetes mellitus in 68 cats. *J. Vet. Intern. Med.* 35: 823–833.
17. Martin, L.G., Owen, T.J., Chen, A.V. et al. (2016). Clinical characteristics and outcome in dogs treated with transsphenoidal hypophysectomy for non-functional sellar masses. *J. Vet. Intern. Med.* 30–1941.
18. van Bokhorst, K.L., Galac, S., Kooistra, H.S. et al. (2021). Evaluation of hypophysectomy for treatment of hypersomatotropism in 25 cats. *J. Vet. Intern. Med.* 35: 834–842.
19. den Hertog, E., Braakman, J.C., Teske, E. et al. (1999). Results of non-selective adrenocorticolysis by o,p'-DDD in 129 dogs with pituitary-dependent hyperadrenocorticism. *Vet. Rec.* 144: 12–17.
20. Bruyette, D.S., Ruehl, W.W., Entriken, T. et al. (1997). Management of canine pituitary-dependent hyperadrenocorticism with l-deprenyl (Anipryl). *Vet. Clin. North Am. Small Anim. Pract.* 27: 273–286.
21. Lien, Y.H. and Huang, H.P. (2008). Use of ketoconazole to treat dogs with pituitary-dependent hyperadrenocorticism: 48 cases (1994–2007). *J. Am. Vet. Med. Assoc.* 233: 1896–1901.
22. Alenza, D.P., Arenas, C., Lopez, M.L. et al. (2006). Long-term efficacy of trilostane administered twice daily in dogs with pituitary-dependent hyperadrenocorticism. *J. Am. Anim. Hosp. Assoc.* 42: 269–276.
23. Neiger, R., Ramsey, I., O'Connor, J. et al. (2002). Trilostane treatment of 78 dogs with pituitary-dependent hyperadrenocorticism. *Vet. Rec.* 150: 799–804.
24. Castillo, V., Theodoropoulou, M., Stalla, J. et al. (2011). Effect of SOM230 (pasireotide) on corticotropic cells: action in dogs with Cushing's disease. *Neuroendocrinology* 94: 124–136.
25. Mellett Keith, A.M., Bruyette, D., and Stanley, S. (2013). Trilostane therapy for treatment of spontaneous hyperadrenocorticism in cats: 15 cases (2004–2012). *J. Vet. Intern. Med.* 27: 1471–1477.
26. Gostelow, R., Scudder, C., Keyte, S. et al. (2017). Pasireotide long-acting release treatment for diabetic cats with underlying hypersomatotropism. *J. Vet. Intern. Med.* 31: 355–364.
27. Goossens, M.M., Feldman, E.C., Theon, A.P. et al. (1998). Efficacy of cobalt 60 radiotherapy in dogs with pituitary-dependent hyperadrenocorticism. *J. Am. Vet. Med. Assoc.* 212: 374–376.

28. de Fornel, P., Delisle, F., Devauchelle, P. et al. (2007). Effects of radiotherapy on pituitary corticotroph macrotumors in dogs: a retrospective study of 12 cases. *Can. Vet. J.* 48: 481–486.

29. Mariani, C.L., Schubert, T.A., House, R.A. et al. (2013). Frameless stereotactic radiosurgery for the treatment of primary intracranial tumours in dogs. *Vet. Comp. Oncol.* 13: 409–423.

30. Goossens, M.M., Feldman, E.C., Nelson, R.W. et al. (1998). Cobalt 60 irradiation of pituitary gland tumors in three cats with acromegaly. *J. Am. Vet. Med. Assoc.* 213: 374–376.

31. Brearley, M.J., Polton, G.A., Littler, R.M. et al. (2006). Coarse fractionated radiation therapy for pituitary tumours in cats: a retrospective study of 12 cases. *Vet. Comp. Oncol.* 4: 209–217.

32. Sellon, R.K., Fidel, J., Houston, R. et al. (2009). Linear-accelerator-based modified radiosurgical treatment of pituitary tumors in cats: 11 cases (1997–2008). *J. Vet. Intern. Med.* 23: 1038–1044.

33. Wormhoudt, T.L., Boss, M.K., Lunn, K. et al. (2018). Stereotactic radiation therapy for the treatment of functional pituitary adenomas associated with feline acromegaly. *J. Vet. Intern. Med.* 32: 1383–1391.

34. Penn, D.L., Burke, W.T., and Laws, E.R. (2018). Management of non-functioning pituitary adenomas: surgery. *Pituitary* 21: 145–153.

35. Ogiwara, T., Nagm, A., Nakamura, T. et al. (2019). Significance and indications of surgery for asymptomatic nonfunctioning pituitary adenomas. *World Neurosurg.* 128: e752–e759.

36. Manojlovic-Gacic, E., Engstrom, B.E., and Casar-Borota, O. (2018). Histopathological classification of non-functioning pituitary neuroendocrine tumors. *Pituitary* 21: 119–129.

37. Rissi, D.R. (2015). A retrospective study of skull base neoplasia in 42 dogs. *J. Vet. Diagn. Investig.* 27: 743–748.

38. Rivenburg, R., Owen, T.J., Martin, L.G. et al. (2021). Pituitary surgery: changing the paradigm in veterinary medicine in the United States. *J. Am. Anim. Hosp. Assoc.* 57: 73–80.

39. Sato, A., Teshima, T., Ishino, H. et al. (2016). A magnetic resonance imaging-based classification system for indication of trans-sphenoidal hypophysectomy in canine pituitary-dependent hypercortisolism. *J. Small Anim. Pract.* 57: 240–246.

40. Teshima, T., Hara, Y., Taoda, T. et al. (2011). Central diabetes insipidus after transsphenoidal surgery in dogs with Cushing's disease. *J. Vet. Med. Sci.* 73: 33–39.

41. Owen, T.J., Martin, L.G., and Chen, A.V. (2018). Transsphenoidal surgery for pituitary tumors and other sellar masses. *Vet. Clin. North Am. Small Anim. Pract.* 48: 129–151.

42. Park, F.M., Blois, S.L., Abrams-Ogg, A.C. et al. (2013). Hypercoagulability and ACTH-dependent hyperadrenocorticism in dogs. *J. Vet. Intern. Med.* 27: 1136–1142.

43. Teshima, T., Hara, Y., Taoda, T. et al. (2008). Cushing's disease complicated with thrombosis in a dog. *J. Vet. Med. Sci.* 70: 487–491.

44. Bryden, S.L., Burrows, A.K., and O'Hara, A.J. (2004). Mycobacterium goodii infection in a dog with concurrent hyperadrenocorticism. *Vet. Dermatol.* 15: 331–338.

45. Hoffman, J.M., Lourenco, B.N., Promislow, D.E.L. et al. (2018). Canine hyperadrenocorticism associations with signalment, selected comorbidities and mortality within North American veterinary teaching hospitals. *J. Small Anim. Pract.* 59: 681–690.

46. Mesich, M.L., Mayhew, P.D., Paek, M. et al. (2009). Gall bladder mucoceles and their association with endocrinopathies in dogs: a retrospective case-control study. *J. Small Anim. Pract.* 50: 630–635.

47. Kipperman, B.S., Feldman, E.C., Dybdal, N.O. et al. (1992). Pituitary tumor size, neurologic signs, and relation to endocrine test results in dogs with pituitary-dependent hyperadrenocorticism: 43 cases (1980–1990). *J. Am. Vet. Med. Assoc.* 201: 762–767.

48. Bertoy, E.H., Feldman, E.C., Nelson, R.W. et al. (1995). Magnetic resonance imaging of the brain in dogs with recently diagnosed but untreated pituitary-dependent hyperadrenocorticism. *J. Am. Vet. Med. Assoc.* 206: 651–656.

49. Bertoy, E.H., Feldman, E.C., Nelson, R.W. et al. (1996). One-year follow-up evaluation of magnetic resonance imaging of the brain in dogs with pituitary-dependent hyperadrenocorticism. *J. Am. Vet. Med. Assoc.* 208: 1268–1273.

50. Kent, M.S., Bommarito, D., Feldman, E. et al. (2007). Survival, neurologic response, and prognostic factors in dogs with pituitary masses treated with radiation therapy and untreated dogs. *J. Vet. Intern. Med.* 21: 1027–1033.

51. Behrend, E.N., Kooistra, H.S., Nelson, R. et al. (2013). Diagnosis of spontaneous canine hyperadrenocorticism: 2012 ACVIM consensus statement (small animal). *J. Vet. Intern. Med.* 27: 1292–1304.

52. Wood, F.D., Pollard, R.E., Uerling, M.R. et al. (2007). Diagnostic imaging findings and endocrine test results in dogs with pituitary-dependent hyperadrenocorticism that did or did not have neurologic abnormalities: 157 cases (1989–2005). *J. Am. Vet. Med. Assoc.* 231: 1081–1085.

53. Hyde, B.R.M.L., Chen, A.V., Guess, S.C. et al. (2016). Clinical characteristics and outcome in dogs treated with transsphenoidal hypophysectomy for non-functional sellar masses. *J. Vet. Intern. Med.* 30 (6): 1941.

54. Menchetti, M., De Risio, L., Galli, G. et al. (2019). Neurological abnormalities in 97 dogs with detectable pituitary masses. *Vet. Q.* 39: 57–64.

55. Duesberg, C.A., Feldman, E.C., Nelson, R.W. et al. (1995). Magnetic resonance imaging for diagnosis of pituitary macrotumors in dogs. *J. Am. Vet. Med. Assoc.* 206: 657–662.

56. Sarfaty, D., Carrillo, J.M., and Peterson, M.E. (1988). Neurologic, endocrinologic, and pathologic findings associated with large pituitary tumors in dogs: eight cases (1976–1984). *J. Am. Vet. Med. Assoc.* 193: 854–856.

57. Ihle, S.L. (1997). Pituitary corticotroph macrotumors. Diagnosis and treatment. *Vet. Clin. North Am. Small Anim. Pract.* 27: 287–297.

58. Lynch, G.L., Broome, M.R., and Scagliotti, R.H. (2006). What is your diagnosis? Mass originating from the pituitary fossa. *J. Am. Vet. Med. Assoc.* 228: 1681–1682.

59. Seruca, C., Rodenas, S., Leiva, M. et al. (2010). Acute postretinal blindness: ophthalmologic, neurologic, and magnetic resonance imaging findings in dogs and cats (seven cases). *Vet. Ophthalmol.* 13: 307–314.

60. Meij, B.P. (2001). Hypophysectomy as a treatment for canine and feline Cushing's disease. *Vet. Clin. North Am. Small Anim. Pract.* 31: 1015–1041.

61. Hullinger, R. (1993). The endocrine system. In: *Miller's Anatomy of the Dog*, 3e (ed. H.E. Evans), 559–585. Philidelphia: WB Saunders.

62. Moore, S.A. and O'Brien, D.P. (2008). Canine pituitary macrotumors. *Compend. Contin. Educ. Vet.* 30: 33–40; quiz 41.

63. Schmid, S., Hodshon, A., Olin, S. et al. (2017). Pituitary macrotumor causing narcolepsy-cataplexy in a dachshund. *J. Vet. Intern. Med.* 31: 545–549.

64. Fleeman, L. and Gostelow, R. (2020). Updates in feline diabetes mellitus and hypersomatotropism. *Vet. Clin. North Am. Small Anim. Pract.* 50: 1085–1105.

65. Greco, D.S. (2012). Feline acromegaly. *Top. Companion Anim. Med.* 27: 31–35.

66. Peterson, M.E. (2007). Acromegaly in cats: are we only diagnosing the tip of the iceberg? *J. Vet. Intern. Med.* 21: 889–891.

67. Kraft, S.L., Gavin, P.R., DeHaan, C. et al. (1997). Retrospective review of 50 canine intracranial tumors evaluated by magnetic resonance imaging. *J. Vet. Intern. Med.* 11: 218–225.

68. Famini, P., Maya, M.M., and Melmed, S. (2011). Pituitary magnetic resonance imaging for sellar and parasellar masses: ten-year experience in 2598 patients. *J. Clin. Endocrinol. Metab.* 96: 1633–1641.

69. Nakamura, T., Schorner, W., Bittner, R.C. et al. (1988). The value of paramagnetic contrast agent gadolinium-DTPA in the diagnosis of pituitary adenomas. *Neuroradiology* 30: 481–486.

70. Macpherson, P., Hadley, D.M., Teasdale, E. et al. (1989). Pituitary microadenomas. Does Gadolinium enhance their demonstration? *Neuroradiology* 31: 293–298.

71. Snyder, J.M., Lipitz, L., Skorupski, K.A. et al. (2008). Secondary intracranial neoplasia in the dog: 177 cases (1986–2003). *J. Vet. Intern. Med.* 22: 172–177.

72. Gutierrez-Quintana, R., Carrera, I., Dobromylskyj, M. et al. (2013). Pituitary metastasis of pancreatic origin in a dog presenting with acute-onset blindness. *J. Am. Anim. Hosp. Assoc.* 49: 403–406.

73. van der Vlugt-Meijer, R.H., Voorhout, G., and Meij, B.P. (2002). Imaging of the pituitary gland in dogs with pituitary-dependent hyperadrenocorticism. *Mol. Cell. Endocrinol.* 197: 81–87.

74. Voorhout, G. (1990). Cisternography combined with linear tomograpghy for visualization of the pituitary gland in healthy dogs. A comparison with computed tomography. *Vet. Radiol. Ultrasound* 31: 68–73.

75. Meij, B., Voorhout, G., and Rijnberk, A. (2002). Progress in transsphenoidal hypophysectomy for treatment of pituitary-dependent hyperadrenocorticism in dogs and cats. *Mol. Cell. Endocrinol.* 197: 89–96.

76. Haussler, T.C., von Puckler, K.H., Thiel, C. et al. (2018). Measurement of the normal feline pituitary gland in brachycephalic and mesocephalic cats. *J. Feline Med. Surg.* 20: 578–586.

77. Klibanski, A. and Zervas, N.T. (1991). Diagnosis and management of hormone-secreting pituitary adenomas. *N. Engl. J. Med.* 324: 822–831.

78. Kippenes, H., Gavin, P.R., Kraft, S.L. et al. (2001). Mensuration of the normal pituitary gland from magnetic resonance images in 96 dogs. *Vet. Radiol. Ultrasound* 42: 130–133.

79. Kooistra, H.S., Voorhout, G., Mol, J.A. et al. (1997). Correlation between impairment of glucocorticoid feedback and the size of the pituitary gland in dogs with pituitary-dependent hyperadrenocorticism. *J. Endocrinol.* 152: 387–394.

80. van der Vlugt-Meijer, R.H., Meij, B.P., van den Ingh, T.S. et al. (2003). Dynamic computed tomography of the pituitary gland in dogs with pituitary-dependent hyperadrenocorticism. *J. Vet. Intern. Med.* 17: 773–780.

81. Pollard, R.E., Reilly, C.M., Uerling, M.R. et al. (2010). Cross-sectional imaging characteristics of pituitary adenomas, invasive adenomas and adenocarcinomas in dogs: 33 cases (1988–2006). *J. Vet. Intern. Med.* 24: 160–165.

82. Fracassi, F., Mandrioli, L., Shehdula, D. et al. (2014). Complete surgical removal of a very enlarged pituitary corticotroph adenoma in a dog. *J. Am. Anim. Hosp. Assoc.* 50: 192–197.

83. Chen, A.V., Owen, T.J., Martin, L.G. et al. (2016). Magnetic resonance imaging characteristics of histopathologically confirmed non-functional sellar masses in dogs. *J. Vet. Intern. Med.* 30: 1939.

84. Auriemma, E., Barthez, P.Y., van der Vlugt-Meijer, R.H. et al. (2009). Computed tomography and low-field magnetic resonance imaging of the pituitary gland in dogs with pituitary-dependent hyperadrenocorticism: 11 cases (2001–2003). *J. Am. Vet. Med. Assoc.* 235: 409–414.

85. Hasegawa, T., Ito, H., Shoin, K. et al. (1984). Diagnosis of an "isodense" pituitary microadenoma by dynamic CT scanning. Case report. *J. Neurosurg.* 60: 424–427.

86. Escourolle, H., Abecassis, J.P., Bertagna, X. et al. (1993). Comparison of computerized tomography and magnetic resonance imaging for the examination of the pituitary gland in patients with Cushing's disease. *Clin. Endocrinol.* 39: 307–313.

87. van der Vlugt-Meijer, R.H., Meij, B.P., and Voorhout, G. (2006). Thin-slice three-dimensional gradient-echo magnetic resonance imaging of the pituitary gland in healthy dogs. *Am. J. Vet. Res.* 67: 1865–1872.

88. Dwyer, A.J., Frank, J.A., Doppman, J.L. et al. (1987). Pituitary adenomas in patients with Cushing disease: initial experience with Gd-DTPA-enhanced MR imaging. *Radiology* 163: 421–426.

89. Taoda, T., Hara, Y., Masuda, H. et al. (2011). Magnetic resonance imaging assessment of pituitary posterior lobe displacement in dogs with pituitary-dependent hyperadrenocorticism. *J. Vet. Med. Sci.* 73: 725–731.

90. Fischetti, A.J., Gisselman, K., and Peterson, M.E. (2012). CT and MRI evaluation of skull bones and soft tissues in six cats with presumed acromegaly versus 12 unaffected cats. *Vet. Radiol. Ultrasound* 53: 535–539.

91. Hermanson, J.W., DeLahunta, A., and Evans, H.E. (2020). *Miller and Evans' Anatomy of the Dog*, 5e, 527. St. Louis: Elsevier.

92. Hermanson, J.W., de Lahunta, A., and Evans, H.E. (2020). The endocrine system. In: *Miller and Evans' Anatomy of the Dog*, 5e, vol. 470, 471. St. Louis: Elsevier.

93. Meij, B.P., Mol, J.A., van den Ingh, T.S. et al. (1997). Assessment of pituitary function after transsphenoidal hypophysectomy in beagle dogs. *Domest. Anim. Endocrinol.* 14: 81–97.

94. Owen, T.J., Chen, A.V., Frey, S. et al. (2018). Transsphenoidal surgery: accuracy of an image-guided neuronavigation system to approach the pituitary fossa (sella turcica). *Vet. Surg.* 47: 664–671.

95. Edate, S. and Albanese, A. (2015). Management of electrolyte and fluid disorders after brain surgery for pituitary/suprasellar tumours. *Horm. Res. Paediatr.* 83: 293–301.

96. Hara, Y., Masuda, H., Taoda, T. et al. (2003). Prophylactic efficacy of desmopressin acetate for diabetes insipidus after hypophysectomy in the dog. *J. Vet. Med. Sci.* 65: 17–22.

97. Black, P.M., Zervas, N.T., and Candia, G.L. (1987). Incidence and management of complications of transsphenoidal operation for pituitary adenomas. *Neurosurgery* 20: 920–924.

98. Nemergut, E.C., Zuo, Z., Jane, J.A. Jr. et al. (2005). Predictors of diabetes insipidus after transsphenoidal surgery: a review of 881 patients. *J. Neurosurg.* 103: 448–454.

99. Papanek, P.E. and Raff, H. (1994). Chronic physiological increases in cortisol inhibit the vasopressin response to hypertonicity in conscious dogs. *Am. J. Phys.* 267: R1342–R1349.

100. Papanek, P.E., Sladek, C.D., and Raff, H. (1997). Corticosterone inhibition of osmotically stimulated vasopressin from hypothalamic-neurohypophysial explants. *Am. J. Phys.* 272: R158–R162.

101. Sawyer, W.H., Acosta, M., and Manning, M. (1974). Structural changes in the arginine vasopressin molecule that prolong its antidiuretic action. *Endocrinology* 95: 140–149.

102. Kimbrough, R.D. Jr., Cash, W.D., Branda, L.A. et al. (1963). Synthesis and biological properties of 1-desamino-8-lysine-vasopressin. *J. Biol. Chem.* 238: 1411–1414.

103. Nichols, R. and Hohenhaus, A.E. (1994). Use of the vasopressin analogue desmopressin for polyuria and bleeding disorders. *J. Am. Vet. Med. Assoc.* 205: 168–173.

104. Richardson, D.W. and Robinson, A.G. (1985). Desmopressin. *Ann. Intern. Med.* 103: 228–239.

105. Krause, K.H. (1986). The use of desmopressin in diagnosis and treatment of diabtes insipidus in cats. *Compend. Contin. Educ. Vet.* 9: 752–758.

106. Greene, C.E., Wong, P.L., and Finco, D.R. (1979). Diagnosis and treatment of diabetes insipidus in two dogs usnig two synthetic analogs of anitdiuretic hormone. *J. Am. Anim. Hosp. Assoc.* 15: 371–377.

107. Burnie, A.G. and Dunn, A.K. (1979). A case of central diabetes insipidus in the cat: diagnosis and treatment. *J. Small Anim. Pract.* 24: 569–573.

108. Rado, J.P., Marosi, I., and Fisher, J. (1977). Comparison of the antidiuretic effects of single intravenous and intranasal doses of DDAVP in diabetes insipidus. *Phamacology* 15: 40–45.

109. Feldman, E.C. and Nelson, R.W. (2004). Water metabolism and diabetes insipidus. In: *Canine and Felins Endocrinology and Reproduction*, 3e, 2–44. St. Louis: Saunders.

110. Nicohols, R. (2000). Clinical use of the vasopressin analogue DDAVP for the diagnoisis and treatment of diabetes insipidus. In: *Kirk's Current Veterinary Therapy XIII Smal Animal Practice* (ed. J.D. Bonagura), 325–326. Philadelphia: WB Saunders.

111. Yee, A.H., Burns, J.D., and Wijdicks, E.F. (2010). Cerebral salt wasting: pathophysiology, diagnosis, and treatment. *Neurosurg. Clin. N. Am.* 21: 339–352.

112. Costa, M.M., Esteves, C., Castedo, J.L. et al. (2018). A challenging coexistence of central diabetes insipidus and cerebral salt wasting syndrome: a case report. *J. Med. Case Rep.* 12: 212.

113. Kiran, Z., Sheikh, A., Momin, S.N. et al. (2017). Sodium and water imbalance after sellar, suprasellar, and parasellar surgery. *Endocr. Pract.* 23: 309–317.

114. Lin, J.J., Lin, K.L., Hsia, S.H. et al. (2009). Combined central diabetes insipidus and cerebral salt wasting syndrome in children. *Pediatr. Neurol.* 40: 84–87.

115. Guerrero, R., Pumar, A., Soto, A. et al. (2007). Early hyponatraemia after pituitary surgery: cerebral salt-wasting syndrome. *Eur. J. Endocrinol.* 156: 611–616.

116. Hara, Y., Teshima, T., Taoda, T. et al. (2010). Efficacy of transsphenoidal surgery on endocrinological status and serum chemistry parameters in dogs with Cushing's disease. *J. Vet. Med. Sci.* 72: 397–404.

117. Plumb, D. (2015). *Diazoxide, Oral.* Ames, IA: Wiley-Blackwell.

118. St-Jean, M., Lim, D.S.T., and Langlois, F. (2021). Hypercoagulability in Cushing's syndrome: from arterial to venous disease. *Best Pract. Res. Clin. Endocrinol. Metab.* 35: 101496.

119. Manetti, L., Bogazzi, F., Giovannetti, C. et al. (2010). Changes in coagulation indexes and occurrence of venous thromboembolism in patients with Cushing's syndrome: results from a prospective study before and after surgery. *Eur. J. Endocrinol.* 163: 783–791.

120. Kastelan, D., Dusek, T., Kraljevic, I. et al. (2009). Hypercoagulability in Cushing's syndrome: the role of specific haemostatic and fibrinolytic markers. *Endocrine* 36: 70–74.

121. Akaza, I., Yoshimoto, T., Tsuchiya, K. et al. (2010). Endothelial dysfunction aassociated with hypercortisolism is reversible in Cushing's syndrome. *Endocr. J.* 57: 245–252.

122. Kol, A., Nelson, R.W., Gosselin, R.C. et al. (2013). Characterization of thrombelastography over time in dogs with hyperadrenocorticism. *Vet. J.* 197: 675–681.

123. Feldman, B.F., Rasedee, A., and Feldman, E.C. (1986). Haemostatic abnormalities in canine Cushing's syndrome. *Res. Vet. Sci.* 41: 228–230.

124. Jacoby, R.C., Owings, J.T., Ortega, T. et al. (2001). Biochemical basis for the hypercoagulable state seen in Cushing syndrome; discussion 1006–7. *Arch. Surg.* 136: 1003–1006.

125. Pace, S.L., Creevy, K.E., Krimer, P.M. et al. (2013). Assessment of coagulation and potential biochemical markers for hypercoagulability in canine hyperadrenocorticism. *J. Vet. Intern. Med.* 27: 1113–1120.

126. Stuijver, D.J., van Zaane, B., Feelders, R.A. et al. (2011). Incidence of venous thromboembolism in patients with Cushing's syndrome: a multicenter cohort study. *J. Clin. Endocrinol. Metab.* 96: 3525–3532.

127. Soni, P., Koech, H., Silva, D. et al. (2020). Cerebral venous sinus thrombosis after transsphenoidal rresection: a rare complication of cushing disease-associated hypercoagulability. *World Neurosurg.* 134: 86–89.

128. Boswood, A., Lamb, C.R., and White, R.N. (2000). Aortic and iliac thrombosis in six dogs. *J. Small Anim. Pract.* 41: 109–114.

129. Respess, M., O'Toole, T.E., Taeymans, O. et al. (2012). Portal vein thrombosis in 33 dogs: 1998–2011. *J. Vet. Intern. Med.* 26: 230–237.

130. Hardie, E.M., Vaden, S.L., Spaulding, K. et al. (1995). Splenic infarction in 16 dogs: a retrospective study. *J. Vet. Intern. Med.* 9: 141–148.

131. Myers, J.A., Lunn, K.F., and Bright, J.M. (2014). Echocardiographic findings in 11 cats with acromegaly. *J. Vet. Intern. Med.* 28: 1235–1238.

132. Borgeat, K., Niessen, S., Scudder, C. et al. (2015). Feline hypersomatotropism is a naturally occurring, reversible cause of myocardial remodeling. *J. Vet. Intern. Med.* 29: 1263.

133. Kenny, P., Scudder, C., Keyte, S. et al. (2015). Treatment of feline hypersomatotropism. efficacy, morbiditiy and mortality of hypophysectomy. *J. Vet. Intern. Med.* 29: 1271.

134. Meij, B.P., Voorhout, G., van den Ingh, T.S.G.A.M. et al. (2001). Transsphenoidal hypophysectomy for treatment of pituitary-dependent hyperadrenocorticism in 7 cats. *Vet. Surg.* 30: 72–86.

135. Niebauer, G.W. (2003). Hypophysectomy. In: *Textbook of Small Animal Surgery* (ed. D. Slatter), 1677–1694. Philadelphia: WB Saunders.

136. Theon, A.P. and Feldman, E.C. (1998). Megavoltage irradiation of pituitary macrotumors in dogs with neurologic signs. *J. Am. Vet. Med. Assoc.* 213: 225–231.

137. Hansen, K.S., Zwingenberger, A.L., Theon, A.P. et al. (2019). Long-term survival with stereotactic radiotherapy for imaging-diagnosed pituitary tumors in dogs. *Vet. Radiol. Ultrasound* 60: 219–232.

138. Spugnini, E.P., Thrall, D.E., Price, G.S. et al. (2000). Primary irradiation of canine intracranial masses. *Vet. Radiol. Ultrasound* 41: 377–380.

139. MagalhAes, T.R., BenoIt, J., Néčov, S. et al. (2021). Outcome after radiation therapy in canine intracranial meningiomas or gliomas. *in vivo* 35: 1117–1123.

140. Van Asselt, N., Christensen, N., Meier, V. et al. (2020). Definitive-intent intensity-modulated radiation therapy provides similar outcomes to those previously published for definitive-intent three-dimensional conformal radiation therapy in dogs with primary brain tumors: a multi-institutional retrospective study. *Vet. Radiol. Ultrasound* 61: 481–489.

21

Surgical Management and Intraoperative Strategies for Tumors of the Skull
Jonathan F. McAnulty

University of Wisconsin-Madison, Madison, WI, USA

Surgical removal of tumors of the skull presents numerous challenges due to the proximity of vital structures, the potential for significant complications, and the delicacy of proximate structures that may sustain injury during dissection. Although a majority of bony tumors of the skull affect the maxilla [1], this discussion will focus on the challenges, both technical and medical, of bony tumors of the cranium. There are a variety of tumor types that have been reported to affect the cranium including infrequent chrondroma, chrondrosarcoma, squamous cell carcinoma, fibrosarcoma, or other tumor types with osteosarcoma and multilobular osteochrondrosarcoma (MLO) comprising the majority of the tumors encountered [1–6]. In retrospective series, MLO tumors appear to occur somewhat more often in the skull than osteosarcoma although definitive data on the relative frequency of these tumor types is not available.

Osteosarcoma and Multilobular Osteochrondrosarcoma of the Cranium

Osteosarcoma of the cranial bones is a malignancy that presents with proliferative and osteolytic lesions and has been suggested to exhibit a somewhat different biological behavior compared to appendicular osteosarcomas with respect to the incidence of distant metastasis as a cause of death [1]. This may in part be due to their location, where difficulty in achieving large margins of resection due to proximity to critical structures makes local recurrence more frequent (80% of cases in one report) and often a cause of death or euthanasia, possibly before metastasis is detected [1]. Osteosarcomas tend to occur in middle-aged pure-bred

dogs and frequently do not have pulmonary metastasis, the most common site of distant spread, at the time of diagnosis. Surgical excision with or without adjuvant therapies provides the best outcome in terms of survival time with median survival times reported at 329 days for osteosarcomas of the head, although calvarial lesions had a greater hazard of local recurrence or progression [1, 7, 8].

MLO tumors (synonymous terms used over time for this lesion include chondroma rodens, multilobular osteoma, multilobular chondroma, multilobular tumor of bone, multilobular osteosarcoma, cartilage analogue of fibromatosis, calcifying aponeurotic fibroma, and juvenile aponeurotic fibroma) are relatively uncommon tumors arising from the flat bones of the skull with rare reports of such tumors at other sites. MLO tumors occur primarily in middle aged to older, medium- to large-breed dogs, but also can occur in young and small-breed dogs as well as occasionally in other species [9–11].

These tumors generally present as a firm well demarcated swelling on the skull although internal expansion into the cranial cavity or sinuses/nasal cavity may mask the presence of these tumors early in the course of the disease as well as obscure the overall extent of tumor growth. Neurological or other clinical signs can occur, which are mostly dependent on the structures impinged upon by the expanding mass. MLOs are graded on a three-tier histological scale with higher grade lesions showing greater likelihood of local recurrence and distant metastasis [5, 12]. MLOs tend to be slow growing and metastasize later in the course of the disease. Complete excision is the treatment of choice with some studies suggesting adjuvant therapies, such as chemotherapy or radiation, may provide additive benefit to surgical excision [4–8]. Although the database

---

Advanced Techniques in Canine and Feline Neurosurgery, First Edition. Edited by Andy Shores and Brigitte A. Brisson.
© 2023 John Wiley & Sons, Inc. Published 2023 by John Wiley & Sons, Inc.
Companion site: www.wiley.com/go/shores/advanced

for assessment of adjuvant therapy efficacy is not large, early results are encouraging. Dogs with this type of tumor can have an excellent short to intermediate term prognosis following surgical excision but incomplete excision and local recurrence can be problematic. Depending on the histological grade, MLO lesions are likely to recur locally as well as develop metastatic lesions greater than 50% of the time. However, the long timeline for recurrence in most MLO cases, greater than two years median for grade I and II lesions [4, 6, 9, 12], and the improved quality of life during that time makes surgical treatment an attractive option for many clients. It should be noted that the biological behavior of MLOs can be variable and that in a minority of cases the lesions can be considerably more aggressive with more rapid growth and a shorter time to recurrence.

Diagnosis and Characterization

Diagnosis of tumors of the skull is generally not difficult. Imaging will usually provide an accurate presumptive diagnosis for most due to the characteristic appearance of MLO and osteosarcoma lesions [13]. Most calvarial tumors are readily accessible for incisional biopsy for definitive diagnosis. Biopsy procedures should be planned so that the biopsy tract and related incisions are removed as part of any excisional therapeutic procedure. Imaging plays an important role in both diagnosis and therapeutic planning. Computed tomographic (CT) imaging will provide the most information for diagnostic and therapeutic purposes for tumors with proliferative bony characteristics. In some cases, the unique appearance of MLO tumors, sharply marginated masses with a granular mixed bony appearance, can provide a presumptive diagnosis and be advantageous for lesions in difficult to access locations for biopsy [10, 12, 13]. For bony tumors, magnetic resonance imaging (MRI) is less informative. However, in certain scenarios (see sections below regarding occipital tumors affecting the caudal dorsal sagittal or transverse sinuses), MRI can be essential in formulating a therapeutic approach to excision that minimizes patient risks [14–17].

Surgical Planning and Treatment

Surgical excision is the treatment of choice for both MLO lesions and calvarial osteosarcomas. Follow up chemotherapy or radiation therapy may also be warranted for specific case presentations. There are a variety of challenges that will affect the feasibility and difficulty of excision of MLOs. These challenges are directly related to the location of the tumors and the biological behavior of the lesions in any individual patient. These factors will affect the ability to gain margins of excision free of neoplasia and avoid complications related to damage to nearby structures. Achieving wide margins in many calvarial lesions, at least in some parts of an excisional boundary, is frequently impossible due to the proximity to critical structures and lack of tissues that can be sacrificed to obtain such margins. This is likely a significant reason behind the relatively high incidence of local recurrence for these lesions. However, as noted earlier, the slow growth and long timelines for recurrence still make excisional surgery a reasonable option for many clients. Other factors related to the tumor size, location, and behavior affect the probability of severe complications, including death, and the overall resectability of the masses as well as the likelihood of needing adjunctive therapy, such as radiation, that may increase costs of treatment.

Exposure

The difficulty of exposure of these lesions varies from simple to complex as a direct effect of the tumor location on the skull. As a general strategy, the normal bone completely encircling the mass is cleared of all soft tissue attachments prior to commencing cutting the bone. This will allow the surgeon to complete the initial bone cuts and excision as efficiently as possible so that hemorrhagic structures under the bone that may be difficult to access can then be exposed for establishing complete hemostasis. For MLO tumors, the overlying skin is often unaffected unless there is a biopsy tract that needs removal and can be preserved to facilitate closure. Similarly, for mid-calvarial and occipital lesions, the temporalis fascia may remain mostly intact, except at midline where it attaches to the dorsal sagittal crest, due to the temporalis muscle often providing a barrier to the tumor. Similarly, in most such cases the bulk of the temporalis muscle can be preserved. However, deep temporalis muscle fibers are often attached to the tumor surface and a layer of muscle should be excised along with the tumor in those instances. Recurrence in these soft tissues with sharply marginated lesions is rare in the author's experience and is instead usually seen in bone adjacent to the excision. The exception to this concept is in MLO lesions with substantial expansion into the surrounding soft tissues. In those cases, complete excision of tumor remnants in the surrounding musculature is difficult to achieve. It should be noted that access to the normal bone around the base of MLO lesions can be impeded by the tumor itself. MLO lesions not uncommonly expand outside of the skull in a mushroom-like fashion. In some cases, it is necessary to cut off portions of overhanging tumor tissue to effectively access the normal bone underneath and establish a line of excision. In MLO lesions with high bone content, the hemorrhage associated with this maneuver may be relatively minimal. In other lesions, particularly

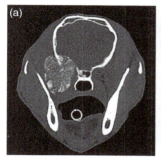 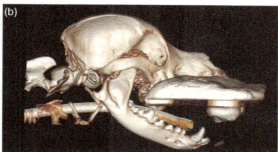 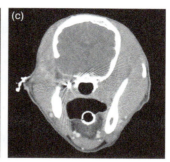

Figure 21.1 (a) Transverse CT image a showing an MLO lesion of the basal skull that presents challenges in access and exposure. A 3D reconstruction (b) of the CT illustrates the challenges in access to the mass due to overlying bony structures. Lesions similar to this presentation may require more complex surgical approaches including incising and retraction or excision of the zygomatic arch and resection of part of the mandible to achieve adequate exposure. (c) shows a transverse CT image of the excision site five weeks after surgery with the zygomatic arch and ramus of the mandible removed. Mandibular function was minimally affected at the time of followup.

those with a higher soft tissue component, hemorrhage can ooze from the cavernous-like cut tissue surface and be significant and continuous. For this reason, the author delays such partial excisional maneuvers until later in the procedure as much as possible. Once made, broad manual pressure with gauze on the cut surface may be the most effective way to reduce blood loss until the en bloc resection is completed.

Tumors on the dorsal calvarium or zygomatic arch are usually simple to access and isolate from surrounding tissues for excision. As tumors arise from more lateralized and ventral locations on the skull, exposure and isolation of the neoplasms becomes more complex. Similarly, tumors affecting the occiput also require complex dissections of overlying soft tissue structures in order to isolate the lesions. It should be noted that these dissections may not necessarily be overtly difficult but can be lengthy and tedious due to the multitude of affected structures, such as the cervical musculature and associated vasculature and the need for meticulous hemostasis. In some instances, overlying structures, such as the zygomatic arch, may need to be moved and either sacrificed or affixed back in place at the end of the procedure in order to obtain adequate exposure. Similarly, for lesions arising from the orbit or toward the base of the skull, the ramus of the mandible may need to be excised to allow access to the lesion. This can be done, particularly above the temporomandibular joint, with minimal functional effects on the patient. Figures 21.1a–c illustrate an example of this approach for an MLO lesion in the caudoventral orbit that was exposed and excised by zygomatic arch excision with removal of the ramus of the mandible above the temporomandibular joint. In this example, the eye was severely proptosed but visual and both the eye and vision were preserved after surgery. For lesions affecting the occiput, careful positioning of the patient to create an angle approaching 90° between the axis of the cervical vertebrae and craniocaudal axis of the skull is needed to facilitate isolation of tumors to the base of the occiput and foramen magnum (Figure 21.2).

Patient positioning may also be advantageously used to reduce blood loss during surgery. In most MLO excisions, bleeding is less often from larger or high pressure vessels which, if encountered, can be quickly controlled. Instead, there is a significant risk of excessive blood loss over the long time periods often required for these surgeries due to low pressure continuous diffuse bleeding from the tumor surface or venous/capillary sources. Positioning

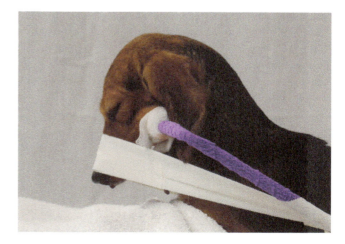

Figure 21.2 Patient positioning. Cadaver specimen demonstration of the author's preferred positioning for skull tumor resections. Positioning of the patient on a highly padded rack contacting the caudal molar teeth allows for elevation of the neck and avoidance of jugular compression. Tilting of the operating table to elevate the skull above the central circulation also assists in reducing low pressure venous congestion that may occur with standard surgical positioning. In this example, the head is rotated to create an approximate right angle at the occipital–cervical junction. This position is advantageous for exposure and resection of lesions affecting the occiput. A broad base of tape on the dorsal muzzle is used to secure this positioning.

the patient with the head elevated relative to the body and avoiding compression of the jugular veins helps to avoid venous congestion and reduces the rate of bleeding from diffuse low pressure sources in the surgical field [14]. In many cases, use of a supportive rack allows both proper positioning and avoidance of venous compression (Figure 21.2).

Challenges in Skull Tumor Resection

Resection of MLO lesions can present various challenges depending on the location of the lesion. In some areas, solutions to specific problems have not been completely described and remain areas for further investigation and innovation. Cutting of the bone around these lesions is usually done with either high speed burrs or ultrasonic or piezoelectric bone scalpel devices. Wetting of the area being cut with normal saline to prevent heat induced tissue injury is standard practice. Burring of the bone tends to be slower than cutting with advanced bone scalpel devices. However, the greater width of a burr excision line, referred to as the kerf, is advantageous for angled introduction of periosteal elevators under the bone to tease the underlying dura mater with the entrained dorsal sagittal sinus off the inner calvarial and tumor surface. In some cases, using a bone scalpel, it may be useful to enlarge the cutting kerf by making two parallel cuts approximately 0.25–0.5 cm apart to more easily allow introduction of an elevator under the calvarial bone without having to exert upward traction on the bone prematurely. In the author's experience, the dura is easily elevated off the underside of MLO lesions with occasional exceptions in cases with unusual presentations of more diffuse disease (Figure 21.3).

Parietal Calvarial and Dorsal Frontal Bone Lesions

Resections of lesions involving the dorsal calvarium can be some of the least challenging resections within the spectrum of locations where MLO or other bony lesions may arise. Dorsal calvarial lesions are generally straightforward to isolate on their external surface by retracting and elevating the soft tissues away from the lesion and normal bone to expose an area for bone incision. The dura and dorsal sagittal sinus can be elevated off the underside of the bone and lesion relatively easily, usually without significant damage to the dura. Perforations of the dura are preferentially repaired by suturing or, for larger defects, use of a fascial or other patch can be implemented. Repair of perforations is preferred although modest dural perforations may be tolerated. Elevation of the dura in the mid-dorsal calvarium will invariably encounter modest hemorrhage from a cut unnamed diploic vessel that is consistently encountered entering the dorsal surface of the sagittal sinus. This is best controlled with a partial thickness suture of 6-0 polyglyconate or polypropylene in a cruciate pattern.

As lesions arise on the more lateral aspect of the calvarium in the parietal and temporal bones, exposure becomes more difficult. Extensive elevation of the temporalis muscle is possible by incising the temporal fascia at the outer border of the muscle and elevating the muscle off the underlying bone. Elevation of the temporalis can be extensive since the blood supply to the muscle arises at its caudoventral aspect from the occipital branch of the caudal auricular artery and the temporal branch of the superficial temporal artery, which arise from the carotid and maxillary arteries, respectively. Caution should be exercised in elevation of the cranial portion of the temporalis muscle to avoid damage to the palpebral nerve and loss of the ipsilateral palpebral reflex, although in some tumor presentations this may be

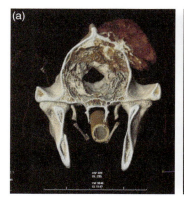
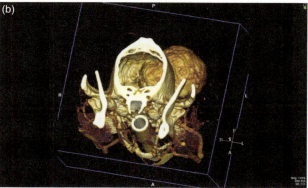

Figure 21.3 MLO lesions are typically sharply marginated masses but can be variable in their presentation and biological behavior. Figure 21.3 shows 3D reconstruction images of two presentations of MLO lesions that may be encountered. (a) shows an MLO lesion with a diffuse spread of fine spiculated lesions within the calvarium. This mass was very adherent to the dura, unlike most MLO lesions, and recurred in a short time period after excision. (b) shows a more typical MLO lesion with protrusion into the cranial cavity and sharply delineated margins.

unavoidable. Lesions of the lateral parietal and temporal bones can be excised similar to those on the dorsal surface down to the dorsal margin of the external auditory meatus. Lesions that extend ventral to this area often invade the middle and inner ear where excision may result in severe vestibular dysfunction and should be considered with caution and planned carefully if an excision is to be attempted.

Lesions arising in the frontal bones present different challenges. Excision of the skull in the caudal frontal bone area typically may include a portion of the cranial parietal bone and, depending on the size and extent of the mass, result in an excision site that spans both the frontal sinus and the cranial cavity. Data regarding the relative risk of infection progressing from the sinus to the meninges or brain is extremely limited. In a small series of cases, this author has not seen any neurologic complications arise attributable to these spaces becoming contiguous where the dura remains intact and the sinus is able to freely drain into the nasal cavity after mass excision. Some surgeons have attempted to create a barrier between these spaces based on concern for bacterial contamination of the cranial cavity, but the benefits of these efforts remain theoretical. Data from a larger case series is needed to ascertain what proportion, if any, of these cases are at risk of significant complications in this situation. In a single case where a prosthetic required removal, this author was able to observe that the dura had formed a substantive fibrotic layer walling off the sinus from the cranial cavity. If this response is general, it would support a relaxed concern about long-term risks of infection ascending into the cranial cavity from the sinus. Another unsolved challenge related to excision of the frontal bone is when the dorsal orbital rim must be removed. This presents issues with the loss of anchoring of the upper eyelids, lid droop, and potential for eye problems. Cranioplasty in this area may present some difficulties which are discussed below in the section on Cranioplasty.

Frontal Bone within the Orbit and Sphenoid Bone Lesions

Most MLO lesions arising in bone within the orbit can be effectively excised. The primary decision in approaching such lesions is whether the eye will be preserved or removed. Depending on the location of the mass and ease of exposure, it may be advantageous to incise and ventrally retract the zygomatic arch with transection of the orbital ligament and remove a portion of the ramus of the mandible to increase exposure. The zygomatic arch can be reaffixed in place, usually by orthopedic wire fixation, or removed if needed. Resection of frontal bone lesions with preservation of the eye is best accomplished by incision along the edge of the orbit and elevating the bulbar sheath (Tenon's capsule) with its encased muscles and neurovascular bundle away

from the bone. Resection can then proceed with gentle retraction of these structures as described for other locations on the skull. In cases where adjunctive radiation therapy is to be considered, it may be prudent to remove the eye to avoid short- and intermediate-term complications due to radiative damage to the eye. In that scenario, associated orbital structures and the eye can be excised prior to excision of the bony mass to facilitate exposure and maneuvering within the orbit. Lesions arising from the sphenoid bones can also be excised down to a line extending from the dorsal margin of the optic canal to the caudal alar foramen. Similarly, access to this area is improved by retracting or removing overlying bony structures as feasible. The cavernous sinus lies within the cranial cavity just medial to these structures. In a limited case series, this proximity has not presented itself as a problem but likely prevents surgery or increases surgical risk with lesions located more medially.

Occipital Bone Lesions

Until recently, occipital lesions represented one of the greatest challenges in the skull for safe excision. In such excisions, the primary risk lies in the potential for acute occlusion of the caudal dorsal sagittal sinus and/or both transverse sinuses with subsequent acute, potentially fatal, cerebral edema. Further considerations during surgery relate to the relatively complex three-dimensional structure of the skull in this area, risk of ongoing hemorrhage during the excision, and potential for extension of pathology along the tentorium cerebelli and deeply between the cerebrum and cerebellum.

Risk assessment in a patient presented for an occipital excision requires determination of the patency of the vessels and blood flow from the dorsal sagittal sinus into the transverse sinuses and whether the anticipated line of excision will affect the confluens sinuum, caudal dorsal sagittal sinus, or both transverse sinuses. This assessment is obtained via specific MRI studies that are able to delineate flow in these vessels (see below regarding time-of-flight MRI imaging). These studies are also compared with CT studies to ascertain the line of resection and determine the steps required to minimize risk in the patient. Based on the results of MRI imaging, there are three scenarios that may be encountered. The scenarios that affect strategic surgical decision making are that of (i) a lateralized occipital lesion where the proposed line of excision will not affect either the confluens sinuum or the flow from the dorsal sagittal sinus to the contralateral transverse sinus. These masses may either have no effect on the ipsilateral transverse sinus or more commonly have growth into the ipsilateral sinus causing spontaneous occlusion of blood flow on one side only. In this case, an excision that removes the ipsilateral transverse sinus and spares the confluens sinuum has little to no risk of cerebral

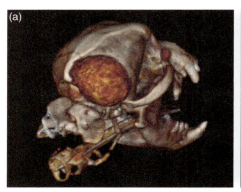
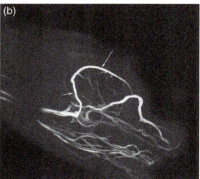

Figure 21.4 Three-dimensional image (a) reconstruction of a CT scan shows encroachment of an MLO lesion on the occipital and temporal bones housing the confluens sinuum and right transverse sinus. Obstruction of flow to both transverse sinuses would indicate that the lesion can be excised without further interventions. Magnetic resonance image using time-of-flight methodology (b) is used to outline the patency of blood flow from the dorsal sagittal sinus (long arrow) to the left transverse sinus (short arrow). In this case, the right transverse sinus is blocked by tumor ingrowth but the left transverse sinus has intact flow and no collateral circulation is seen. In such cases, a gradual occlusion using a balloon catheter will reduce the risk of cerebral edema after excision.

edema [15]. (ii) a midline occipital lesion that has occluded all flow from the dorsal sagittal sinus to both transverse sinuses. In this scenario, substantial blood flow through collateral vessels along the lateral and ventral cerebrum is usually seen on MRI. In such an instance, the occipital skull with the confluens sinuum and portions of both transverse sinuses can be removed with minimal risk of cerebral edema [14]. (iii) an occipital lesion with intact blood flow to at least one transverse sinus where the line of excision will include the confluens sinuum and/or the intact transverse sinus. In this scenario, surgical excision of the lesion will result in an acute obstruction of blood flow draining from the dorsal sagittal sinus and significant edema formation in the brain tissue [16]. In this scenario, a gradual occlusion of the flow of blood from the dorsal sagittal sinus into the confluens sinuum will result in recruitment of collateral vasculature, accommodating the necessary flow of blood and preventing clinically significant cerebral edema. Slow occlusion of these vessels over 24–48 hours can be accomplished using a balloon embolization catheter placed within the dorsal sagittal sinus (see below for methods) [17]. Once this occlusion is complete, resection of the lesion that may include the caudal dorsal sagittal sinus, confluens sinuum, and both transverse sinuses can be completed with a low risk of clinically significant brain edema.

MRI Assessment of Blood Flow to the Transverse Sinuses

MRI imaging is currently the most effective and convenient way to assess the patency of the vessels and flow from the dorsal sagittal sinus to the transverse sinuses. Time-of-flight (TOF) MRI angiography takes advantage of the difference in magnetization between static and flowing tissue (blood) exposed to repetitive radiofrequency pulses. This results in an enhancement of imaging of the dorsal sagittal sinus (DSS) and transverse sinuses when assessing the vasculature for surgical risk (Figure 21.4) [17–19]. In a scenario such as that shown in Figure 21.4, where flow from the dorsal sagittal sinus to the transverse sinus is intact and the line of excision will require removal of the confluens sinuum, slow balloon catheter occlusion of the caudal DSS is recommended. In contrast, Figure 21.5 shows a TOF MR angiogram where tumor ingrowth has obstructed the

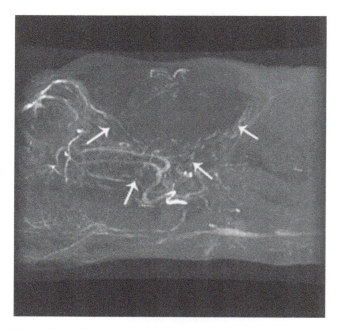

Figure 21.5 Time-of-flight MRI imaging of the dorsal sagittal and transverse sinuses with a midline occipital MLO lesion. No blood flow is seen in the caudal dorsal sagittal sinus or either transverse sinus. Collateral vessels are diffusely distributed around the lesion (arrows). This lesion was excised without additional interventions prior to definitive surgery.

confluens sinuum. In that case, significant collateral circulation around the tumor can be seen and excision of the confluens along with the tumor mass can be performed without additional steps.

Slow Occlusion of Flow from the DSS to the Transverse Sinus Using a Balloon Catheter

In patients where the caudal DSS and/or confluens sinuum will require removal during tumor excision, a slow occlusion of the vessel lumen close to the confluens sinuum over 24–48 hours will recruit collateral circulation and prevent significant edema in the brain tissue that might otherwise occur with an acute cessation of venous sinus blood flow. This is supported by an experimental study documenting a significant reduction in both intracranial pressure and brain edema of dogs when exposed to a gradual occlusion of the caudal DSS over four hours compared to a sudden occlusion [14] as well as by clinical case descriptions [17].

Figure 21.6 shows a schematized view of the procedure. The most appropriate catheter is a Fogarty arterial embolectomy type catheter in a size 2–4 Fr. In smaller dogs, a 4 Fr catheter will be overlarge and the smaller sizes should be used. This type of catheter has a round balloon as opposed to the elliptical shape seen in other balloon catheter devices and therefore has less balloon material on the catheter end to introduce into the vessel. A test inflation of the balloon with saline, which is noncompressible compared to air and will not create a gas embolus if ruptured, is performed and the diameter of the balloon is measured and recorded at increments of injection volume up to its maximum inflation capacity. These measurements are compared to the cross-sectional diameter of the caudal DSS as measured on MRI images to formulate a schedule for incremental inflation over 24 hours. Typically, the catheter is placed and then the first inflation performed a few hours after recovery from anesthesia. Incremental inflation is repeated two to three times at regular intervals over a 24-hour period until the full diameter of the DSS is occluded. If the animal evidences discomfort during an inflation event, it is assumed that inflation is complete and no further balloon inflation is done to avoid overstretching of the wall of the DSS. Further observation for an additional 24 hours provides a large margin of error prior to surgery but excisional surgery has been performed as early as 24 hours after catheter insertion.

For catheter placement, the patient is placed in ventral recumbency and the dorsal skull and cervical region clipped of hair and aseptically prepared for surgery. A prophylactic antibiotic regimen, as per surgeon preference, is administered. An approximately 5 cm skin

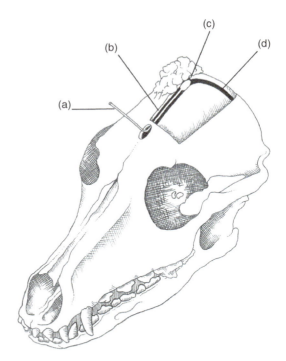

Figure 21.6 Schematic illustration of dorsal sagittal sinus catheterization for balloon occlusion. A Fogarty-style balloon catheter (a) is introduced into the dorsal sagittal sinus (b) through a burr hole in the dorsal midline skull. The catheter is advanced to the foramen impar where the dorsal sagittal sinus enters the bone and divides at the confluens sinuum (c). Gradual occlusion of the patent transverse sinus is achieved by staged inflation of the balloon to the diameter of the caudal dorsal sagittal sinus as measured on MRI imaging. In this illustration, the right transverse sinus is occluded by tumor but excision of the mass will require removal of the confluens sinuum. Illustration by H. M. McAnulty.

incision is made over the sagittal crest and dissection continued to the surface of the skull. Trephination of the skull using a high speed surgical burr is performed on midline at the level of the cranial sagittal crest or bregma or at the expected cranial margin of the tumor excision. Placement of the trephination is ideally cranial to the lesion to be excised in such a position that the trephine hole will eventually be part of the bone excisional boundary at the definitive surgery, but this is not a necessity. Hemorrhage can be controlled with hemostatic foam or bone wax. It should be noted that the bone may be relatively thick in this location creating more difficult angles of insertion for the catheter. For this reason, the cranial border of the trephine hole is beveled with the burr to create an angle of insertion that better approaches parallel to the vessel surface. The DSS will be readily visible through the dural membrane. If the DSS is not identified, the trephine hole can be enlarged laterally in both directions to make the DSS more visible.

A small stab incision is made in the DSS with a #11 scalpel blade and the balloon catheter advanced into the sinus. A small amount of hemorrhage will be encountered during this maneuver which is easily controlled by pressure using a sterile cotton-tipped applicator and then by the catheter once inserted through the venotomy. The catheter is advanced as far caudally as possible until it contacts bone presumed to be the foramen impar where the DSS enters into the occipital bone. This will place the balloon at the caudal extent of the DSS. Measurements of the distances to be traversed can also be obtained from MRI images to assist in estimating catheter positioning if desired. The catheter is then secured in place with encircling sutures such as 5-0 polypropylene and the entrance site into the DSS sealed with a surgical tissue sealant or cyanoacrylate glue. The superficial tissues of the skull are then closed around the protruding catheter and the catheter anchored to the epidermis to prevent dislodgement. An adhesive iodine-containing plastic drape can be placed over the incision and catheter insertion site to maintain sterility. After recovery, balloon inflation can be initiated. In the author's experience, insertion of the catheter and inflation at increments is well tolerated and no neurological signs have been noted in these patients to date during the inflation sequence.

At the time of the excisional surgery, the catheter is left in place. During the course of the occipital resection, the DSS will eventually be transected close to the foramen impar where the DSS enters the occipital bone. At that time, the catheter can either be transected or removed and the distal DSS ligated. The remainder of the catheter is removed from the more cranial DSS and the venotomy incision closed with fine suture such as 6-0 polypropylene.

Extension of Tumor to the tentorium Cerebelli

In some cases with occipital or ventral parietal MLO lesions, the tumor will extend on to the tentorium cerebelli and may extend deeply between the cerebral hemispheres and the cerebellum. In some of these cases, it can be difficult to remove all gross tumor where the tentorium attaches at its base to the parietal and occipital bones and greater attention to removing all visible tumor in this location will be required. It is possible, however, to remove the bulk of the tumor on the tentorium that extends deeply between the cerebrum and cerebellum in most cases. The tentorium cerebelli is a thin bony shelf that is covered by a reflection of the dura mater. Similarly to the scenario with calvarial tumors, the dura can be gently elevated off the tentorium between the hemispheres and cerebellum and once the base of the tentorium is freed via judicious

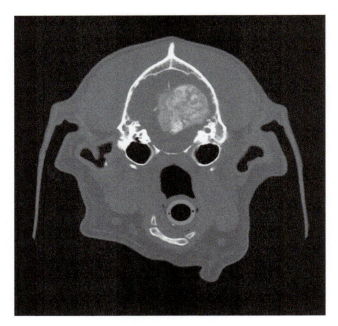

Figure 21.7 Extension and expansion of an MLO lesion on to the tentorium cerebelli. Although these lesions protrude between the cerebrum and cerebellum, gentle elevation of the dura from its surface and detachment of the base of the tentorium allows removal in most cases, although clean excision margins are difficult to obtain in these situations. Hemorrhage is typically controlled by packing between the cerebellum and cerebral hemispheres with hemostatic foam materials.

rongeur or burr excision, the tentorium, with entrained tumor, can be removed (Figure 21.7). In some cases, hemorrhage from deep between the hemispheres and cerebellum may be encountered upon removal of the tentorium. However, in a limited number of such cases performed to date by this author, this hemorrhage may be controlled with slight pressure/coverage of the area or gentle packing of this space with a gelatin hemostatic sponge material. No significant negative impacts directly attributable to these maneuvers have been observed in our patients to date.

Zygomatic Arch and Ramus of the Mandible

Lesions affecting the zygomatic arch or ramus of the mandible are among the most accessible of skull tumors. These lesions typically affect the ability to open the mouth without pain or the eye due to encroachment by the expansile lesion. The cranial zygomatic arch can be removed, along with the caudal maxilla at its cranial base with little effect. Similarly, the caudal zygomatic can be removed along with the temporomandibular joint if necessary and have the patient remain functional. Removal of the ramus of the mandible or the zygomatic arch at a level requiring excision of the temporomandibular joint will result in a shifting of the mandible due to the loss of caudal anchoring and may result in malocclusion issues and repetitive oral trauma requiring dental revision.

Complications and Risks

Aside from tumor recurrence, excessive blood loss is one of the greatest risks of surgeries discussed here. Hemostasis should be meticulous during surgery but at times it will not be possible to stop all hemorrhage until the tumor and cranial vault is removed so that all sources of hemorrhage can be exposed and addressed. Hemorrhage is cumulative over the long time frames for the more complex approaches described here, four to seven hours in many cases, and may need to be addressed by transfusions from matched blood sources. Hemorrhage is largely due to low pressure continuous slow bleeding and can be reduced by patient positioning with the head elevated above the core and avoidance of jugular compression as noted earlier. Further, overall hemorrhage can be reduced by strategic planning of the progression of the procedures so that portions of the surgery that are expected to create more hemorrhage or induce hemorrhage that is difficult to address until after the mass is removed are delayed until later in the procedure. Hemorrhage is controlled in routine manner with bipolar electrocautery and suture ligation. However, significant hemorrhages will also come directly from the bone or from transected transverse sinuses within the bone and are best stopped by bone wax tamponade. Hemorrhage may also be observed from the underside of the calvarium during bone incision. Elevation of the dura off the underside of the bone and placement of hemostatic foam in that space is an effective way of providing slight pressure on these bleeders and keeping the incision line free of blood.

Cerebral edema and other neurological injury are potential risks in the surgeries affecting the calvarium as described here. Cerebral edema (real and anticipated) is frequently addressed by administration of intravenous mannitol during the procedure. However, if a surgical plan is devised that accounts for the blood flow from the DSS to the transverse sinuses, as described above, cerebral edema seldom creates significant problems either intraoperatively or postoperatively, in this author's clinical experiences. In some dogs, postoperative seizures may occur. The cause of these seizures is not known but likely occurs due to the manipulation and possible injury of the brain tissue or the changes in the brain tissue as it expands back into its normal contour. Thus, a seizure watch after surgery is important and if seizures occur they should be controlled using standard anti-seizure interventions. With the exception of a single case, the author has seen no other patients with

calvarial resections as described here to have repetitive recurrent seizure activity once a perioperative period of 2–3 days has elapsed. Thus, for the most part, seizures appear to be a risk primarily in the perioperative period for most patients and that risk decreases significantly as the length of time since surgery increases. However, it should be noted that seizures have been seen to arise at much longer time periods (many months to years) after surgery and are likely related to recurrence of the tumor in the brain or associated structures [20]. For large occipital resections, cerebellar neurological signs such as ataxia and hypermetria are common in the postoperative period. For these excisions, nearly all dogs will have some degree of cerebellar signs, most commonly a hypermetric gait, that persist between 24 hours and 5–7 days. In the author's experience to date, these signs have all resolved within 2 weeks of surgery and posed no significant risk to the patient in the interim.

Soft tissue invasion by the tumors, particularly MLO lesions, can present a significant challenge. In the author's experience, recurrence of MLOs in the adjacent soft tissues after excision of a highly marginated skull lesion is seldom observed. Recurrence most commonly occurs in adjacent bone or by metastasis. However, there are MLO lesions that arise in the skull but also present with significant invasion of the adjacent head and cervical soft tissues. In these cases, it can be technically challenging to excise all of the tumor from the soft tissues. These lesions are often poorly marginated with little structural integrity in the soft tissues. The masses will crumble during dissection and can be assured of removal only by wide excision of normal soft tissues, a maneuver that is not always possible in the cervical and cephalic area. Recurrence within such poorly excised margins is frequent and should be considered a target for adjuvant therapy such as radiation.

Infection is a risk of such procedures although the risk appears to be low when appropriate prophylactic antibiotic regimens are utilized. Rare reports of delayed infection related to polymethylmethacrylate (PMMA) implants used for cranioplasty have been published, some occurring as long as several years after surgery. Reports of infection in both animals and humans when autologous or heterologous bone grafts, calcium phosphate, or hydroxyapatite implants used for cranioplasty are present in the literature [21–25]. One concern raised regarding infection is in situations where a prosthetic is utilized for cranioplasty that spans over the nonsterile nasal sinus or nasal cavity. Currently, there is insufficient evidence to suggest that this scenario represents an enhanced risk of infection. It should be noted that for prosthetics created with PMMA, inclusion of powdered cephalosporin or aminoglycoside antibiotics into the polymer mix, as is standard practice for many orthopedic procedures, is routine and may exert a preventative effect on device related infection.

Cranioplasty

Reconstruction of the cranium after excision, referred to as cranioplasty, is an area that has drawn a considerable amount of attention and innovation in both veterinary and human medicine. The goals of cranioplasty are to provide a protective covering for the brain, provide an attachment point for cervical muscles (in occipital resections) and, in some cases, to recreate a more normal cranial contour and avoid obstruction of sinus drainage into the nasal cavity. The ideal prosthetic is able to be manufactured in real time after the excision is completed so it can be customized to the defect, fits the defect tightly to enhance anchoring to the skull, is made of inert materials that do not resorb or promote infection, and can be modeled to mimic the contours of the normal skull and provide soft tissue attachments if desired. There is currently no single method for meeting all of these criteria so some degree of compromise by the surgeon is necessary.

The need for prosthetic cranioplasty after a partial craniectomy will depend on the location of the craniectomy on the skull and the size of the defect remaining after excision of the bone. In some cases, a relatively limited craniectomy that will be effectively covered by the temporalis muscle and fascia upon closure may not need any prosthetic implant at all or soft materials such porcine submucosa or polypropylene mesh can be utilized [26]. In large craniectomy excisions, substantial portions of the brain may be left unprotected under a thin superficial layer of tissue or the brain may actually protrude above the line of excision, increasing exposure to incidental trauma. In those cases, which will include nearly all occipital bone resections, a prosthetic implant, most often of a rigid construction, is warranted. Further, it may be advantageous for occipital implants to be fashioned in a manner that the implant is firmly attached to the skull and the detached cervical musculature can be anchored to the implant in addition to nearby soft tissue structures. This allows restoration of the muscular attachment along the nuchal crest and thus transfer of forces effectively to the head to restore relatively normal cervico-cephalic movement and function. In one dog, failure to restore these anchor points and reliance on attachment to the temporalis fascia was observed to result in an abnormal head carriage when running [17].

Cranioplasty prosthetics are prone to an array of complications [27]. Prosthetics comprised of processed bone grafts can have problems with infection and resorption of the bone [21]. For more rigid cranioplasty prosthetics in veterinary patients, most appear to favor using PMMA, three dimensionally (3-D) printed materials, or titanium mesh. Titanium mesh is relatively easy to work with but will not have the structural rigidity of PMMA or 3-D printed prosthetics and may be best used where large areas of the calvarium that are to be covered are relatively flat and mostly require a semi-rigid barrier without convex contouring [8, 28]. For larger defects, convex contouring of the prosthetic to approximate the original cranial cavity is warranted. Follow-up imaging at the author's institution has shown that brain tissue compressed by expansile tumors will rebound and fill the cranial cavity in a relatively normal conformation Cranioplasty for larger defects where the brain may protrude above the line of excision or in areas that are 3-D complex, such as the occiput, may be best treated by more rigid materials. Three-dimensional printing of prosthetics has mostly focused on use of either hydroxyapatite-based materials or titanium [20, 22–24, 28, 29]. Titanium appears to be favored in this technology and excellent descriptions of the workflow in manufacturing such a prosthetic are available in the literature [23]. PMMA generates a substantial amount of heat during the polymerization process and thus is not recommended to be formed in situ where it is able to contact the brain tissues. A cast and molding technique has been described where a PMMA prosthetic can be formed to custom fit the calvarial defect away from the patient and then placed after the material has cooled [25]. The PMMA prosthetic, once created, may also be augmented by cementing polypropylene mesh (Figure 21.8) to the prosthetic for attachment of

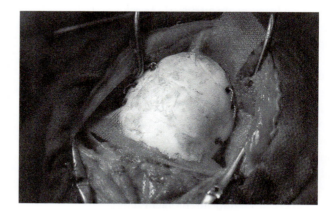

Figure 21.8 Polymethylmethacrylate cranioplasty with mesh strips for a large occipital MLO lesion. Cranioplasty for large excisions or those with significant potential for exposure of the brain to external trauma is warranted. Various preferred methods are available for cranioplasty. Shown here is a custom molded polymethylmethacrylate prosthetic created using a cast and mold technique with attached strips of polypropylene mesh for suturing of cervical muscles and other relevant soft tissues. The prosthetic is anchored to the calvarial bone with wire in this example. The mesh is trimmed to fit as needed as the closure progresses.

soft tissues such as the cervical musculature. The method is a two-step process where a cast of the defect is created and this is used as a mold to create the final prosthetic. The advantages of this method is that the prosthetic can be custom formed to fit the defect and, if done with proper attention to detail, will fit the calvarial defect in a lock-and-key manner to promote substantial anchoring. The disadvantages of the method are that it will require at least two, and perhaps three if mesh is attached to the material afterward, preparation mixtures of PMMA with associated costs and potential exposure to fumes escaping the vacuum systems into the operating room. Creation of the prosthetic can add an hour or more to the operative time. Regardless of the material, prosthetics are directly attached to the skull to augment their anchoring by using either orthopedic screws or sutures or wire placed through holes drilled in the surrounding bone.

There remain a number of open questions regarding the optimal approach to cranioplasty after craniectomy. The ideal materials and methods to create the prosthetics requires more data to assess outcomes and complications. It is also not known what are the relative risk of complications, such as infection, if the prosthetic crosses from the calvarium over to the frontal sinus. Further, techniques for cranioplasty involving the orbital rims need to be refined. In a prior report, cranioplasty in this area resulted in infection and ulceration at the leading edge of the prosthetic which continued to recur at the receding edge of the prosthetic even after the wounds were treated and the prosthetic shortened [25]. In that case, the working hypothesis was that a pressure point at the leading edge of the prosthetic combined with a non-sterile sinus environment promoted recurrent infection and fistulation. Further refinement of methods in this difficult area and further case experience is needed to ascertain the feasibility of prosthetic reconstruction of this part of the skull.

In summary, complex resections of large portions of the skull may be performed with careful planning and appropriate skill levels with relatively minimal negative effects on the individual patient. Such procedures require a detailed plan and development of new skills for many surgeons but are well within the difficulty level of most specialty trained surgeons.

 Video clips to accompany this book can be found on the companion website at: www.wiley.com/go/shores/advanced

References

1. Selmic, L.E., Lafferty, M.H., Kamstock, D.A. et al. (2014). Outcome and prognostic factors for osteosarcoma of the maxilla, mandible, or calvarium in dogs: 183 cases (1986–2012). *J. Am. Vet. Med. Assoc.* 245 (8): 930–938.
2. Kim, H., Nakaichi, M., Itamoto, K., and Taura, Y. (2007). Primary chondrosarcoma in the skull of a dog. *J. Vet. Sci.* 8 (1): 99–101.
3. Łojszczyk, A., Łopuszyński, W., Szadkowski, M. et al. (2021). Aggressive squamous cell carcinoma of the cranium of a dog. *BMC Vet. Res.* 17 (1): 144.
4. Straw, R.C., LeCouteur, R.A., Powers, B.E., and Withrow, S.J. (1989). Multilobular osteochondrosarcoma of the canine skull: 16 cases (1978–1988). *J. Am. Vet. Med. Assoc.* 195 (12): 1764–1769.
5. Dernell, W.S., Straw, R.C., Cooper, M.F. et al. (1998). Multilobular osteochondrosarcoma in 39 dogs: 1979–1993. *J. Am. Anim. Hosp. Assoc.* 34: 11–18.
6. Vancil, J.M., Henry, C.J., Milner, R.J. et al. (2012). Use of samarium Sm 153 lexidronam for the treatment of dogs with primary tumors of the skull: 20 cases (1986–2006). *J. Am. Vet. Med. Assoc.* 240 (11): 1310–1315.
7. Sweet, K.A., Nolan, M.W., Yoshikawa, H., and Gieger, T.L. (2020). Stereotactic radiation therapy for canine multilobular osteochondrosarcoma: eight cases. *Vet. Comp. Oncol.* 18 (1): 76–83.
8. Holmes, M.E., Keyerleber, M.A., and Faissler, D. (2019). Prolonged survival after craniectomy with skull reconstruction and adjuvant definitive radiation therapy in three dogs with multilobular osteochondrosarcoma. *Vet. Radiol. Ultrasound* 60 (4): 447–455.
9. Jacobson, S.A. (1971). Chondroma rodens. In: *The Comparative Pathology of Tumors of Bones, Part III: Chondroblastic Tumors* (ed. S.A. Jacobson), 102–109. Springfield, IL: Charles C. Thomas.
10. Diamond, S.S., Raflo, C.P., and Anderson, M.P. (1980). Multilobular osteosarcoma in the dog. *Vet. Pathol.* 17: 759–780.
11. Fukui, K. and Takamori, Y. (1986). Multilobular osteoma (chondroma rodens) in a pekingnese. *Vet. Rec.* 118: 483.
12. Avallone, G., Rasotto, R., Chambers, J.K. et al. (2021). Review of histological grading Systems in Veterinary Medicine. *Vet. Pathol.* 58 (5): 809–828.
13. Hathcock, J.T. and Newton, J.C. (2000). Computed tomographic characteristics of multilobular tumor of bone involving the cranium in 7 dogs and zygomatic arch in 2 dogs. *Vet. Radiol. Ultrasound* 41 (3): 214–217.

14. Gallegos, J., Schwarz, T., and McAnulty, J.F. (2008). Massive midline occipitotemporal resection of the skull for treatment of multilobular osteochondrosarcoma in two dogs. *J. Am. Vet. Med. Assoc.* 233 (5): 752–757.

15. Bagley, R.S., Harrington, M.L., Pluhar, G.E. et al. (1997). Acute, unilateral transverse sinus occlusion during craniectomy in seven dogs with space-occupying intracranial disease. *Vet. Surg.* 26 (3): 195–201.

16. Tuzgen, S., Canbaz, B., Kaya, A.H. et al. (2003). Experimental study of rapid versus slow sagittal sinus occlusion in dogs. *Neurol. India* 51 (4): 482–486.

17. McAnulty, J.F., Budgeon, C., and Waller, K.R. (2019). Catheter occlusion of the dorsal sagittal sinus-confluens sinuum to enable resection of lateral occipital multilobular osteochondrosarcoma in two dogs. *J. Am. Vet. Med. Assoc.* 254 (7): 843–851.

18. Chen, L., Shaw, D.W.W., Dager, S.R. et al. (2021). Quantitative assessment of the intracranial vasculature of infants and adults using iCafe (intracranial artery feature extraction). *Front. Neurol.* 12: 668298.

19. Broussolle, T. and Berhouma, M. (2021). On the importance of a thorough analysis of pre-operative imaging: variations of posterior fossa venous sinus anatomy. *Neurochirurgie* 67 (5): 518–519.

20. Hayes, G.M., Demeter, E.A., Choi, E., and Oblak, M. (2019). Single-stage craniectomy and cranioplasty for multilobular Osteochondrosarcoma managed with a custom additive manufactured titanium plate in a dog. *Case Rep. Vet. Med.* 2: 6383591.

21. Zhu, W., Wu, J., Zhao, H. et al. (2020). Establishment and characteristic analysis of a dog model for autologous homologous cranioplasty. *Biomed. Res. Int.* 22: 5324719.

22. Koller, M., Rafter, D., Shok, G. et al. (2020). A retrospective descriptive study of cranioplasty failure rates and contributing factors in novel 3D printed calcium phosphate implants compared to traditional materials. *3D Print Med.* 6 (1): 14.

23. James, J., Oblak, M.L., Zur Linden, A.R. et al. (2020). Schedule feasibility and workflow for additive manufacturing of titanium plates for ranioplasty in canine skull tumors. *BMC Vet. Res.* 16 (1): 180.

24. Itokawa, H., Hiraide, T., Moriya, M. et al. (2007). A 12 month in vivo study on the response of bone to a hydroxyapatite-polymethylmethacrylate cranioplasty composite. *Biomaterials* 28 (33): 4922–4927.

25. Bryant, K.J., Steinberg, H., and McAnulty, J.F. (2003). Cranioplasty by means of molded polymethylmethacrylate prosthetic reconstruction after radical excision of neoplasms of the skull in two dogs. *J. Am. Vet. Med. Assoc.* 223 (1): 67–72, 59.

26. Sheahan, D.E. and Gillian, T.D. (2008). Reconstructive cranioplasty using a porcine small intestinal submucosal graft. *J. Small Anim. Pract.* 49 (5): 257–259.

27. Zaed, I. and Tinterri, B. (2020). Comparison of complications in cranioplasty with various materials: a systematic review and meta-analysis. *Br. J. Neurosurg.* 31: 1.

28. Langer, P., Black, C., Egan, P., and Fitzpatrick, N. (2018). Treatment of calvarial defects by resorbable and non-resorbable sonic activated polymer pins and moldable titanium mesh in two dogs: a case report. *BMC Vet. Res.* 14 (1): 199.

29. Lal, B., Ghosh, M., Agarwal, B. et al. (2020). A novel economically viable solution for 3D printing-assisted cranioplast fabrication. *Br. J. Neurosurg.* 34 (3): 280–283.

22

Surgical Management of Intracranial Meningiomas

R. Timothy Bentley

Purdue University, West Lafayette, IN, USA

Introduction

Meningiomas are the most common primary brain tumor of dogs (especially non-brachycephalic breeds) and cats [1, 2], and they are the most responsive to surgery. Gross-total resection (GTR) refers to the complete removal of a brain tumor, as assessed by a combination of intraoperative inspection and postoperative Magnetic Resonance Imaging (MRI) [3]. In cats, as in humans, meningiomas tend to be low grade and surgery alone is often curative [1, 2]. In dogs, surgical biopsy often results in a low grade, yet meningiomas may recur despite GTR [2, 4]. Necropsy may reveal that when the histological features of a canine meningioma itself are worthy of a low grade, there is microscopic invasion of the adjacent brain surface [2, 5].

Meningiomas are believed to arise from the arachnoid cap cells within arachnoid villi [1, 2], and as such they are located deep to the dura mater and attached to its underside (Figure 22.1). They are superficial to the pial surface of the brain. Particularly in cats, the meningioma may be very well encapsulated and peel off the pial surface of the brain very easily. In dogs, meningiomas can be much more adherent to the brain surface, even invasive [2]. The subarachnoid space containing cerebrospinal fluid (CSF) is deep to the meningioma, but it is typically collapsed, with the meningioma tight against the brain surface. When incising the dura *adjacent* to a meningioma, CSF should leak out, but when incising the dura immediately over a meningioma often no CSF appears.

The vascular supply of meningiomas appears to arise from a combination of the overlying dura mater and the pial surface of the brain [6–8]. In humans, it is often dural and pial. In cats, it is often dural. In dogs, it is often pial. This may correlate to the ease with which many feline meningiomas can be physically removed from the brain surface at surgery and/or their lower rate of postoperative recurrence [2]. This also pertains to the recurrence rate as in many canine meningiomas, a majority of the vasculature arises from the pia, and thus has a close association with the brain parenchyma.

Most meningiomas occur in the rostral cranial fossa, which is the location most amenable to surgery. Caudal fossa meningiomas are less common, but cerebellar tumors in particular can be operable (see section Suboccipital craniectomy below, and Chapter 24 Surgery of the Caudal Fossa in this book). Middle fossa meningiomas are also less common but can be operable [see Chapter 20 Surgical Management of Sellar Masses in this book]).

Anatomy

The dura mater is a single surgical layer; however, it is comprised of two layers: the outer periosteal layer and the inner meningeal layer. These two layers divide around venous sinuses such as the dorsal sagittal sinus (DSS). These veins are valve-less and must be ligated on *both sides* of any intended incision. The dura mater is fused with the periosteum of the skull (there is no epidural fat). The epidural space is a potential space that can be filled with hematoma postoperatively.

The falx cerebri sits within the longitudinal fissure, immediately under the skull and between the two cerebral hemispheres. It attaches rostrally to the internal frontal crest (frontal bone), the crista galli (the midline ridge in the cribriform plate, ethmoid bone), and the presphenoid bone.

Advanced Techniques in Canine and Feline Neurosurgery, First Edition. Edited by Andy Shores and Brigitte A. Brisson.
© 2023 John Wiley & Sons, Inc. Published 2023 by John Wiley & Sons, Inc.
Companion site: www.wiley.com/go/shores/advanced

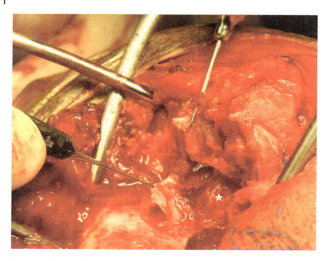

Figure 22.1 Caudal cerebellar meningioma in a dog. The white dura mater (Bishop-Harmon forceps) is being reflected back from the cerebellum, revealing a meningioma (asterisk) and the cerebellar vermis. Note that the meningioma is stuck to the underside of the dura mater. The defect in the dura (durectomy) is purposefully being made larger than the meningioma.

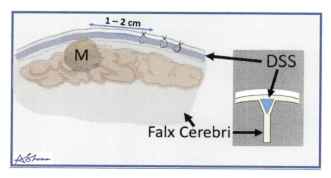

Figure 22.2 Placement of three ligatures around the dorsal sagittal sinus (DSS) before incising the rostral falx. Note that ligatures can only be placed around the rostral one-third of the DSS, unless a preoperative angiogram has documented occlusion of the DSS by a meningioma in caudal two-thirds of the falx. To remove a meningioma and all associated dura mater from the rostral falx, the DSS must be ligated. First, durotomy is performed on both sides of the falx cerebri (or a durectomy on the side of the tumor). If possible, the intended falcine incision (white arrow) should be 1–2 cm caudal to the meningioma (M). At least one simple and one transfixing (or three simple) sutures must be placed caudal to the intended incision. At least one suture should be placed rostral to the intended incision. The falx can then be pre-cauterized (bipolar) and incised (e.g. Metzenbaum scissors). For a rostral falcine meningioma, either additional ligatures can be placed rostral to the tumor (with multiple sutures rostral to the incision). Or the falx can simply be removed from its attachment to the rostral skull (internal frontal crest, crista galli, and the presphenoid bone) using pre-cautery (bipolar) and scissors. Lifting up the caudal edge of the falcine strip facilitates access to the falcine attachment to the skullbase. Inset: the falx cerebri is immediately ventral to the skull. The DSS is within the dorsal falx cerebri, and fully enveloped by dura mater in the normal subject.

It is continuous with the membranous tentorium cerebelli caudally. The DSS is within the dorsal part of the falx (Figure 22.2), fully enclosed within the falcine dura. The DSS flows from rostral to caudal, becoming progressively wider in diameter as it accepts dorsal cerebral veins (vv. cerebri dorsales) and diploic veins from the skull. Ventral to the falx is the vein of the corpus callosum (v. corporis callosi), which joins with other veins to form the straight sinus (sinus rectus). The straight sinus enters the DSS at the level of the occipital lobes. Caudal to the occipital lobes, the DSS passes through the periosteal dura mater to enter the foramen for the DSS (syn. impar foramen) where it is about 3 mm in diameter in dogs. The DSS ends at the confluence of the sinuses (confluens sinuum) located inside the caudal skull, which is drained by the paired transverse sinuses. The straight sinus sometimes joins the confluence within the skull, rather than joining the DSS in the falx. Each transverse sinus runs laterally in the transverse canal (fully enclosed in bone) then in the transverse groove (incompletely enclosed in bone), then continues as the temporal sinus after giving off the sigmoid sinus. The single DSS and paired transverse sinuses provide the only venous drainage of the dorsal cerebral hemispheres. Surgically, the rostral third of the DSS can be ligated (e.g. rostral to the cruciate sulcus or ventral to the frontal nasal sinus). The caudal two thirds cannot be acutely occluded, nor can the confluence within the bone, without risking venous stroke of both dorsal cerebral hemispheres. The caudal third of the falx also contains the straight sinus. If the caudal falx cerebri is traumatized leading to hemorrhage (e.g. debriding a meningioma away from the falx), it cannot be ligated. Pressure must be applied to the falx (e.g. gelatin sponge) until the bleeding arrests. The surgeon must hope that the sinuses do not thrombose. The dura *cannot* be elevated from the caudal skull on the midline (the vertical bone caudal to the occipital lobes), as this would tear the DSS between the dura mater and the foramen for the DSS. One transverse sinus can be occluded, but *not* both. For extremely ventral hemispheric exposure, the temporal sinus can be occluded within the temporal bone using bone wax.

Surgical locations of rostral fossa meningiomas include convexity tumors, on the surface of one cerebral hemisphere [9]. Falcine tumors, arising from the falx cerebri, are especially common in the fronto-olfactory region [1]. Variations of meningiomas recognized in human neurosurgery include parasagittal (to one side of the dura [9], e.g.

Table 22.1 Main approaches to the cranial vault for the extirpation of meningiomas in dogs and cats [4, 12, 13].

Approach	Indications	Modifications
Transfrontal craniotomy	Meningiomas ventral to frontal nasal sinus *Olfactory bulbs; rostral frontal lobe Rostral falx cerebri*	1. Purdue diamond
Rostrotentorial (lateral) craniotomy/craniectomy	Convexity meningiomas and parasagittal meningiomas *Parietal, temporal, caudal frontal lobes Middle – caudal falx cerebri*	1. Combined with transfrontal 2. Split temporalis muscle (to access skullbase) 3. Transzygomatic (see Chapter 25)
Bilateral rostrotentorial craniotomy	Falcine meningiomas that have occluded DSS flow *Middle – caudal falx cerebri*	
Suboccipital craniectomy	Caudal cerebellar meningiomas (see Chapter 24)	1. Combine with C1 laminectomy
Transsphenoidal hypophysectomy	Pituitary fossa meningiomas (see Chapter 20)	

contacting both the dorsal dura and the falcine dura), olfactory groove (the depression in the ethmoid bone for the olfactory bulb), and sphenoid wing (the ridge of the sphenoidal bone on the skullbase that is highly developed in humans, separating the anterior and middle cranial fossae). Of these, parasagittal and olfactory groove meningiomas are frequently operated in dogs and cats, but often classified simply as falcine meningiomas. Sphenoidal wing meningiomas necessitate a different surgical approach in humans (e.g. pterional craniotomy), but in dogs and cats most would be accessed through a rostrotentorial or transzygomatic approach (see Chapter 25 Transzygomatic Approach to Ventrolateral Craniotomy/Craniectomy in this book) and would often be classified simply as convexity meningiomas. This ridge of bone is poorly developed in dogs and cats and referred to simply as the sphenofrontal suture rather than the sphenoidal wing. As such, adoption of the sphenoidal wing terminology used in humans does not seem appropriate.

Tentorial meningiomas may be accessible by a caudal rostrotentorial craniectomy and working under the occipital lobe or a transtentorial craniectomy [10]; note the transverse sinus anatomy. It is possible to have multiple meningiomas, especially in cats, and it may be appropriate to remove two or more in a single surgery [11]. Uncommon locations include intraventricular meningiomas in cats, and the optic nerve (which is sheathed by dura mater rather than epineurium) [1].

A summary of the surgical approaches to the differing locations of intracranial meningiomas is shown in Table 22.1.

Transfrontal Craniotomy (Bilateral Transfrontal Craniotomy)

This provides access to the olfactory bulbs, the rostral frontal lobes and up to one third of the falx cerebri. Typically, the upper plate of the frontal bone is removed (and replaced during closure), then the lower plate of the frontal bone is removed (and not replaced) to access the cranial vault [4, 14].

Technique

A dorsal midline skin incision is made, starting rostral to the medial canthi and ending over the external sagittal crest. The subcutaneous frontalis muscle is sharply incised on midline. A vein often exits through a small midline foramen in the nasal bone; it can be cauterized or bone-waxed. The sharp midline incision is continued to the periosteum. The periosteum and subcutaneous tissues are elevated (e.g. Freer elevator) in a lateral direction, to either side of the incision.

A diamond-shaped bone flap is now removed from the upper plate of bone, to enter the frontal sinus [4]. The outline of this bone flap is the diamond shape of bone, rostral to the temporalis muscles. It is a flat segment of bone bordered by the left and right frontal crests, the zygomatic processes, and the orbits. It is primarily the squamous part of the frontal bone, but the rostral section is nasal bone.

A sagittal saw (e.g. 3–5 mm blades, E-pen) can be used to cut the bone flap at a 45° angle [4]. This angulation allows

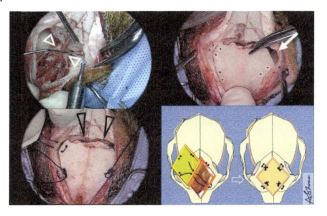

Figure 22.3 A conventional diamond-shaped bone flap for a transfrontal craniotomy. Note the wide access to the olfactory bulbs (white triangles) but the narrow access to the frontal lobes. Additional bone is being burred away to improve access to the left frontal lobe, resulting in a bone gap at closure (white arrow). In this brachycephalic cat skull conformation, the caudal half of the diamond is reduced in size and made even smaller by burring bone to pass osteotomes (black triangles). Matching pairs of 1 mm burr holes were made in a small ledge created by making the bone flap slightly less wide than the frontal sinus itself. Note that none of the horizontal mattress sutures (0 PDS) are tied down until the suture has been passed through *all* the burr holes. Bone sutures are often placed on all 4 sides of a bone flap, but suturing three sides is acceptable. Note that the rostral bone sutures were placed by first passing both ends of the suture *down* through the skull and then *up* through the bone flap. This leaves the knots dorsal to the bone flap and medial to sagittal saw incision. In this case, the caudal suture was placed by passing the suture ends *down* through the bone flap and *up* through the skull, but this can be very awkward. In extremely small patients with very thin plates of bone, it is especially important to make the sagittal saw cut at a steep angle (far from vertical). The bone flap would fall down into the frontal sinus if vertical cuts were made.

the bone flap to sit in position during closure (Figure 22.3). Leaving a small ledge laterally facilitates closure (see below). Once this cut has been made, the plate of bone will be rigidly held in place by the many osseous septa within the frontal sinus, and especially by the midline septum (septum sinuum frontalium) that divides the frontal sinus into left and right compartments. A small burr (e.g. 3 mm) can be used on the external sagittal crest and the most caudal corner of the diamond-shaped flap to gain access to the septum. Next, a small osteotome is driven down the midline, passing ventral to the bone flap and roughly parallel with it in a rostro-ventral direction, to destroy the midline septum (Figures 22.4 and 22.5). Often, it becomes impossible to drive the osteotome any further rostrally. Even smaller osteotomes can now be used either side of midline, to crack the osseous septa that connect the upper and lower plates of frontal bone. As the bone flap becomes progressively more mobile, the first osteotome can be driven further down the midline septum and the bone flap will come free.

The osseous septa are removed with rongeurs from the underside of the bone flap, as are the septa remaining within the sinus. The bone flap is kept clean and secure (e.g. a bowl of flush) until closure. Ectoturbinates 2 and 3 extend into the most rostral aspect of the fontal sinus. To access the most rostral cranial vault (olfactory bulbs), these can be removed with rongeurs. The resulting mucosal hemorrhage is controlled by packing gauzes or lap sponges rostrally in the frontal sinus. Ectoturbinate removal maximizes frontal sinus drainage postoperatively, minimizing mucocele formation. The cribriform plate itself can even be resected unilaterally, but it is usually possible to resect even the most rostral meningiomas through a bone defect that ends immediately caudal to the cribriform plate, reaching behind an intact cribriform plate. Intraoperative mucosal hemorrhage and postoperative hyposmia arise from cribriform plate resection, severely impacting postoperative appetite.

The mucoperiosteum is removed from the entire frontal sinus, to reduce postoperative mucocele (e.g. dry gauze is driven over every surface and into every crevice using a Freer elevator).

A burr (e.g. 3 mm, E-pen or Surgairtome) is used to remove the inner plate of the frontal bone, entering the cranial vault. This second bone flap will also be diamond-shaped, but it can be discarded. Ipsilateral to the tumor, it is often beneficial to make this bone flap as wide as possible. To do so, burr exactly where the horizontal bone over the brain meets the vertical bone that makes up the lateral aspects of the frontal sinus. The bone will be of varying thickness as it follows the underlying gyri and sulci, and there are larger indents of bone, on the midline over the falx cerebri (frontal suture), and between the frontal lobe and the olfactory bulb. When encountering spots with thicker bone, it can be useful to change the direction of burr movement. Briefly stop moving the burr parallel to the bone cut being made and oscillate it perpendicularly until the ridge of thicker bone gives way. For example, burr rostro-caudally through the midline frontal suture at the caudal most point of the diamond but be especially careful not to damage the dura mater and underlying DSS.

It is usually possible to remove the inner plate of the frontal bone in a single piece, taking care to patiently and carefully work it free from the dura mater. Some surgeons first divide the bone in two, burring down the midline over the falx cerebri, to increase mobilization. The older the patient, the more the dura mater and periosteum will have become fused, frustrating attempts to remove the bone flap without tearing the dura mater. For meningioma surgery, if

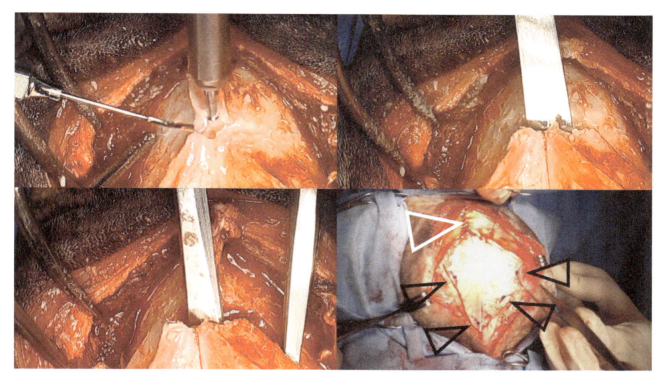

Figure 22.4 Using osteotomes to elevate a Purdue diamond. A Purdue diamond bone flap was made with a sagittal saw. Just enough bone is being burred away from the caudal edge of the diamond and the external sagittal crest to pass a small osteotome into the septum sinuum frontalium. When this osteotome would not advance any further, an even smaller osteotome was driven either side of midline, to crack the many osseous septa within the frontal sinus. The first osteotome was again advanced, cracking the bone flap free. Osteotomes are driven rostro-ventrally, parallel with the underside of the bone flap. At closure, bone sutures have been placed at multiple locations (black triangles). A suture was also placed in the third side of the bone flap (Figure 22.5). The left and right temporalis muscles have been apposed to one another where the external sagittal crest was sacrificed (white triangle), and the bilateral incisions in the temporalis fascia alongside the frontal crests are now being sutured.

necessary, a segment of torn dura can be removed along with the bone flap, as the dura needs to be removed anyway. Iris scissors can facilitate this. Resultant dural bleeding can be controlled with bipolar cautery. However, it is *not* permitted to accidentally tear or purposefully incise the midline dura mater while elevating the bone flap. This would cause hemorrhage from the DSS.

The dura mater is opened by making a stab incision (e.g. #11 blade or a bent needle, Figure 22.6) then performing a durectomy (e.g. iris scissors and DeBakey forceps). The widest possible margin of normal dura should be excised (maximum 1–2 cm). To prevent iatrogenic trauma to healthy brain, the initial stab incision can be made over the tumor itself, then scissors used to create a durectomy larger than the tumor. For a convexity tumor, the dura mater is opened unilaterally, preserving the falx cerebri and DSS. For a falcine tumor, a "falcine strip" can be removed (see below).

The meningioma can now be removed (see section Meningioma resection). Lateral to the cribriform plate are one to two ethmoidal foramina (ethmoid bone), allowing passage of the ethmoidal vessels and nerve through the skull. These can be ablated during meningioma/dura resection, if necessary.

Usually, olfactory bulb meningiomas are unilateral, separated from the contralateral olfactory bulb by an intact falx. It is often necessary to retract the olfactory bulb or debride the ipsilateral cribriform plate to remove such meningiomas. If the tumor involves the falx, resect a "falcine strip," but protect the contralateral olfactory bulb and cribriform plate that are exposed upon doing so. With meningiomas covering the entire unilateral cribriform plate, complete ablation of one olfactory nerve is indicated, as adequate olfaction and appetite will be present postoperatively.

Closure

The surgical site is copiously lavaged. A dural substitute (see section Substitutes for resected dura mater) is placed but gelatin sponge (e.g. Gelfoam®) is *never* left in the frontal sinus. The lower plate of frontal bone is not replaced.

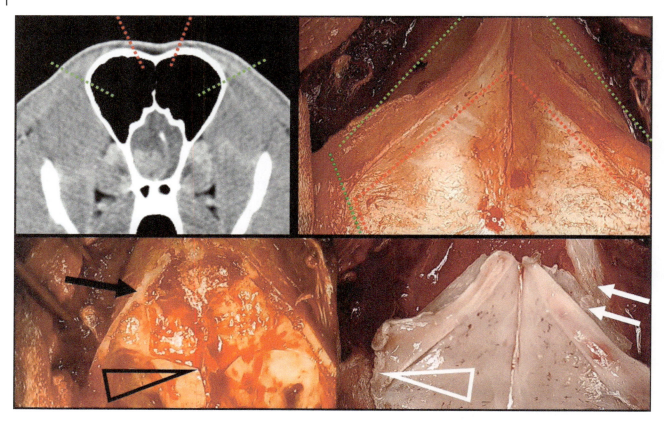

Figure 22.5 Bilateral Purdue diamond. Top left: a CT image of a dolichocephalic dog demonstrates that a conventional diamond-shaped bone flap is created medial to the temporalis muscles (red lines) and provides narrow access to the frontal lobes. A Purdue diamond bone flap (green lines) is much wider. It is made by elevating the temporalis muscle, then incising the bone at its widest point. Top right: intraoperative photograph after bilaterally elevating the temporalis muscles. The dashed lines again demonstrate the bone cuts made for a traditional diamond (red) compared to a Purdue diamond (green). Bottom left: the access to the cranial vault after removing a bilateral Purdue diamond. The remaining bone making up the wall of the caudal right frontal sinus (black arrow) will be sacrificed as part of the craniectomy, to access the right frontal lobe. Note the remnant of the frontal sinus septum (black triangle). Bottom right: replacing the bone flap after a combined transfrontal and right rostrotentorial craniectomy. Bone sutures will be placed on both rostral edges of the diamond, and a single suture will be placed on the caudal-left edge (white arrows indicate suitable burr hole locations). Note that the temporalis muscle fascia has been preserved on the frontal crest bilaterally, except where it was incised to be able to make the bone cut (white triangle). The fascia will be used for routine re-apposition of the temporalis muscles, further securing the bone flap (see Figure 22.4). Compare the lower-left image to the size of a traditional diamond bone flap. The exposure of the caudo-lateral frontal sinus with a Purdue diamond is considerably greater.

There are multiple techniques to replace the upper bone flap. The simplest is to make matching burr holes (e.g. 1 mm) in the skull and bone flap, then place bone sutures (e.g. size 0 PDS). Horizontal mattress sutures are recommended. As in Figure 22.3, it is much easier to pass suture *down* through the skull and *up* through the moveable bone flap. Sutures are temporarily secured with hemostats. Once sutures have been passed through *all* burr holes they are tied off. Typically, sutures are placed in all four sides of the diamond. If additional bone removal prevents this, sutures must be placed in three sides of the diamond.

While using the sagittal saw during the approach, usually a small ledge is purposefully left lateral to the bone incision to facilitate burr hole placement during closure. However, a cut made at the extreme lateral edge of the frontal sinus improves access. If there is insufficient ledge to create a simple burr hole, an L-hole can be made (see Figure 22.7).

A simple continuous suture is placed in the frontalis muscle (e.g. 3-0 synthetic absorbable suture). The subcutis and skin are closed routinely.

Modifications

Purdue Diamond Modification. The frontal nasal sinus has three parts (lateral, medial, rostral). The lateral part is large and makes up the caudal and lateral boundaries of the sinus. It begins under the squamous part of the frontal bone and continues caudally under the frontal crests (syn. orbitotemporal crest). Especially in dolichocephalic dogs, it continues well under the temporalis muscle. Frontal lobe convexity

22 Surgical Management of Intracranial Meningiomas | 229

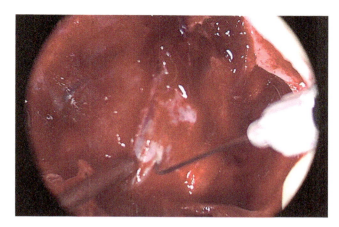

Figure 22.6 A 23-gauge needle is bent 90°, then used to make the initial penetration through the left dura. The DSS is visible as a purple venous structure, immediately under the Frazier suction tip.

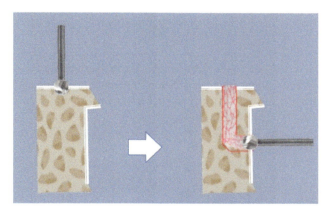

Figure 22.7 Placing an L-hole when an insufficient ledge has been left in the upper plate of frontal bone to place a standard bone suture. First drive a 1 mm burr vertically into the skull, just lateral to the sagittal saw cut. Second, burr horizontally, through the wall of the frontal sinus and aiming for the base of the first burr hole. The suture can be passed into the first burr hole, exiting through the second burr hole.

meningiomas under this lateral part of the sinus are not well accessed by a conventional transfrontal craniotomy. The standard diamond-shaped bone flap provides very wide access to the olfactory bulbs. Moving caudally from there, the opening in the sinus becomes narrower as the brain becomes wider: the standard diamond bone flap only provides midline access to the frontal lobes. To take advantage of the lateral frontal sinus, a Purdue diamond bone flap is created (Figure 22.5) [13]. The fascia of the temporalis muscle is incised just lateral to its insertion on the frontal crest. The temporalis muscle is elevated to expose the bone housing the lateral frontal sinus. This bone is cut at its most lateral aspect with a sagittal saw. One simple interrupted 1-0 synthetic absorbable suture is placed here through burr holes in the bone at closure. The temporalis fascia is then closed using absorbable synthetic suture in a simple continuous pattern, further immobilizing the bone flap.

A Purdue diamond is of no benefit to an olfactory falcine meningioma. A unilateral Purdue diamond is extremely advantageous to a lateral frontal lobe convexity meningioma, ventral to where the frontal sinus is covered by temporalis muscle. A bilateral Purdue diamond improves access to the falx of the caudal frontal lobes.

Unilateral Transfrontal Craniotomy. A unilateral approach can be performed (e.g. a meningioma lateral to the frontal lobe/olfactory bulb where no falcine resection is indicated). It is easier, however, to retract the brain medially when a bilateral approach has been made: bone dorsal to the falx cerebri and contralateral hemisphere prevents brain retraction. It is also easier to manipulate instruments through a bilateral craniotomy, as compared to the narrow corridor of a unilateral craniotomy.

Brachycephalic Dogs. Note that in brachycephalic dogs, the frontal sinus may be much reduced in size and, in some cases, it does not contain any air-filled spaces at all (only medullary bone). In these cases (rather than entering through two layers of bone), it is necessary to perform a craniectomy of a single sheet of bone with a burr. If more ventral access is necessary (e.g. olfactory meningiomas on the skullbase), first a craniectomy is performed between the eyes. Burring is then continued in a ventral direction, progressively exposing more ventral dura mater. The bone will progressively thicken until the air-filled nasal cavity is penetrated. Bone removal is now sufficient – further bone removal will cause hemorrhage from the vascular mucosa of the nose and damage the cribriform plate, damaging olfaction. In this skull shape, the surgeon can easily reach behind an intact cribriform plate to access the skullbase.

The Falx Cerebri and the Dorsal Sagittal Sinus (DSS)

In all cats and dogs, the DSS can be sacrificed within the rostral one-third of its length (see section Anatomy, above). Ligation of the caudal two-thirds of the DSS risks venous stroke of the dorsal aspect of both cerebral hemispheres. Accordingly, it is safe to ligate the DSS that is exposed by a transfrontal craniotomy (anywhere between the cribriform plate and the caudal aspect of the frontal nasal sinus). Caudal to the frontal sinus (e.g. ventral to the ext. sag. crest of the parietal or occipital bones) the DSS should not be ligated or sacrificed, *unless there has been preoperative vascular imaging* documenting that the DSS has already been occluded by the meningioma (venous phases of MR or CT angiograms). While surgical ligation of the caudal two-thirds of a *patent* DSS is *not* permissible, when flow is steadily occluded by a tumor, there is time for collateral circulation to develop. In such cases, an angiogram should be added to the MRI, or an immediately preoperative CT performed. These decide between removing a "falcine strip" (for an occluded DSS) versus dissecting a parasagittal meningioma away from an intact falx cerebri (for a patent DSS), leaving the DSS intact.

Typically, the ligation of dorsal cerebral veins *(v. cerebri dorsales)* that empty into the DSS is minimized (e.g. only one per side). The number of dorsal cerebral veins that can be ligated without impairing venous drainage has not been studied, and in human patients these may be reconstructed to allow resection of large parasagittal meningiomas [15].

The Falcine Strip Procedure. The entire portion of the falx cerebri and DSS that is accessible through a transfrontal craniotomy (olfactory bulbs and rostral frontal lobes) can be safely resected. A portion of the falx including a falcine meningioma can thus be resected en masse, after suturing the falcine strip and DSS at the caudal aspect and suturing or cauterizing the falcine strip at its rostral aspect.

In order to remove a *falcine strip*, first the dura mater is incised either side of midline. Typically, a durectomy is performed on the side of the meningioma, to one side of the falx. On the other side, a durotomy is made just lateral to the DSS, longer than the section of falx to be removed (Figure 22.8). Caudal to the tumor, three sutures are placed through the falx cerebri to ligate the DSS using 3-0 synthetic absorbable suture. One transfixing suture and one single suture are placed caudal to the intended incision, and one simple suture rostral to the intended incision (Figures 22.1, 22.8–22.10). Alternatively, four simple sutures can be placed, incising between the first and second sutures. The falx cerebri and enclosed DSS can now be incised between these sutures, by pre-cautery (bipolar) followed by Metzenbaum/iris scissors. This frees up the caudal end of the falcine strip.

The rostral end of the falcine strip is freed up by repeating the suturing process rostrally, or more commonly by completely removing the entire attachment of the falx cerebri to the rostral skull. When removing the attachment of the falx to the skull, aggressive pre-cautery of the falx before incision replaces the need for suturing, as the DSS has negligible diameter immediately caudal to the cribriform plate. The falx cerebri attaches to the midline of the underside of the rostral frontal bone (frontal crest), to the cribriform plate (crista galli) and to the most rostral aspect of the skullbase (sphenoid bone). Progressively working from dorsal to ventral or vice versa, the entire attachment of the falx to these rostral skull structures is pre-cauterized then incised. This is performed by carefully passing bipolar electrocautery then iris or Metzenbaum scissors between the two hemispheres. Remaining tags of falx are again cauterized and then rongeured away. Conclude hemostasis by cauterizing/bone-waxing on the midline of the cribriform plate, where the DSS arises from veins draining the osseous nasal septum.

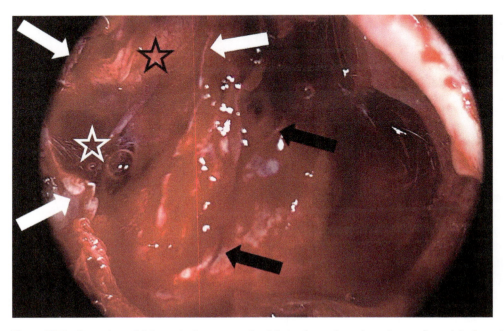

Figure 22.8 Preparing a falcine strip for sutures after bilateral transfrontal craniotomy for a right frontal cystic meningioma. White arrows: margins of the extensive right-sided durectomy, ipsilateral to the tumor. The durectomy reveals the right frontal lobe (black star), rostral to which is the large cavity created by opening the cystic meningioma (white star). Black arrows: a left-sided rostro-caudal durotomy has been made alongside the falx cerebri. The falx cerebri is now prepared for ligation of the DSS and removal of a "falcine strip."

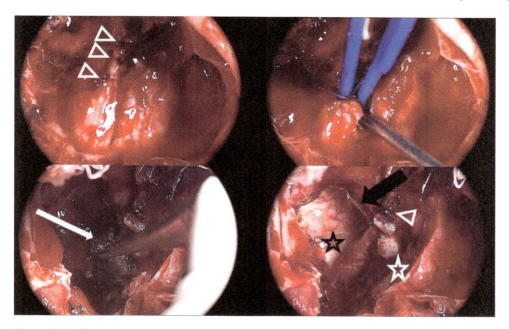

Figure 22.9 Same case as Figure 22.8. Three DSS ligatures have been placed (white triangles), the caudal one being a transfixing suture. Bipolar electrocautery (blue instrument) then scissors are used to incise the falx, from the DSS to the skullbase. The falcine strip is then removed by pre-cauterizing and incising all attachments to the rostral skull. After removal of the meningioma itself, the dura of the skullbase and lateral cranial vault is cauterized until charred remnants can be elevated from the bone (white arrow). The pial surface of the chronically compressed right frontal lobe is visible (black star). There is no falx between it and the left hemisphere. The two caudal DSS sutures (white triangle) are still in the falx cerebri. The edge of the large right durectomy can be seen (black arrow). The left durotomy has been reflected against bone (white star) – this will be placed back over the left hemisphere. These dural edges will anchor a temporalis fascia graft (Figure 22.14).

For an olfactory meningioma, dural margins and any remaining tumor on the skullbase are removed by retracting the ipsilateral olfactory bulb laterally using the side of a Frazier suction tip. Note that an olfactory falcine meningioma is surrounded by dura mater on three sides – the dorsal dura is removed during the initial durectomy, the medial dura is removed within the falcine strip, and lastly the ventral dura is ablated by elevating/cauterizing the skullbase dura. Skullbase dura mater contralateral to tumor should also be ablated to achieve what margin is possible, while fully preserving the olfactory bulb.

A *falcine strip* can be removed from the caudal two-thirds of the falx cerebri (caudal frontal lobes, parietal and occipital lobes), but *only* if occlusion of the DSS by the meningioma has been documented by vascular imaging preoperatively (see section Anatomy). A bilateral rostrotentorial craniotomy is performed and the dura is incised to both sides of the falx (this may include a durectomy on the side of a parasagittal tumor). As above, three or more sutures are placed at both of the intended incisions in the falx. The caudal incision must have two of these sutures (including one transfixing) *caudal* to it. The rostral incision must have two of these sutures (including one transfixing) *rostral* to it. Many falcine tumors of the caudal or middle falx cerebri can alternatively be accessed via a unilateral rostrotentorial approach and debrided from the falx cerebri while preserving the DSS; for example, if preoperative imaging documents flow through the DSS. In human patients, reconstruction of the superior sagittal sinus (SSS) has been described to facilitate parasagittal meningioma resection (e.g. patching the SSS with a temporalis fascia graft or bypassing it with a radial artery or internal saphenous vein graft) [15] but such aggressive resection is controversial and has not been described in small animals.

Rostrotentorial Craniectomy/ Craniotomy (Lateral Craniectomy/ Craniotomy)

This provides access to the lateral convexity of the hemisphere, save for the rostral extent that is accessed via a transfrontal approach (above). Access is provided to parasagittal meningiomas, convexity meningiomas, and to a limited degree skullbase pyriform meningiomas.

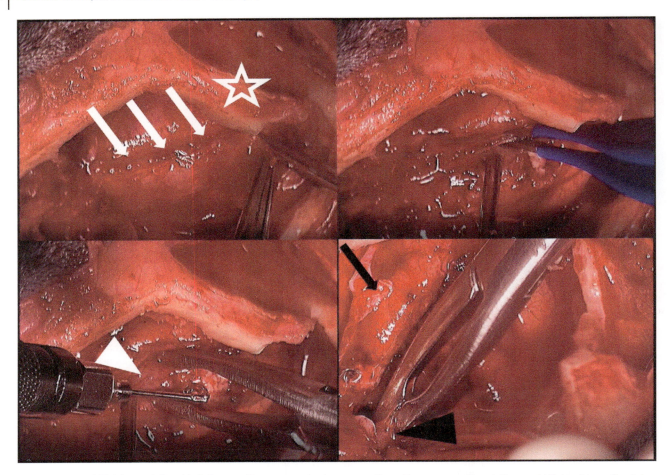

Figure 22.10 A "falcine strip" and left fronto-olfactory meningioma resection, after a conventional diamond bilateral transfrontal craniotomy. The DSS is easily visible as a purple venous structure (white arrows) under the intact dura mater. Sutures are being placed in it caudally. A left durectomy was performed as close to the DSS as possible without incising it. A right durotomy was performed and the dura reflected (black arrow), exposing normal right frontal lobe. Pre-cautery (blue bipolar instrument) and incision is then performed on the falx, caudal to the tumor on the left. The purple tumor (white triangle) is removed with rongeurs. Note that it is possible to reach forward to the cribriform plate and remove the tumor (black triangle), working behind an intact cribriform plate. Note that in this case, a standard diamond bone flap was removed from the upper plate of the frontal bone, rather than a Purdue diamond. After bilateral temporalis muscle elevation, the bone of the caudal left nasal sinus was sacrificed to improve access. The bone of the caudal right nasal sinus (white star) was later also removed to further improve visualization.

Technique

The skin is incised in a curvilinear fashion, following the frontal crest and the external sagittal crest (Figure 22.11). Incision of the terminal branches of the facial (rostral auricular plexus) and trigeminal (zygomatico-temporal nerve) nerves causes no clinically apparent deficit. A midline skin incision is an alternative, but this hampers temporalis muscle elevation as far rostro-laterally as the zygomatic process.

Thin, bilateral subcutaneous muscles are sharply incised (the frontalis and interscutularis muscles, which may appear as one continuous muscle belly that becomes thicker caudally). Deep to the interscutularis muscle, the occipitalis muscle is incised just lateral to its origination from the external sagittal crest.

The fascia of the temporalis muscle is incised just lateral to its attachment to the frontal crest and the external sagittal crest. For more rostral tumors, the incision can be continued as far as the zygomatic process of the frontal bone. For more caudal tumors, a 90° turn can be taken so that the fascial incision turns to follow the nuchal crest. For very ventral lesions, it may be necessary to extend the incision both rostrally and caudally. The temporalis muscle is then elevated from the lateral skull (frontal and parietal bones,

22 Surgical Management of Intracranial Meningiomas | 233

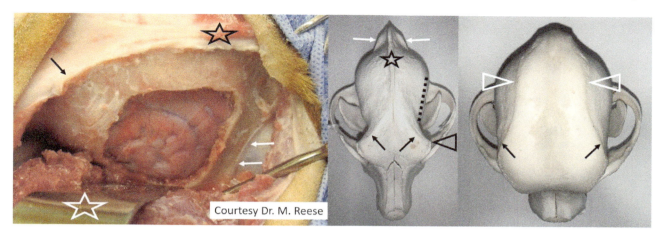

Figure 22.11 A left rostrotentorial craniectomy on a normal dog cadaver. *Source:* Courtesy of Dr. Michael Reese, DACVIM (Neurology). The single midline external sagittal crest (black stars) continues rostrally as the paired frontal crests (black arrows). The nuchal crest is visible (white arrows). The fascia of the temporalis muscle must be incised from zygomatic process (black triangle) to the nuchal crest to achieve such ventral muscle elevation and bone exposure. A Meyerding or malleable retractor (white star) can help visualize the ventral cranial vault. The normal dura mater can be seen covering the lateral cerebrum. At this stage, if more ventral access is required, further bone can be removed (e.g. double-action rongeurs, sliding one tip between the bone and the dura mater). The frontal sinus is the rostral surgical landmark for the lateral cranial vault. The middle landmark is where the skull runs caudally in a straight line (black line). The caudal landmark is the curve of the skull around the occipital lobe. Comparing these three landmarks on a dorsal plane MR image to the surgical view of the skull from above allows localization of the correct area to create a bone flap. In a normal Boston terrier skull, note that paired temporal lines (white triangles) replace the single external sagittal crest. The dorsal skull between these lines is not covered by temporalis muscle.

continuing ventrally as necessary). The temporalis muscle can be elevated from the frontal sinus until the retrobulbar muscles are exposed, and as far caudally as the nuchal crest. The temporalis muscle is retracted with Gelpi or Lonestar retractors. To place Gelpi retractors, stab incisions in the contralateral temporalis muscle fascia are useful. If necessary, to increase ventral exposure (e.g. piriform lobe), the temporalis fascia can also be split vertically, creating a T-shaped incision. The temporalis muscle is then divided vertically with monopolar cautery. Alternatively, a transzygomatic approach is performed (see Chapter 25 Transzygomatic Approach to the Temporal Lobe).

The necessary bone flap is then created. Where possible, the bone flap is larger than the durectomy, and the durectomy is larger than the meningioma, so ensure adequate muscular elevation. Except in brachycephalic dogs who do not have an external sagittal crest, the skull is much thicker dorsally, immediately adjacent to the crest. To decide the borders of the bone flap (Figures 22.11 and 22.12), compare external skull structures with dorsal and transverse plane MR images (e.g. T1-weighted post-contrast). Note the frontal sinus, the flat lateral skull wall, and the bone curving around the occipital lobe to decide the rostral–caudal borders. The external skull forms two planes: an initial slope coming down from the external sagittal crest, then an almost vertical wall more ventrally. Typically, the bone flap starts on the diagonal slope, and continues as far down the lower, vertical wall as necessary for the individual tumor.

After elevating the bone flap, the middle meningeal artery is exposed. It is cauterized or ligated ventrally. A durectomy is performed with either a #12 or #11 scalpel blade and iris scissors. The meningioma and associated dura mater can now be removed (see section Meningioma resection).

Anatomic Variation. In some cats and dogs (e.g. Boston terriers), instead of a midline external sagittal crest there are paired temporal lines (Figure 22.11). The surgical approach is largely the same. To access parasagittal tumors, the bone flap will span dorsal and ventral to the temporal line. Remain unilateral while burring, or if crossing midline take care not to traumatize the dura mater over the DSS.

Closure: Craniectomy vs Craniotomy

After placing a dural substitute (see section Substitutes for resected dura mater), a gelatin sponge or synthetic mesh (Figure 22.12) is placed in the bone defect or the bone flap is replaced. The temporalis muscle fascia is closed in a simple continuous suture using an absorbable synthetic 2-0

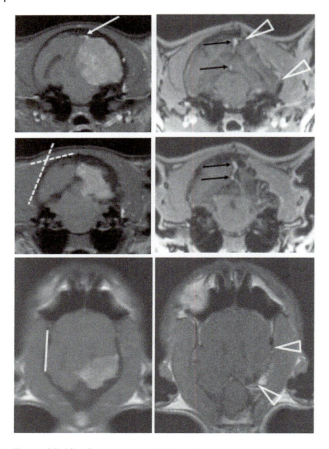

Figure 22.12 Preoperative (left) and six-months postoperative (right) post-contrast T1-weighted fat saturated images of a feline rostrotentorial craniectomy. A convexity meningioma (top images) makes contact with the caudal falx cerebri in a parasagittal location (middle images). Note the preoperative hyperostosis, compared to the contralateral occipital bone. Abnormal bone and all associated dura should be resected, where possible. To plan the edges of the bone flap (white triangles), in the transverse plane the skull slopes diagonally, then turns to be almost vertical (white dashed lines). In the dorsal plane (bottom images) the skull curves inwards from the frontal sinus, then runs caudally in a straight line (white solid line), then curves around the occipital lobe. In this case, the rostral edge of the bone flap should be halfway along this straight line. Caudally, the bone flap must allow access behind the occipital lobe without burring near the transverse sinus or confluens sinuum. The dural removal included the "dura tail" present preoperatively (white arrow) by incising the dura immediately lateral to the falx cerebri. The dura of the falx cerebri itself was preserved, to preserve the DSS. The meningioma was debrided from the falx until grossly normal dura mater was visible: in this one region associated dura was *not* resected. Note the preservation of flow through the DSS and straight sinus postoperatively (black arrows). A temporalis fascia graft was used to replace the large dural defect. The boney defect was easily covered by temporalis muscle during routine closure.

suture material. Simple continuous sutures (2-0 or 3-0) are placed in the occipitalis muscle then the subcutaneous muscles (frontalis and interscutularis muscles). Skin closure is routine.

It is not essential to reconstruct the skull [14] anywhere the bone defect can be covered by temporalis muscle. This facilitates Simpson Grade I surgical resection (see Table 22.2), which includes removal of any abnormal bone. Replacing the bone flap can have downsides: extended surgical/anesthesia time, costly implants that may complicate postoperative infection, artifacts surrounding screws/plates on postoperative imaging, and finally the significant cost of titanium screws and plates. Replacing the bone does, however, better preserve normal anatomy (e.g. should recurrence warrant re-operation) and is done to according to the surgeon's preference.

If the bone defect cannot be completely covered by routine closure of the temporalis, it may be possible to stretch the temporalis fascia over the bone defect. For example, in a Boston terrier with a parietal craniectomy that spans the temporal line: a continuous horizontal mattress suture (e.g. 2-0 absorbable synthetic suture) is placed between the temporalis fascia and the contralateral temporalis fascia, stretching the fascia over the bone defect. A tension-relieving incision in the ipsilateral temporalis fascia can facilitate this. Rostral and caudal to the bone defect, the temporalis fascia is closed routinely along the temporal line.

Combined Rostrotentorial–Transfrontal Approach

A rostrotentorial approach can be combined with a transfrontal approach for aggressive exposure of lesions that involve the lateral and rostral cerebral hemisphere (Figure 22.5). This includes a meningioma that is located ventral to the temporalis muscle *and* ventral to the frontal sinus. Midline incisions are made in the skin, and the frontalis and interscutularis muscles. The occipitalis muscle and the temporalis fascia are incised ipsilaterally, and the temporalis muscle elevated. A sagittal saw is used to remove a diamond-shaped bone flap that is set aside until closure, as described above. A Purdue diamond is recommended, otherwise the caudal wall of the frontal sinus and the frontal crest must be sacrificed to access the cranial vault.

A craniectomy is now performed, e.g. extending from the parietofrontal suture to the falx cerebri. Durectomy and

Table 22.2 Simpson classification of meningioma resection in humans [3, 16–18].

Simpson Grade	Tumor	Associated dura mater	Abnormal bone	Reported recurrence rates[a] (%)
"Grade 0"	Gross-total resection	Complete removal with 2 cm dural margin	Complete removal	≥ 0
Grade I	Gross-total resection	Complete removal	Complete removal	5–9
Grade II	Gross-total resection	Coagulated		19–22
Grade III	Gross-total resection			29–31
Grade IV	Subtotal resection			35–39
Grade V	Decompression/biopsy only			–

a) Recurrence rates (around five years) reported for human meningiomas after surgery.

meningioma resection are performed (see section Meningioma resection). The upper bone flap is replaced as above, including re-apposing the temporalis muscle fascia. Closure of the occipitalis muscle, frontalis and interscutularis muscles, and skin is routine.

Suboccipital Craniectomy (See Also Chapter 24 Surgery of Caudal Fossa Tumors)

This provides access to the caudal cerebellum and, if necessary, the dorsal foramen magnum [19].

Technique

The patient is positioned with the head downwards, to flex the atlanto-occipital (AO) joint. A dorsal midline skin incision is made from the external sagittal crest to C2. The median raphe is sharply incised. A T-shaped incision is made as follows, to elevate the biventer and rectus capitus dorsalis muscles. The paired biventer muscles are separated on the midline. A second incision is made just below the nuchal crest. Enough tendinous origination is left on the nuchal crest to allow closure, especially on the midline (ventral to the external occipital protuberance). The muscle bellies are separated down the midline and elevated laterally to expose a triangle of nearly vertical supraoccipital bone caudal to the cerebellum. If necessary, the rectus capitis dorsalis muscles are also elevated from the arch of C1 and from one or both sides of the C2 spinous process. This facilitates exposure of the ventral bone that slopes down to form the roof of the foramen magnum. The dorsal

AO membrane may be visible and should not be confused with the dura mater. Muscle elevation can also continue laterally as necessary; the final bone triangle need not be symmetrical for a lateralized tumor. The ventrolateral occipital bone contains a foramen that will bleed if exposed; this can be bone-waxed. It is the mastoid foramen and contains only the occipital emissary vein. The muscle elevation can even be continued ventrolaterally over exoccipital bone until the dorsal aspect of the occipital condyle and AO joint capsule are exposed. The musculature is retracted with Gelpi retractors.

A bone flap is removed from the supraoccipital bone (e.g. 3 mm burr, E-pen, or Surgairtome), along with exoccipital bone if further ventrolateral exposure is necessary. Bone thickness is very uneven. The vermis sits within the vermiform impression: the midline bone is thin. The bone is much thicker just lateral to the vermis, where each internal occipital crest makes an indent between the vermis and the cerebellar hemisphere. Upon encountering such internal bone ridges, it can be advantageous to move the burr perpendicular to the outline of the bone flap being created. For example, moving the burr vertically, to wear down the internal occipital crest between the vermis and the hemisphere.

A maximal durectomy is performed, removing as much of the dura associated with the meningioma as possible (Figure 22.13). If the tumor continues laterally or caudally, the boney defect can be further enlarged with rongeurs and additional dura mater removed. However, the boney defect should not be enlarged dorsal to the cerebellum, to prevent iatrogenic harm to the confluence of the sinuses (see section Anatomy). The meningioma is removed (see section Meningioma resection). Removing the meningioma may

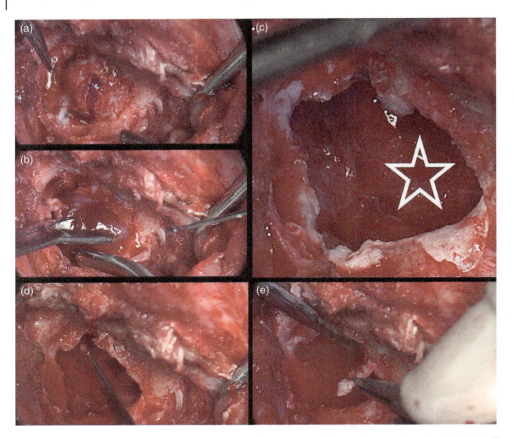

Figure 22.13 Cerebellar meningioma resection after suboccipital craniectomy in a dog. In (a), the first vertical incision in the white dura mater exposes a purple meningioma. In (b), the dural incision has been expanded to an initial durectomy, and the purple tumor is being biopsied. In (c), after using biopsies and suction to remove tumor, the normal vascular pial surface of the cerebellum (star) is exposed. In (d), a house curette is used to debride the dura that is out of sight dorsal to the cerebellum, taking care not to traumatize the sulcus for the transverse sinus. Finally, in (e), all accessible dura mater is resected.

provide access to remove additional associated dura. Dura lateral to the cerebellum can be cauterized by retracting the cerebellum medially. There may be additional meningioma in the roof of the cerebellar fossa, under the intact bone where visualization is limited. This can be blindly palpated and debrided with the spoon end of a Gross ear hook and spoon (Figure 22.11). The roof of the cerebellar fossa can be palpated on the midline, as the confluence of the sinuses and the transverse sinuses are housed within solid bone (transverse canal). Take care debriding laterally, where the transverse sinuses are incompletely enclosed in bone (sulcus for the transverse sinus, syn. transverse groove).

Closure

The dura is not closed: all dura superficial to the meningioma should be resected (see section Substitutes for resected dura mater). The bone flap is not replaced [19] in suboccipital craniectomies in humans or small animals, as the boney defect is covered by thick cervical musculature. The biventer and rectus capitis dorsalis muscles are closed in two suture lines forming a "T." A cruciate suture (synthetic absorbable 2-0) where the two lines of the "T" meet, under the external occipital protuberance, helps to unite the thick tendon and both sides of the musculature. Two simple, continuous sutures (synthetic absorbable 2-0) then complete the "T," one re-attaching muscle to the nuchal crest and the other re-apposing muscles on the dorsal midline. If there is not enough tendinous tissue remaining on the nuchal crest, tension-relieving sutures are placed from the temporalis muscle fascia to the dorsal cervical muscular fascia. The median raphe is closed in a simple continuous suture (synthetic absorbable 2-0). The subcutis and skin are closed routinely.

Meningioma Resection and Instrumentation

Meningioma tissue is often firmer and more fibrous than normal brain tissue. It often resists suction and even attempts to destroy it with bipolar electrocautery. It is typically between purple to grey in color. It can have paler, more fibrous regions.

Where possible, the defect in the bone is larger than the defect in the dura, and the defect in the dura is larger than the tumor. This allows a margin of normal dura to be resected within the durectomy. Additionally, the plane between the meningiomas and the brain surface is visualized. This plane is now followed, peeling the tumor back from the brain (Figure 22.10). Working through smaller boney corridors, the tumor must be resected from the "inside-out" (Figure 22.13). Meningioma is progressively removed until the surface of the brain is exposed. It is thus essential to recognize the appearance of the normal pial surface, where normal vasculature runs over an otherwise white tissue.

In some cases, the meningioma is peeled away from the brain simply by applying traction, e.g. while biopsying with rongeurs. In other cases, a dissection plane is created between the pia and the meningioma, using a Gross hook-and-spoon, fine nerve root retractors, etc. Neurosurgical (cotton) patties can be pushed gently into the plane between brain and tumor. Only if necessary, attachments between the pia and meningioma can be obliterated with bipolar electrocautery [4]. Be cognizant that the microcirculation of the cerebrum/cerebellum is derived from the pia mater.

A 2 cm margin of dura mater has been recommended in human meningioma surgery with recurrence rates as low as 0% (see section Simpson classification) [16]. However, a dural margin of 2 cm in all directions can be extremely hard to achieve within the small cranial vault of a dog or cat. In practice, it is common to remove some of the associated dura, then remove the tumor, which provides access to yet more dura. As a final step, all associated dura is either coagulated or better yet removed, including a margin up to 1–2 cm. This also aids hemostasis prior to closure.

Rongeurs (Lempert, pituitary). These can take sizeable biopsies where the surgeon is able to directly visualize what tissue (tumor vs. brain) is being grasped. Single-action rongeurs are widely available and included in most veterinary neurosurgery packs. Double-action rongeurs are not required for tumor biopsy. Cup-shaped pituitary rongeurs can limit the crush artefact to the perimeter of the biopsy, which can help with accurate histology and harvesting viable cells for culture, and they can be easier to control than single-action rongeurs. Rongeurs will make meningioma tissue bleed.

Suction. While using rongeurs to biopsy the tumor, typically the surgeon's non-dominant hand would be continuously suctioning. This may continue until the bulk of the pathological tissue has been removed.

Bipolar electrocautery. Remaining associated dura mater (and margin) can be cauterized and then ideally removed. If necessary, attachments to the pia mater can be obliterated, and bleeding from the brain surface can be controlled. The surgeon's non-dominant hand controls suction while an assistant provides flush.

Micro-instruments can be used to create a dissection plane between the tumor and brain tissue, e.g. the spoon of a Gross ear hook and spoon, or a House curette. Neurosurgical patties can be used this way, and also for hemostasis.

Cavitron ultrasonic surgical aspirator (CUSA). This has been reported to increase remission rates over conventional surgery [12, 20]. It utilizes a combination of ultrasonic waves and suction to fragment and remove pathologic tissue. In theory, healthy tissue and vasculature resists the ultrasonic waves, resulting in preferential removal of pathologic tissue and preservation of normal structures.

Around one quarter of canine meningiomas are "cystic" or "polycystic" on MRI [1, 9]. In some of these cases, it may be possible to considerably decompress a meningioma simply by entering the cyst-like cavity and suctioning away fluid that is clear to grey (Figure 22.9).

Simpson Classification of Meningioma Resection in Humans (Table 22.2)

This has remained one of the most powerful prognostic indicators in human meningioma since the 1950s [17]. Grade I requires that, if a venous sinus is involved, it is also excised. This is not always possible. Grade II resections are most common in human neurosurgery, followed by Grade I. In other words, it is typical to aim for complete removal of the tumor with dural resection or coagulation. The term "Simpson Grade 0" resection was coined in the 1990s [16].

In dogs and cats, for meningiomas of the cerebral convexity or rostral falx cerebri [12], it is reasonable to aim for complete removal of all associated dura and any abnormal bone. In other locations, removal of all associated dura can be impossible or risk significant morbidity (e.g. the caudal falx cerebri).

Substitutes for Resected Dura Mater

Given that resection of the dura mater associated with the tumor may improve remission rates, the dura mater should be removed if possible. The dura superficial to the tumor is replaced with a substitute: brain should *not* be left in

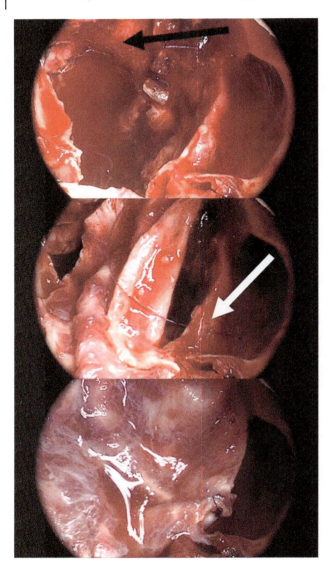

Figure 22.14 Placement of a temporalis fascial graft (same case as Figures 22.8 and 22.9) Top: A large right-sided (left side of image) cavity is present after resecting a cystic meningioma. The previous ligatures in the DSS are visible, and an additional suture (black arrow) is being placed in the dural caudal to the resection cavity, ready for the temporalis fascial graft. Middle: the fascial graft is being secured with a second suture through the left dura (white arrow). Bottom: The fascial graft has been fully secured by a total of four simple interrupted sutures. Note that muscular tags on the ventral aspect of the fascia are visible, as the graft is placed *upside-down* to prevent devitalized muscle from contacting the brain. The graft is considerably larger than the dural defect.

Options include grafts of the temporalis muscle fascia or subcutaneous fat (e.g. dorsal head or dorsal neck) [12], gelatin sponge (e.g. Gelfoam®) [14], or synthetic dural substitutes. To harvest grafts, the preoperative area of skin preparation will need to be large enough. A fascial graft should be *larger* than the dural defect (Figure 22.14). It is placed upside-down (the side that was against the temporalis muscle is placed facing upwards) so that devitalized muscle does not contact the brain. Gelatin sponge can be placed against the brain as long as it is moistened first (but *cannot* be left in the frontal sinus, below). Many surgeons will use a synthetic dural graft (Biodesign® Dural Graft, Vetrix® BioSIS, DuroGen®). The extracellular matrix within these grafts is progressively invaded and vascularized by the patient's own tissues. They are intended to be rehydrated in sterile flush *prior* to implantation, after which they handle much better. If trimming to size, ensure to always allow for overlap and avoid tension.

Dural Substitutes for Transfrontal Craniotomies. Gelatin sponge is not often left in the frontal sinus; however, some neurosurgeons have done so in the past and have not reported any issues. It can rarely act as a foreign body and possibly harbor infection [21, 22], and takes six weeks to be absorbed by the body.

Pneumocephalus has been reported as a complication of this surgery [23]. One option to prevent this is to use temporalis fascia and very carefully apply skin-glue to make a perfect airtight seal between the fascia and bone, after the initial suturing. This author likes to purposefully not make an airtight seal, which if done imperfectly might function as a one-way valve (allowing air into the cranial vault but not back out again). A fascial graft *larger* than the dural defect is sutured to the dura mater with three to five sutures. The graft is adequately immobilized, but it will have loose edges and won't be airtight (Figure 22.14). The graft will eventually be incorporated into granulation tissue and fibrosis, becoming a watertight seal that does not allow CSF leakage. Subcutaneous fat can be used rather than temporalis fascia.

Cerebrospinal Fluid Leaks. Persistent CSF leaks are the bane of human patient neurosurgeons, e.g. olfactory groove meningiomas, and yet appear extremely rare in dogs and cats. CSF leaks are not reported from most approaches (rostrotentorial, transtentorial, etc.). It is possible to have CSF-rhinorrhea following a transfrontal craniectomy. It may be associated with slower neurological recovery. If CSF is dripping from the nares postoperatively, then the communication with the nostrils allowing for *outwards* passage of CSF may allow *inwards* passage of bacteria. A one-week perioperative antibiotic course is indicated.

contact with muscle or the air of the frontal sinus. Deeper dura does not need substituting; for example, the dura removed from the skullbase under an olfactory meningioma, or the falcine dura resected within a "falcine strip."

Complications and Mitigation Strategies

Intracranial meningioma surgery has higher morbidity and mortality in cats, with complications affecting around 18% of patients [1, 2, 24, 25], and perioperative death/euthanasia occurring in 6% even in a more recent study [26]. Infratentorial surgeries are also associated with increased mortality [11].

Aspiration pneumonia occurs in as many as one-quarter of dogs after craniotomy [27] and might be especially common in transfrontal or infratentorial procedures. Preoperative maropitant and postoperative fasting should be considered. In transfrontal procedures, surgical flush and debris will likely enter the pharynx, so packing of the pharynx and careful checking of endotracheal tube cuff inflation should be considered.

Transfrontal approaches have other specific concerns. Pneumocephalus is possible [23] (see section Closure of transfrontal craniotomy), and nasal cannulae should be avoided if possible while managing pneumonia. Limited experience suggests they are safe. Have the head in a snout-down position if administering local anesthetics prior to cannula placement and ensure to never insert the cannula past the level of the medial canthus. Medications should not be administered intranasally (e.g. diazepam for seizures or phenylephrine for postoperative epistaxis). Do not place naso-esophageal feeding tubes.

Patients undergoing cerebral surgery should receive anti-convulsant medications [12]. Many forebrain tumor cases are already experiencing seizures: anti-convulsants should be continued peri- and postoperatively [4]. Seizure free cases should be started on anticonvulsant medications preoperatively. Both phenobarbital and levetiracetam are advantageous in the perioperative period, having enteral and parenteral formulations. Postoperative hypoalbuminemia will potentiate phenobarbital's sedative qualities, but this resolves with recovery from surgical blood loss. Patients who have *never* had seizures can begin to be tapered from anti-convulsant medications 6–12 months postoperatively, especially if complete remission is documented by MRI.

 Video clips to accompany this book can be found on the companion website at: www.wiley.com/go/shores/advanced

References

1. Motta, L., Mandara, M.T., and Skerritt, G.C. (2012). Canine and feline intracranial meningiomas: an updated review. *Vet. J.* 192: 153–165.
2. Sessums, K. and Mariani, C. (2009). Intracranial meningioma in dogs and cats: a comparative review. *Compend. Contin. Educ. Vet.* 31: 330–339.
3. Cossu, G., Messerer, M., Parker, F. et al. (2016). Meningiomas' management: an update of the literature. In: *Neurooncology – Newer Developments* (ed. A. Agrawal). InTech Open.
4. Uriarte, A., Moissonnier, P., Thibaud, J.L. et al. (2011). Surgical treatment and radiation therapy of frontal lobe meningiomas in 7 dogs. *Can. Vet. J.* 52: 748–752.
5. Commins, D., Atkinson, R., and Burnett, M. (2007). Review of meningioma histopathology. *Neurosurg. Focus.* 23: 1–9.
6. Friconnet, G., Hugo, V., Ala, E. et al. (2019). MRI predictive score of pial vascularization of supratentorial intracranial meningioma. *Eur. Radiol.* 29: 3516–3522.
7. Ong, T., Bharatha, A., Alsufayan, R. et al. (2021). MRI predictors for brain invasion in meningiomas. *Neuroradiology* 34: 3–7.
8. Material, C. and Selection, P. (1997). The importance of pial blood supply to the development of peritumoral brain edema in meningiomas. *J. Neurosurg.* 87: 368–373.
9. Sturges, B.K., Dickinson, P.J., Bollen, A.W. et al. (2008). Magnetic resonance imaging and histological classification of intracranial meningiomas in 112 dogs. *J. Vet. Intern. Med.* 22: 586–595.
10. Forterre, F., Fritsch, G., Kaiser, S. et al. (2006). Surgical approach for tentorial meningiomas in cats: a review of six cases. *J. Feline Med. Surg.* 8: 227–233.
11. Forterre, F., Tomek, A., Konar, M. et al. (2007). Multiple meningiomas: clinical, radiological, surgical, and pathological findings with outcome in four cats. *J. Feline Med. Surg.* 9: 36–43.
12. Ijiri, A., Yoshiki, K., Tsuboi, S. et al. (2014). Surgical resection of twenty-three cases of brain meningioma. *J. Vet. Med. Sci.* 76: 331–338.
13. Bentley, R.T. and Thomovsky, S.A. (2016). Evaluation of a modified transfrontal craniotomy technique in 8 dogs. *J. Vet. Intern. Med.* 30: 1940.
14. Suñol, A., Mascort, J., Font, C. et al. (2017). Long-term follow-up of surgical resection alone for primary

intracranial rostrotentorial tumors in dogs : 29 cases (2002–2013). *Open Vet. J* 7: 375–383.

15. Sindu, M. and Alvernia, J. (2006). Results of attempted radical tumor removal and venous repair in 100 consecutive meningiomas involving the major dural sinuses. *J. Neurosurg.* 105: 514–525.

16. Kinjo, T., Al-Mefty, O., and Kanaan, I. (1993). Grade zero memoval of supratentorial convexity meningiomas. *Neurosurgery* 33: 394–399.

17. Simpson, D. (1957). The recurrence of intracranial meningiomas after surgical treatment. *J. Neurol. Neurosurg. Psychiatry* 20: 22–39.

18. Nanda, A., Bir, S.C., Maiti, T.K. et al. (2017). Relevance of Simpson grading system and recurrence-free survival after surgery for World Health Organization Grade I meningioma. *J. Neurosurg.* 126: 201–211.

19. Dewey, C.W., Berg, J.M., Barone, G. et al. (2005). Foramen magnum decompression for treatment of caudal occipital malformation syndrome in dogs. *J. Am. Vet. Med. Assoc.* 227 (8): 1270–1275.

20. Greco, J., Aiken, S., Berg, J. et al. (2006). Evaluation of intracranial meningioma resection with a surgical aspirator in dogs: 17 cases (1996–2004). *J. Am. Vet. Med. Assoc.* 229 (3): 394–400.

21. Kang, G.C., Surg, M., Sng, K.W. et al. (2009). Modified technique for frontal sinus obliteration using calvarial bone and Tisseel glue. *J. Craniofac. Surg.* 20: 528–531.

22. Kang, D., Park, S., Park, J.C. et al. (2004). Neurosurgical approaches to and through the frontal sinus using osteoplastic frontal sinusotomy. *J. Korean Neurosurg. Soc.* 36: 107–113.

23. Garosi, L., Penderis, J., Brearley, M. et al. (2002). Intraventricular tension pneumocephalus as a complication of transfrontal craniectomy: a case report. *Vet. Surg.* 31: 226–231.

24. Gordon, L., Thacher, C., Matthiesen, D., and Joseph, R. (1994). Results of craniotomy for the treatment of cerebral meningioma in 42 cats. *Vet. Surg.* 23 (2): 94–100.

25. Gallagher, J., Berg, J., and Knowles, K. (1993). Prognosis after surgical excision of cerebral meningiomas in cats: 17 cases (1986–1992). *J. Am. Vet. Med. Assoc.* 203: 1437–1440.

26. Cameron, S., Rishniw, M., Miller, A.D. et al. (2015). Characteristics and survival of 121 cats undergoing excision of intracranial meningiomas (1994–2011). *Vet. Surg.* 44: 772–776.

27. Fransson, B.A., Bagley, R.S., Gay, J.M. et al. (2001). Pneumonia after intracranial surgery in dogs. *Vet. Surg.* 30: 432–439.

23

Lateral Ventricular Fenestration

Andy Shores

Mississippi State University, Mississippi State, MS, USA

Introduction

Endoscopic third ventriculostomy (ETV) is a well-established surgical procedure for hydrocephalus treatment [1] in infants [2] and adults [3]. And while the size of our veterinary patients essentially prevents the performance of this endoscopic technique, the same principle is possible with fenestration or marsupialization of the lateral ventricle. This technique was reported in a presentation in 2015 and included five patients [4]. Fairly recent research on canine hydrocephalus suggests we have a lot to learn about the pressure changes in patients with non-obstructive hydrocephalus and that normotensive communicating hydrocephalus does exist [5]. We also have learned from some recent papers that a reduction in volume of the cerebral ventricles does correlate with improvement in at least come clinical signs [6]. When considering these facts and the complications that can be associated with ventriculoperitoneal (VP) shunting in veterinary patients, this technique should be considered as an alternative to VP shunts in specific circumstances, especially when size/age related factors and client economic restraints are a consideration. This chapter will describe the technique and give the author's recommendation for indications. In addition, potential complications will be discussed.

Rationale

Shunting of CSF into another cavity is used to treat hydrocephalus and other disorders that cause secondary obstructive hydrocephalus and increased intracranial CSF accumulation [7]. Conventional valve shunting for treatment of hydrocephalus has been associated with complications, as high as 22% in one study [8] and over 30% in a more recent publication [9]. Reported complications include dislodgement, occlusion, infections, ventricle collapse, and subdural hematoma. The necessity for shunt revision surgery is reported [9]. In humans, complication frequency is related to young age and was 32% in a study of 14 000 patients and 23.8% in a study of over 1700 cases [10].

Because of the level of complications associated with ventriculoperitoneal shunts and possibly a higher rate of complications in very young dogs and cats, the author sought a different method of treating hydrocephalus in small animals. Human infants may be preferentially treated with endoscopic assisted third ventricle fenestration into the subarachnoid space through the basilar cistern. The size of the young canine or feline ventricular system, however, is prohibitively small for this procedure and often for any type of VP shunt system. An alternative procedure (lateral ventricle fenestration) was initially designed with these factors in mind. The procedure initially had successful short-term outcomes in five patients, but three were lost to long-term follow-up. In a domestic short-haired kitten (10 weeks old) and a Labrador puppy (14 weeks old), following an obstructive hydrocephalus diagnosis using advanced imaging, clinical signs resolved or improved over a period of six months. Follow-up imaging demonstrated patency of the fenestrations and reduced ventricle sizes [4]. Follow-up conversations with these owners at six years post fenestration revealed that both these patients were alive, had no perceived neurologic deficits, and were seizure free. The same technique has continued to be performed by the author without adverse events and by many others in the United States, Europe, and South America. The technique is quick, not complicated, and has had a high level of success (improvement) in most patients.

Advanced Techniques in Canine and Feline Neurosurgery, First Edition. Edited by Andy Shores and Brigitte A. Brisson.
© 2023 John Wiley & Sons, Inc. Published 2023 by John Wiley & Sons, Inc.
Companion site: www.wiley.com/go/shores/advanced

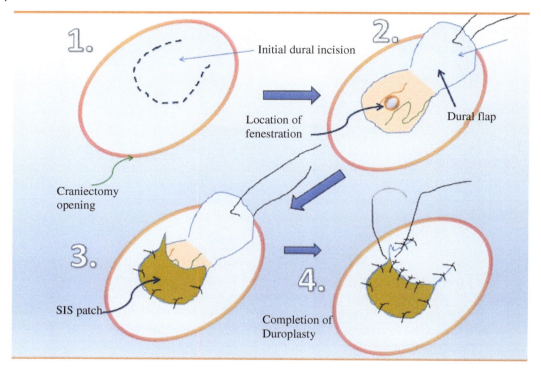

Figure 23.1 A graphic representation of the lateral ventricular fenestration technique. 1. The dotted line shows the shape of the initial dural incision. 2. The dural flap has been created and secured with a stay suture. The fenestration is made into the ventricle through a gyrus. 3. The SIS *patch* has been fashioned to suture to the dura. The goal is to create a *dome-like* structure over the fenestration. 4. The completed duroplasty.

Technique

A graphic overview of the technique is illustrated in Figure 23.1. The objective of this procedure is the creation of a conduit of communication between the lateral ventricle and the subarachnoid space proximal and rostral to the lateral apertures. Patients are placed in sternal recumbency with the head and neck slightly extended and with no pressure on the area of the jugular veins. The cranium is sterilely prepped and draped (Figure 23.2). A curved (approximately 4 cm) skin incision is made to the right or left of midline (or bilaterally if both ventricles are to be fenestrated), extending from above the zygomatic process, dorsally toward midline, and caudally toward occipital protuberance, using a #10 scalpel blade or electroscalpel. Monopolar and bipolar electrocautery are used for hemostasis. The subcutaneous tissues and temporalis muscle are bluntly dissected to expose the external calvarium. A small rostrotentorial craniectomy is performed. Often the opening only needs to be a 3–4 × 3–4 cm square or rectangle using a nitrogen-powered or electric drill (Figure 23.3). The placement of the craniectomy should be 50–60° off the dorsal midline of the skull (Figure 23.4). The exposed dura is carefully incised in a specified manner (Figure 23.5) using a #12 scalpel and reflected using 5-0 stay sutures (Figure 23.6).

The most common site for the ventriculostomy (fenestration) is at the ectosylvian gyrus as this should correlate with the 50–60° point off the dorsal midline. Next, the gyrus is incised longitudinally using a #11 scalpel blade to enter the lateral ventricle. An uninflated, 4 Fr. anal sac catheter[1] (Figure 23.7) or small Foley catheter is introduced into the defect and inflated with 0.5 cc sterile saline. It is then extracted while inflated to create the ventriculostomy. Cerebospinal fluid (CSF) will drain freely from the site. The surgeon may notice a slight *deflation* of the cortex. The stoma or fenestration is freed from any debris or blood using a cellulose eye spear (Figure 23.8). Often the slightly everted ventricular lining can be visualized as a thin, white membrane. A 4-ply SIS[2] patch is shaped to the size of the dural defect and then sutured to the dura (Figure 23.9). Polypropylene mesh is sutured to the underlayer of the temporalis muscle, extending over the craniectomy, using 4-0 absorbable synthetic monofilament suture in an interrupted pattern (Figure 23.10). This is used to prevent muscle adhesion to the dura/SIS patch construct. The subcutaneous tissue is opposed with 3-0 absorbable synthetic monofilament suture, and an intradermal suture pattern used to oppose the skin with 3-0 absorbable synthetic monofilament suture. The incision is covered with a sterile non-stick pad followed by an adhesive bandage.

Potential Complications

Complications can occur with any procedure that drains the CSF from an enlarged ventricle with a thin layer of cortex. These include collapse of the ventricle, hemorrhage (subdural, epidural), CSF leakage under the temporalis muscle layer, and hemorrhage into the ventricle that may lead to additional obstructions or inflammation. Making the entry through a gyrus and at a point 50–60° off the midline can prevent most of these or at least limits their possibility.

Discussion

This procedure, performed correctly, can be a successful way to manage hydrocephalus, especially in younger, small animals. In general, it is recommended for use in those patients that already have a very thin rim of cortical tissue as seen in Figure 23.11. Strict adherence to the illustrated dural incision pattern and the dural patch using multilayer SIS increases the chance of success. In addition, the

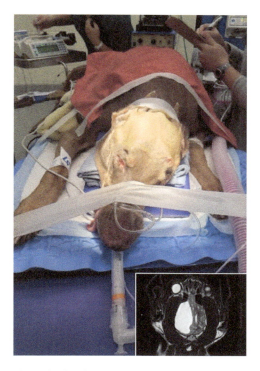

Figure 23.2 This patient is seven months old and was diagnosed with unilateral hydranencephaly (insert – T2 weighted dorsal MRI). Patient is placed in sternal recumbency with the head tilted slightly to the left to facilitate the ventricular fenestration on the right at approximately 60° off midline.

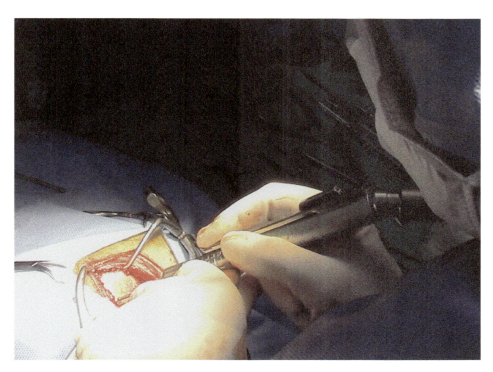

Figure 23.3 A small craniectomy through the parietal bone is being performed using a nitrogen powered drill. Often the opening only needs to be a 3–4 × 3–4 cm square or rectangle.

244 | *Advanced Techniques in Canine and Feline Neurosurgery*

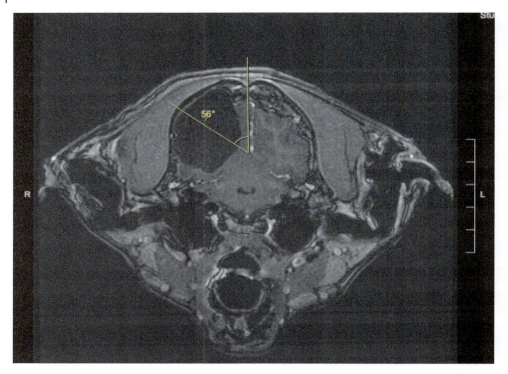

Figure 23.4　Transverse T1+C image showing the approximate entry point for the craniectomy at 56° off midline.

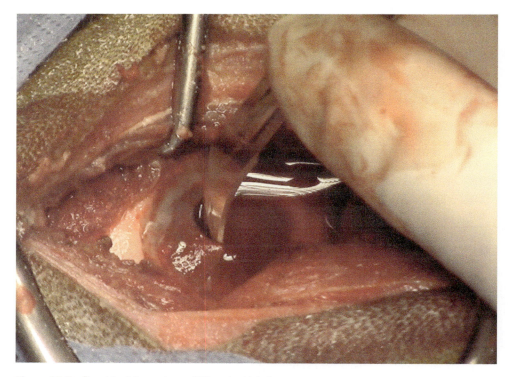

Figure 23.5　Dural incision using a #12 scalpel blade.

23 *Lateral Ventricular Fenestration* | 245

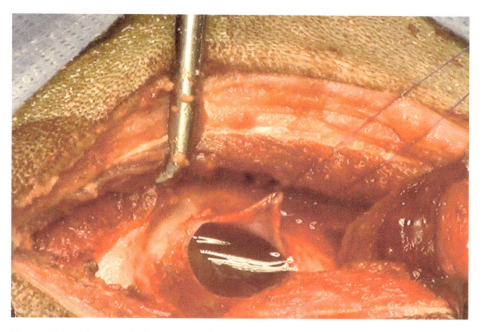

Figure 23.6 After completing the dural incision, a stay suture in placed in the dural flap.

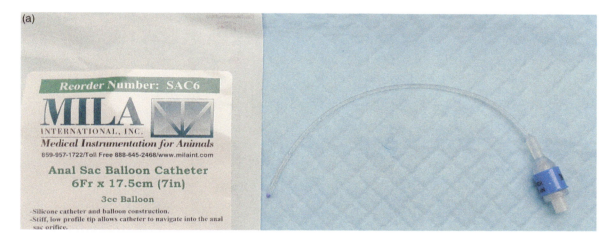

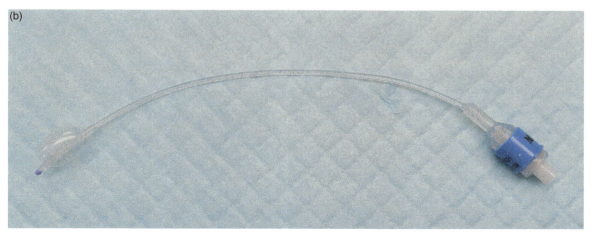

Figure 23.7 The *anal sac balloon catheter* is preferred over the Foley type catheters because the length of the tip past the cuff is much shorter. (a) The catheter with uninflated cuff, and (b) catheter with an inflated cuff (2–3 cc volume).

246 *Advanced Techniques in Canine and Feline Neurosurgery*

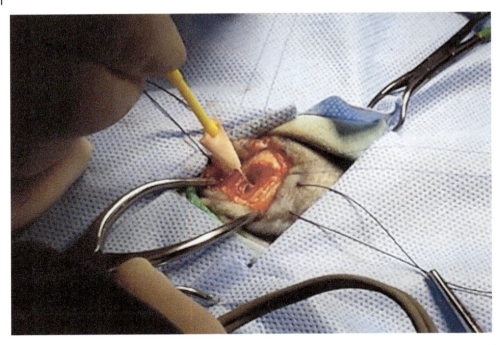

Figure 23.8   A cellulose eye spear is used to remove blood or tissue debris around and in the ventricular stoma (fenestration).

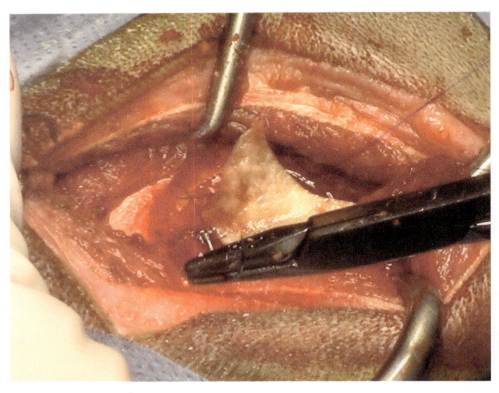

Figure 23.9   A 4-ply SIS[b] patch is shaped to the size of the dural defect and then sutured to the dura.

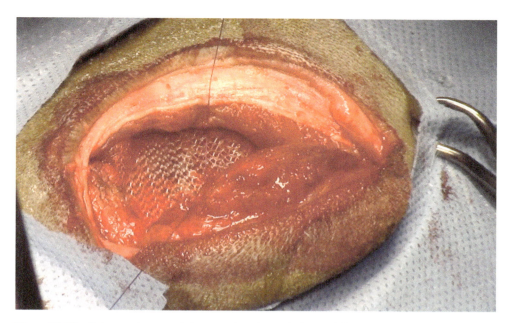

Figure 23.10 Polypropylene mesh is sutured to the underlayer of the temporalis muscle, extending over the craniectomy, using 4-0 absorbable synthetic monofilament suture in an interrupted pattern.

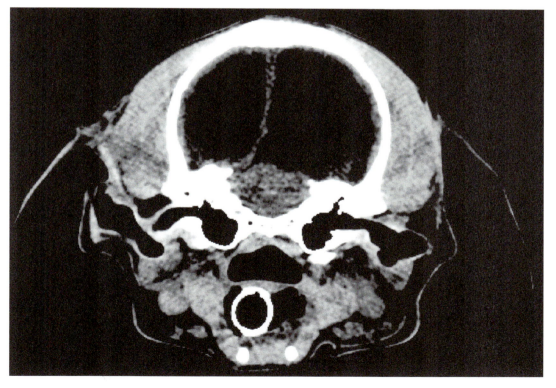

Figure 23.11 This is an image (transverse CT) of a young (four-month-old) mixed-breed dog with congenital hydrocephalus. Notice the thin rim of cortical tissue. This presentation would be considered an ideal patient for performing a lateral ventricular fenestration.

procedure has been used in patients where funding is too limited to include the use of available VP shunts. Some work has been done to develop a stent to place in the fenestration to further ensure maintenance of the flow of CSF into the subarachnoid space surrounding the parenchyma, but this addition needs further study. This procedure is relatively easy to perform and requires minimal operating time. The use of this procedure does not preclude the placement of a VP shunt later should this be deemed necessary. Complications of VP shunting can include shunt obstruction, pain, shunt infection, disconnection, excessive shunting, kinking, and peritoneal infection or obstruction [9]. When the lateral fenestration procedure is used as outlined in this chapter, virtually all these complications are avoided.

Most contraindications for VP shunting are also of no or minimal concern with lateral ventricular fenestration. Those contraindications include a high CSF protein concentration, increased erythrocyte count in the CSF, and intraabdominal/peritoneal inflammation [11].

Obviously, this technique is not a panacea, nor does it completely replace the idea of VP shunting; however, it remains a viable alternative that is less expensive, designed primarily for the younger patients, and carries with it very few possibilities for complications. Additional applications include its use when there is failure/obstruction of VP shunts.

 Video clips to accompany this book can be found on the companion website at: www.wiley.com/go/shores/advanced

References

1. Boaro, A., Mahadik, B., Petrillo, A. et al. (2021). Efficacy and safety of flexible versus rigid endoscopic third ventriculostomy in pediatric and adult populations: a systematic review and meta-analysis. *Neurosurg. Rev.* https://doi.org/10.1007/s10143-021-01590-6. Epub ahead of print. PMID: 34173114.
2. Demerdash, A., Rocque, B.G., Johnston, J. et al. (2017). Endoscopic third ventriculostomy: a historical review. *Br. J. Neurosurg.* 31 (1): 28–32. https://doi.org/10.1080/02688697.2016.1245848. Epub 2016 Oct 22. PMID: 27774823; PMCID: PMC5922250.
3. Xiao, L., Xu, C., Liu, Y. et al. (2019). The surgical results of endoscopic third ventriculostomy in long-standing overt ventriculomegaly in adults with papilledema. *Clin. Neurol. Neurosurg.* 183: 105366. https://doi.org/10.1016/j.clineuro.2019.05.014. Epub 2019 May 14. PMID: 31174900.
4. Shores, A., Kornberg, S., Beasley, M. et al. (2015). Fenestration of the lateral ventricle in the management of obstructive hydrocephalus in young small animals. *J. Vet. Intern. Med.* 29: 1123. ACVIM Forum Research Abstract Program Indianapolis.
5. Kolecka, M., Farke, D., Failling, K. et al. (2019). Intraoperative measurement of intraventricular pressure in dogs with communicating internal hydrocephalus. *PLoS One* 14 (9): e0222725. https://doi.org/10.1371/journal.pone.0222725. PMID: 31560704; PMCID: PMC6764652.
6. Schmidt, M.J., Hartmann, A., Farke, D. et al. (2019). Association between improvement of clinical signs and decrease of ventricular volume after ventriculoperitoneal shunting in dogs with internal hydrocephalus. *J. Vet. Intern. Med.* 33 (3): 1368–1375. https://doi.org/10.1111/jvim.15468. Epub 2019 Apr 8. PMID: 30957934; PMCID: PMC6524126.
7. Hoerlein, B.F. and Gage, E.D. (1978). Hydrocephalus. In: *Canine Neurology: Diagnosis and Treatment* (ed. B.F. Hoerlein), 733–760. Philadelphia: WB Saunders.
8. Biel, M., Kramer, M., Forterre, F. et al. (2013). Outcome of ventriculoperitoneal shunt implantation for treatment of congenital internal hydrocephalus in dogs and cats: 36 cases (2001–2009). *J. Am. Vet. Med. Assoc.* 242 (7): 948–958. https://doi.org/10.2460/javma.242.7.948. PMID: 23517207.
9. Gradner, G., Kaefinger, R., and Dupré, G. (2019). Complications associated with ventriculoperitoneal shunts in dogs and cats with idiopathic hydrocephalus: a systematic review. *J. Vet. Intern. Med.* 33 (2): 403–412. https://doi.org/10.1111/jvim.15422.
10. Merkler, A.E., Ch'ang, J., Parker, W.E. et al. (2017). The Rate of Complications after Ventriculoperitoneal Shunt Surgery. *World Neurosurg.* 98: 654–658. https://doi.org/10.1016/j.wneu.2016.10.136. Epub 2016 Nov 5. PMID: 27826086; PMCID: PMC5326595.
11. Coates, J.R., Axlund, T.W., Dewey, C.W., and Smith, J. (2006). Hydrocephalus in dogs and cats. *Comp. Contin. Ed. Prac. Vet. NA* 28 (2): 136.

24

Surgery of the Caudal Fossa

Beverly K. Sturges

University of California, Davis, CA, USA

The caudal fossa, housing the brainstem and cerebellum, offers unique surgical challenges and rewards due to the location and the critical nature of the structures contained within it. As is true of all cranial surgery, an intimate knowledge of regional anatomy, both outside of the calvarium as well as within the calvarium, is essential for surgical success. This is often challenging due to major variations in anatomy between species as well as between breeds and individuals. Although this chapter focuses on the standard surgical approaches to the caudal fossa, some of what is presented is based on experience and/or anecdote from the author and others providing critique and mentorship over the years.

Anatomy

The caudal–cranial fossa is separated from the cranial–cranial fossa, or supratentorial compartment, by the tentorium cerebelli dorsally; thus, the caudal fossa forms the infratentorial compartment. It is bounded rostrally by the dorsum sellae and ends caudally at the foramen magnum. The dorsal, lateral, and caudal aspects are formed by the occipital bone, being delineated from the temporal fossa (of the occipital bone) by the nuchal crest. The caudal fossa forms a compact and rigid compartment with limited compliance of the parenchymal structures protected within, which include the cerebellum, pons, medulla oblongata, nuclei of cranial nerves V–XII, and the ascending and descending tracts of the spinal cord. It is also where outflow of cerebrospinal fluid (CSF) from the third ventricle into the fourth ventricle and lateral apertures reside. Together the neural structures within the caudal fossa support most vital functions of the body, level of consciousness, and coordination and modulation of activity from the relay of information to and from all parts of the body.

The contents of the caudal fossa are supplied by multiple pairs of arteries: the caudal cerebellar arteries arising from the basilar artery to supply the caudal part of the cerebellum and the rostral cerebellar arteries, supplying the rostral portion of the cerebellum, branch from the caudal communicating artery coming off the terminal internal carotid artery. Other branches from the basilar artery supply other parts of the brainstem. Since the arterial supply to the structures within the cauda fossa is located ventrally with close perforation into parenchyma, disruption of major arterial vessels is rare in most caudal fossa surgery. Venous structures are encountered frequently, though, and detailed knowledge of their location is essential for successful surgery in this region. The ventral venous sinus system contains the basilar sinus that lies on the floor of the occipital bone and eventually joins the internal ventral vertebral venous plexus. The dorsal venous sinus system of the brain consists of the dorsal sagittal sinus which, via the confluence of the sinuses (confluens sinuum), gives rise to the transverse sinuses that run ventrolaterally within the occipital bone. Along their course the transverse sinuses receive major veins from other parts of the brain before branching and exiting the skull ventrally to join the peripheral venous system. These vascular structures, by their proximity to the limits of occipital craniectomy, are given consideration whenever approaching the caudal fossa (Figure 24.1) [1].

Muscles originating from the cervical vertebrae compose most of the musculature of the craniodorsal cervical region. Superficially, the broad, flat superficial muscles of the cervicoauricular–occipital muscle complex are fused on dorsal midline and represent the initial layer in surgical dissection. The deeper paired dorsal muscles attaching to the caudal occipital bone provide essential support to the head and contribute to controlled movement of the occipital–atlanto–axial (OAA) joints. These include the

---

Advanced Techniques in Canine and Feline Neurosurgery, First Edition. Edited by Andy Shores and Brigitte A. Brisson.
© 2023 John Wiley & Sons, Inc. Published 2023 by John Wiley & Sons, Inc.
Companion site: www.wiley.com/go/shores/advanced

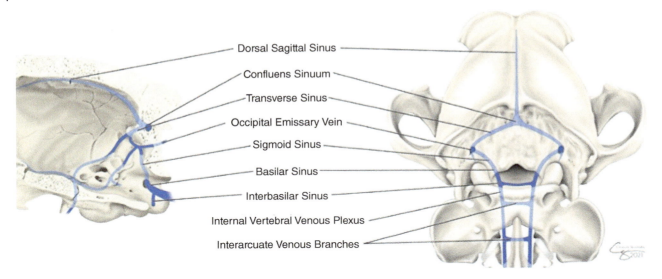

Figure 24.1 Venous system of the caudal fossa. Venous sinuses of the caudal fossa, medial aspect. The dorsal system of venous sinuses begins with the dorsal sagittal sinus running caudally from within the falx cerebri to empty into the confluence of the sinuses (confluens sinuum) within the occipital bone and branches into paired transverse sinuses. These run laterally within the osseous canal, dividing into the sigmoid and temporal sinuses ventrally. The temporal sinuses exit via the retroarticular foramen to the maxillary veins and, then, the jugular veins. The basilar sinus branches off the sigmoid sinus and runs through the condyloid canal (condyloid vein) before joining the internal ventral vertebral venous sinus as it exits the foramen magnum. The condyloid vein may be ruptured if drilling too ventral in the occipital bone. The ventral interbasilar sinus connects the right and left basilar sinuses at the foramen magnum. It lies on the floor and sides of the occipital bone, is irregularly defined, and often has many fingerlike connections to the lateral and ventral meninges of the caudal brainstem. Occasionally there is also a dorsal interbasilar sinus with similar meningeal connections. When removing masses alongside the brainstem, especially when they are invading meninges, hemorrhage may become profuse from rupture of these sinuses. The occipital emissary veins, fed by the transverse and sigmoid sinuses, exit ventrolaterally on the caudal aspect of the skull via the mastoid foramen. During lateral muscle elevation, these may be encountered causing hemorrhage. Anatomic variations in intracranial dural venous sinus anatomy are common in dogs and should be taken into consideration during surgical planning.

semispinalis capitis (biventer and complexus), and rectus capitis dorsalis (major and minor) muscles. Ligamentous structures also provide support and flexibility of the head at the occipital–atlantal joint. *The dorsal atlanto-occipital (AO) membrane, extending between the dorsal edge of the foramen magnum and the arch of C1, is of particular importance when approaching this region* [2].

Indications for Surgery

The clinical presentation of small animals with caudal fossa disease depends on the location and acuity of the lesion as well as the impact of the pathology on cerebrospinal fluid flow dynamics. Chronic, progressive lesions of the caudal fossa generally cause cranial nerve dysfunction (CNs V, VII, VIII, IX, X, XII), cerebellar and vestibular signs (ataxia, tremor, motor dyscoordination), alterations in mental state, sensorimotor deficits in the limbs, and potentially cardiac and respiratory abnormalities. If CSF outflow from the fourth ventricle is severely compromised due to obstruction or swelling, clinical signs may be more consistent with developing intracranial hypertension including marked alteration of consciousness, abnormal posturing, altered respiration, etc.

The surgical indications for caudal fossa surgery primarily include the following:

A) Neoplasms – primary brain tumors affecting the cerebellum, cerebellomedullary junction, and dorsal caudal brainstem are common indications; neoplasms of the rostral cervical spinal cord extending into the brainstem and osseous tumors arising from the occipital bone occur infrequently.

B) Congenital/developmental malformations – Chiari-like malformation and other occipital dysplasias occur commonly in many breeds of dogs; quadrigeminal diverticula, epidermoid, and dermoid cysts occur rarely.

C) Trauma – physical trauma to the back of the head may result in depressed skull fractures and/or hematoma causing compression, vascular disruption, and/or CSF outflow obstruction in the fourth ventricle.

D) Biopsy – any pathology affecting the cerebellum or caudal occipital bone.

E) Drainage – Abscesses (bacterial or fungal), epidural empyema, and granulomas are infrequently encountered.

Preoperative Assessment and Anesthetic Management

Dogs and cats undergoing caudal fossa surgery require the same preoperative assessment as other cranial surgical patients (refer to Chapter X). The presence of cranial nerve deficits resulting in dysphagia, loss of gag reflex, and/or laryngeal nerve dysfunction increase the risk for aspiration and require specific precautions at the time of extubation and in the early postoperative period. Typically, a baseline assessment including CBC, serum biochemical profile, urinalysis, and imaging assessment of the thoracic and abdominal structures is done prior to surgery. Baseline blood gases prior to premedication is recommended for assessment of ventilatory function prior to surgery and is useful for postoperative comparison. Premedication for craniotomy should be directed at the individual patient's level of anxiety, baseline neurological status, and other comorbidities. Dogs and cats with caudal fossa pathology may be especially sensitive to the respiratory depressant effects of benzodiazepines and opioids and may be at increased risk of excessive sedation and aspiration. Sedatives should be titrated to effect using small doses of medication. In patients that are particularly neurologically impaired, withholding sedation until the patient is instrumented for monitoring, and in a setting allowing immediate airway management, is desirable. The choice of anesthetic agents, hemodynamic, and ventilatory management and physiologic monitoring are similar for other cranial surgeries in small animals. Overarching goals include the maintenance of hemodynamic stability and cerebral perfusion pressure while avoiding increases in intracranial pressure.

Surgical Positioning

Patients are positioned in sternal recumbency with the head flexed as close to perpendicular to the longitudinal axis of the vertebral column without affecting patency of the endotracheal tube (Figure 24.2). The level of the brain should be maintained higher than the level of the heart and direct pressure on jugular veins is strictly avoided since this can interfere with venous outflow and increase intracranial pressure. In some instances, it is useful to tilt the head away from the side of the lesion if it is lateralized. Once positioned, the patient is secured firmly in place using a combination of sandbags, tape, inflatable sandbags, or other positioning devices. A mouth gag is used to prevent compression of the tongue during surgery, which can lead to lingual swelling and postoperative airway obstruction; in more severe situations it can result in ischemia and necrosis of the tongue. The head is shaved and prepped from the eyebrows to the mid-cervical region and a surgical prepping solution (3M™ DuraPrep™) is applied to the shaved skin and allowed to dry before placing an iodophor-impregnated

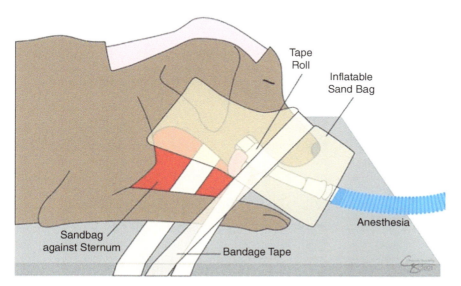

Figure 24.2 Positioning for caudal fossa surgery. Proper positioning is important for accessing the caudal fossa. The patient's head is strongly flexed, as close to 90° as possible without compromising the endotracheal tube. Jugular compression and lingual compression are avoided to prevent complications from venous drainage from the brain and postoperative airway obstruction respectively. A small sandbag placed between the manubrium and the mandibles is useful in larger dogs to wedge the head against before securing into position. A mouth gag is needed to prevent the tongue from swelling. This can also be done simply by using a roll of tape around the endotracheal tube in the mouth and pulling the tongue out laterally behind the tape roll (inset). A small U-shaped inflatable sandbag is very helpful for holding the head and anesthesia-related equipment in non-dislodgeable orientation.

plastic incision drape (3M™ Ioban™) over the area. This improves the adhesion of the iodophor-impregnated plastic incision drape to the skin while the combination of the two provide long-lasting antimicrobial persistence. Both bony and soft tissue anatomy of the caudal fossa is uniquely specific to every patient and must be carefully evaluated preoperatively since it heavily influences surgical positioning, approach, instrumentation, and overall success of the procedure. This is especially applicable in dogs with occipital dysplasia/malformation, dolicocephalic breeds with an occipital bone that is rostrally offset from a prominent external occipital protuberance, and large dogs with heavy muscling of the head and neck.

Surgical Approach(es) to the Caudal Fossa

Midline Occipital Approach [3–5]

The midline approach through the occipital bone provides a good view of the cerebellar vermis, the medial portion of the cerebellar hemispheres, and the caudodorsal part of the brainstem. With retraction of the cerebellar vermis, the obex and fourth ventricle are also visualized. It is often combined with C1 partial or complete laminotomy to increase access to the area when pathology affects the cervicomedullary junction (C1 spinal cord segment and caudal brainstem). In small animals, it is the most straightforward approach and is frequently used to decompress Chiari-like malformations (Figure 24.3), remove caudal cerebellar convexity masses, smaller, midline fourth ventricular masses and tumors affecting the cervicomedullary junction (C1), and caudal brainstem (Figure 24.4).

A dorsal midline skin incision is made from 2 cm rostral to the external occipital protuberance to approximately the level of C3 vertebrae. Using an electrocautery pencil, subcutaneous fat tissue and superficial cervical musculature are incised together on midline following the dorsal median raphe (Figure 24.5). Gelpi or other self-retaining retractors are placed to retract tissue at the cranial and caudal aspect of the surgical site and repositioned as needed. From here, the spinous process of C2 and the external occipital protuberance are palpable landmarks that may be used to envision midline as dissection and elevation of deeper musculature is performed to eventually expose the caudal occipital bone, the arch of the C1 and the rostral portion of the spinous process of C2. First, the paired semispinalis capitis biventer *cervicis* muscles are separated on midline and retracted revealing the deeper paired rectus capitis dorsalis muscles (Figure 24.6). These are also divided on midline from the level of the

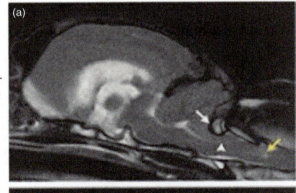

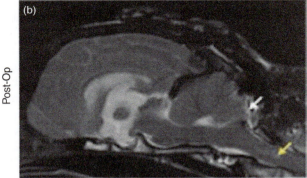

Figure 24.3 Midline occipital craniectomy to decompress caudal occipital malformation. Mid-sagittal T2W images from a six-month-old Ocelot kitten. (a) Severe malformation of the caudal occipital bone (white arrow) reducing the volume of the caudal fossa is resulting in marked cerebellar compression, foraminal herniation (arrowhead), and obstructive hydrocephalus with involvement of olfactory bulb, and syrinx formation (yellow arrow). Neurologically, this kitten was weakly ambulatory and markedly ataxic with positional vertical nystagmus. (b) Immediate postop image using midline occipital craniectomy affords decompression of the cerebellar vermis (white arrow), resolution of reduction in obstruction of CSF outflow, and partial resolution of syrinx. The kitten became neurologically normal within a few days.

occipital bone to the C2 vertebrae. The insertions of the caudal portion of the rectus capitis dorsalis (major and minor) muscles onto the atlas and axis are removed by incising the fascial attachment dorsally and periosteally elevating the insertion of the muscle from the cranial half of the C2 spinous process and the arch of C1. The cranial aspects of the rectus capitis dorsalis muscles are elevated from the caudal aspect of the occipital bone and the nuchal crest using a combination of periosteal elevation, electrocautery, and/or sharp dissection. Monopolar and/or bipolar electrocautery and/or bone wax are used to control hemorrhage from the elevated muscles which may be significant in some dogs. Profuse hemorrhage may be encountered when elevating muscles from the ventrolateral portion of the occiput where the occipital emissary vein emerges from the mastoid foramen. This is especially

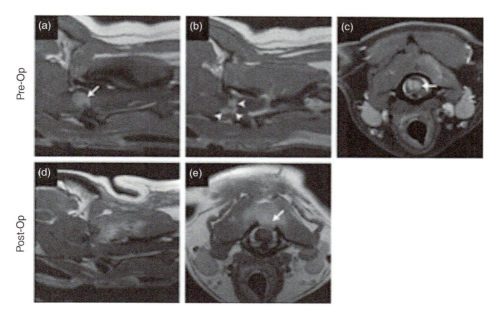

Figure 24.4 Midline occipital craniectomy combined with C1 laminotomy to excise intradural mass. T1W post-contrast MR images from a 5yo English Springer Spaniel. (a) Mid-sagittal image showing a contrast enhancing mass affecting the first spinal cord segment and caudal brainstem. (b) A para-sagittal image illustrating enlarged, contrast-enhancing nerve roots adjacent to the mass consistent with a peripheral nerve sheath tumor. An enlarged nerve root also extended cranially in the foramen magnum (c) Transverse view showing mass effacing most of spinal cord. (d and e) A midline occipital craniectomy and a dorsal laminectomy of C1 afforded a good surgical corridor for resection of the mass along its entire length.

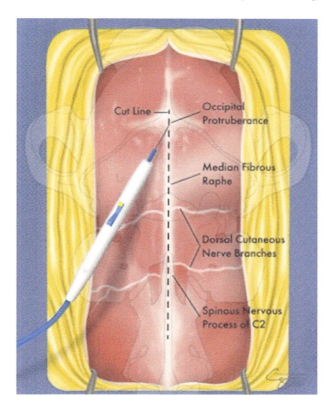

Figure 24.5 Superficial muscle dissection. The broad expanse of flat superficial muscles, lying below skin and subcutaneous fat, is fused on dorsal midline and represent the first layer in surgical dissection (dotted line).

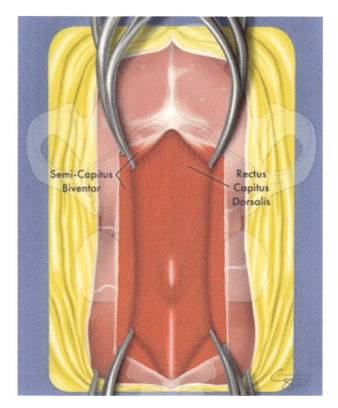

Figure 24.6 Deep muscle dissection. The paired semispinalis capitis (*biventer cervicis*) muscles are divided on midline and retracted laterally maintaining their attachment to the nuchal crest as far as possible. Paired underlying rectus capitis dorsalis muscles are then divided on midline as well and elevated from their attachments to the occipital bone, C1 and the cranial portion of C2.

common in large breed dogs with muscular head and neck regions. Once muscle elevation is completed, the caudal portion of the occiput, the arch of the atlas, and the cranial half of the axis (spinous process and lamina) and the dorsal atlanto-AO membrane should be exposed (Figure 24.7).

The actual size of the occipital craniectomy is based on the goal(s) of the procedure, and once determined, either a nitrogen-powered air drill or an electric drill is used to burr away the occipital bone. There is marked normal variation in occipital bone thickness over the caudal cerebellum and bone directly overlying the caudal cerebellar vermis is especially thin, often without an identifying medullary cavity. In some instances where occipital bone dysplasia is present, the bone may be unusually thin, or even absent,

and use of small Lempert rongeurs may be a safer and easier alternative. Laterally and dorsally, the occipital bone becomes more robust, usually with an identifiable medullary cavity; dense cortical bone forms the dorsal rim of the (normal) foramen magnum. The surgical limits of the bony defect are ultimately dictated by essential structures in the area that should be avoided as far as possible. On midline, the dorsal sagittal sinus flows into the transverse sinuses within the occipital bone at the confluence of the sinuses which are situated approximately 1/2–2/3 of the distance between the external occipital protuberance and the dorsal rim of the foramen magnum. It is particularly important to avoid violation and/or occlusion of this confluence for risk of lethal acute cerebral edema. The lateral limits of the craniectomy are defined by the location of the transverse sinuses dorsolaterally and the occipital condyles ventrolaterally. Partial or complete laminectomy of the arch of C1 may be performed depending on the surgical corridor needed. The lateral vertebral foramina of the atlas define the lateral surgical limits on C1 (Figure 24.7). When decompressing the caudal cerebellum, as in animals with Chiari-like malformations, the limits of the craniectomy are typically narrow and centered over the cerebellar vermis primarily. However, wider approaches are frequently needed to access tumors associated with the tentorium or more rostral cerebellum, in the cerebellomedullary angle, or in the fourth ventricle.

The dorsal AO membrane is made of dense connective tissue running between the occipital bone and the arch of C1. This fibrous membrane is dissected from the underlying dura mater using a combination of fine forceps (vascular forceps or Bishop–Harmon forceps), bipolar cautery on a low setting and/or #11 scalpel blade to "peel" it back laterally on each side. Bleeding is controlled using bipolar electrocautery. The underlying dura mater is opened with a nick incision on midline. Using a right-angle probe, the dura is tented up and the incision extended along the length of the craniectomy using a #11 blade or titanium micro scissors ending in a Y or H shaped incision at either end. The meninges are reflected and preserved. The cerebellar vermis, and medial portion of the hemispheres in wider approaches, is visualized along with the dorsal caudal brainstem and junction with the craniodorsal cervical spinal cord. From this point on nervous tissues are handled as delicately as possible frequently using lint-free cellulose patties/spears to protect and keep them moist or by using continuous saline drip lavage. Gentle traction on the cerebellar vermis with incision into the transparent tissue overlying the obex allows good visualization into the fourth ventricle. Adhesions in this area are commonly encountered with chronic compressive or inflammatory conditions and may need to be gently broken down using a combination of sharp and

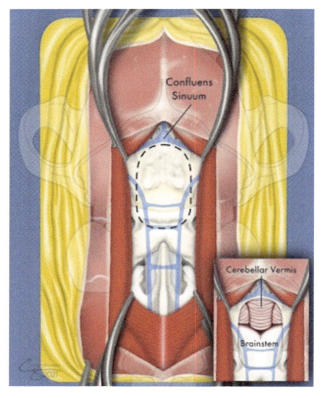

Figure 24.7 Completed dissection with craniectomy outline (and inset). The limits of the craniectomy are ultimately dictated by essential anatomy:
a. Dorsal: by the confluens sinuum on midline, 1/2–2/3 of the way between the dorsal rim of the foramen magnum and the external occipital protuberance.
b. Dorsolateral: by the transverse sinuses, ventral to the nuchal crest.
c. Ventrolaterally: by the occipitoatlantal joints (occipital condyles).
d. Ventral: by the foramen magnum.
Laminotomy of the rostral aspect of the atlas is often combined with occipital craniectomy with the lateral foramina on the base of the wings representing the lateral limits and a variable caudal limit, generally limited to ½ to ¾ the craniocaudal length of the C1 arch, although the entire arch may be removed when necessary.

blunt dissection. Titanium micro dissector instruments (Rhoton™) are especially useful for this purpose.

Surgical notes:

1) The *biventer cervicis* muscles should be preserved at their attachment as far as possible to avoid alterations in normal head carriage following surgery. If they are elevated from the occiput to gain surgical access, leaving a centimeter of tendinous tissue for re-apposition is recommended. Mild but permanent alteration in the postural angle of the head relative to the vertebral column may occur when both *rectus capitis* and *biventer cervicis* muscles are removed completely bilaterally.

2) In some dogs, interarcuate venous branches running dorsally between the left and right internal vertebral venous plexi are very well developed, appearing as circumferential venous structures surrounding C1/C2 spinal cord segments. As the dorsal AO membrane is dissected off the dura, these thin-walled sinuses are easily ruptured, especially when attempting to get more lateral to the spinal cord – e.g. nerve root or meningeal resections. This may be associated with significant bleeding which can obscure visualization or lead to postop hematoma formation. It is helpful to recognize and cauterize these structures on approach, before performing durotomy, to prevent hemorrhage from occurring.

3) Ensure that the dorsal AO membrane is completely released/removed before completing occipital bone removal. This prevents it from acting as a constricting band at the cervicomedullary junction if swelling of the cerebellum is likely to occur, as is common in situations of chronic cerebellar herniation, cerebellar edema, large fourth ventricular masses, etc.

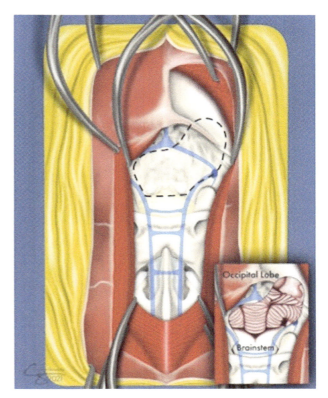

Figure 24.8 Lateralized occipital approach with occlusion of the transverse sinus (and inset). The midline approach may be modified to increase lateral exposure. The biventer cervicis muscle is elevated at its insertion on the occipital bone and the temporalis muscle is partially reflected rostrally. The craniectomy (dotted line) is extended dorsolaterally over the nuchal crest to expose and occlude the transverse sinus before approaching the osseous tentorium. The craniectomy may be extended further rostrally to include the caudal parietal bone if needed, to get better access for masses situated more ventrally.

Extended Lateral Approach with Occlusion of The Transverse Sinus [3, 6]

The attachment of the tentorium osseum to the inner surface of the cranium is formed by the juncture of the parietal, interparietal, and occipital bones. The nuchal crest represents the external feature of the skull that roughly marks its attachment to the inner aspect of the skull. A more lateralized exposure into the caudal fossa may be achieved by removing additional occipital bone laterally and occluding the transverse sinus (Figure 24.8). This may safely be done unilaterally, alone or in combination with a caudal rostrotentorial craniectomy depending on the desired surgical corridor. Indications for this extended approach to the caudal fossa include:

a) Removing masses attached to or arising from the tentorium. For example, meningiomas commonly arise from the infratentorial meningeal lining; while the bulk of the tumor may be removed fairly easily with a midline approach, meningeal tissue giving rise to the tumor may be left behind on the ventral aspect of the tentorium. Occluding the transverse sinus allows for wider tumor and meningeal resection as well as partial tentoriectomy if needed (Figure 24.9).

b) Accessing masses situated more deeply alongside the brainstem and/or into the cerebellomedullary angle, typical of choroid plexus tumors (Figure 24.10).

c) Increasing ease and safety of cerebellar retraction with enhanced visualization of (large) intraventricular masses and/or cerebellar tumors extending into the fourth ventricle (Figure 24.11).

The transverse sinuses are large venous structures with a thin epithelial lining, running within the occipital bone.

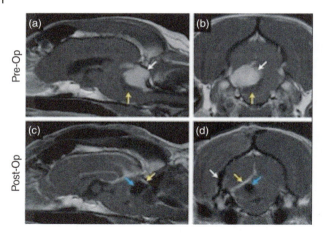

Figure 24.9 A lateralized approach with occlusion of transverse sinus to excise a tentorial mass. Mid-sagittal and transverse T1W post-contrast MR images from a 5 yo FS German short-haired Pointer. (a and b) A caudal fossa meningioma arising from the tentorium cerebelli (white arrow) with an associated cystic structure ventrally (yellow arrow) resulting in effacement of the fourth ventricle. (c and d) Images obtained following a lateralized approach with occlusion of the transverse sinus; transient air in the tumor cavity (blue arrow) and tentorial contrast enhancement (yellow arrow) are typical immediate postsurgical findings that resolve in time.

Advanced imaging is used extensively in people as a means of characterizing intracranial venous structures, but rare reports exist in veterinary medicine. Understanding and characterizing the relevant vascular anatomy of the confluence and transverse sinuses, using intracranial magnetic resonance (MR) venography prior to mass removal, is helpful in determining patency of vascular structures prior to surgical resection (Figure 24.12). In the case of a multilobular tumor of bone that may involve large portions of the occiput and a potential that the confluence and/or a transverse sinus will be violated during mass removal, this is especially critical. If blood flow is intact through the dorsal sagittal sinus into the transverse sinuses, preoperative occlusion of the dorsal sagittal sinus and confluens sinuum has been reported [7] with successful tumor excision thereafter. In some cases, compressive effects from the mass itself leads to alternative venous drainage (Figure 24.13), which can both help and hinder surgical excision.

Using a larger-sized burr, the bone overlying the transverse sinus is removed to expose the sinus. Fine-tipped bipolar electrocautery (0.4 mm wide, non-stick) is used to effectively cauterize the sinus at proximal and distal ends. If the transverse sinus has been inadvertently ruptured during bone removal, sinus hemorrhage is controlled with electrocautery, bone wax, or minute rolled, (cigar-shaped) pieces of absorbable gelatin compressed

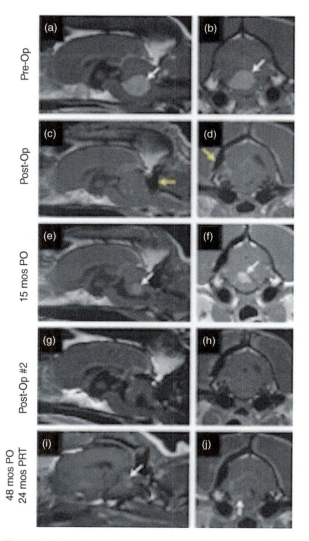

Figure 24.10 A lateralized approach with occlusion of transverse sinus to remove intraventricular mass. Mid-sagittal and transverse T1W post contrast MR images from 3 yo MC Shepherd dog mix. (a and b) Choroid plexus carcinoma (white arrows) extending from lateral aperture into the fourth ventricle. (c and d) Mass removed with typical contrast enhancement of the tentorium visualized. A PMMA plate was formed to reconstruct the cranial defect (yellow arrows). (e and f) Recheck images obtained 15 months later shows regrowth of the mass. (g and h) A second resection was performed through previous craniectomy site and closed using the same PMMA plate. Radiation therapy was performed after the second debulking surgery. (i and j) Recheck image obtained 48 months post first surgery and 24 months post radiation showing early regrowth of the mass in the same area. There were also multiple metastases throughout the entire length of the spinal cord (not shown) at this time.

sponge (Gelfoam®) placed in the ends of the tentorial canal. Once the sinus is occluded, a portion of the osseous tentorium extending between the cerebellum and occipital lobe may be burred away if needed.

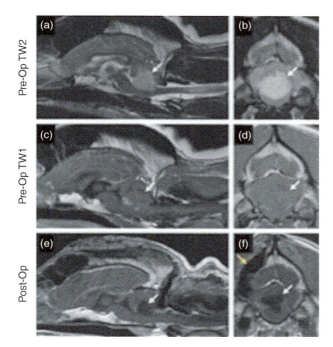

Figure 24.11 A lateralized approach with occlusion of transverse sinus to remove a cerebellar mass extending intraventricularly. Mid-sagittal and transverse MR images from a 6 yo German Shepherd dog. (a and b) T2W images showing a hyperintense mass arising from the cerebellum extending into the fourth ventricle (white arrows). (c and d) T1W post contrast images reveal that the mass is minimally contrast-enhancing, subsequently diagnosed as a cerebellar astrocytoma (white arrows). The fourth ventricle is mostly occluded by the mass. (e and f) Postoperative imaging shows a typical air-filled tumor cavity. A PMMA plate is seen covering the surgical defect. It might be possible to remove this mass without transverse sinus occlusion; however, the risk of complication from inadequate hemostasis would likely be greater. (This patient is presented on video).

Alternatively, Lempert rongeurs may be used for this but there is risk of "grabbing" deeper venous structures and creating significant hemorrhage that may be difficult to control.

At the ventrolateral extent of this dissection, it is possible to violate the occipital emissary vein draining from the sigmoid and transverse sinuses. This bleeding may be copious and will obscure visualization if not controlled. Careful cauterization and/or packing off the area with various hemostatic agents (e.g. gelatin foam, oxidized regenerated cellulose, etc.) is usually effective although it is preferable to avoid this hemorrhage by identifying the vessels first and pre-emptively occluding them.

When excising tumor tissue, ultrasonic aspiration or controlled suction may be used for the entire mass. In some situations, though, tumor excision is achieved more safely and more completely by first identifying the plane

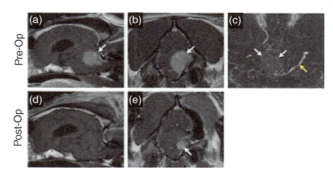

Figure 24.12 A lateralized approach with occlusion of transverse sinus and partial tentoriectomy to remove mass in cerebellomedullary angle. Mid-sagittal and transverse T1W post-contrast MR images from a 7 yo MC Boxer. (a and b) A meningioma is situated in the cerebellomedullary angle with tentorial contact dorsally and dural extension ventrally. (c) An MRV time of flight MR sequence clarifies that the transverse sinus is patent on the unaffected side (yellow arrow) but occluded by the mass (white arrows) on the affected side. (d and e) Images obtained following surgery show a mass that has been incompletely excised. Meningiomas in this location, with significant meningeal invasion adjacent to the brainstem, are particularly difficult to resect completely due to hemorrhage obscuring visualization and risking hematoma formation from penetration of basilar sinuses and/or interbasilar venous structures invading meninges.

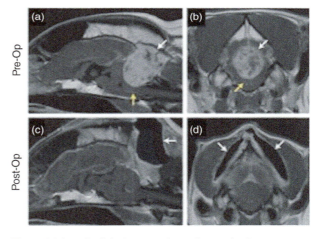

Figure 24.13 Occipital approach used to excise bony mass. Mid-sagittal and transverse T1W post contrast MR images from a 6 yo FS Golden Retriever. (A–C) Preoperative mid-sagittal, transverse, dorsal plane images of a multilobular tumor of bone (white arrows) causing marked compression of the cerebellum and fourth ventricular effacement (yellow arrows). The mass is likely affecting the confluens sinuum and proximal transverse sinuses bilaterally. Rostroventral portions of the osseous tentorium can be seen (arrowheads). The patency of the venous structures could not be determined prior to surgery from imaging. (d and e) In surgery it was noted that the normal confluens sinuum and the transverse sinuses had been occluded by the tumor. Large abnormal vascular structures were visualized ventral to the mass likely reflecting development of collateral drainage pathways from a slowly developing tumor. The caudal portion of the skull was reconstructed with PMMA, including a large external occipital protuberance to maintain the normal aesthetic presentation of the dog.

of dissection between normal and affected tissues and then meticulously following the dissection plane around the mass while placing gentle traction on it using tumor ring tip forceps. Once the mass is freed up from surrounding normal tissue, it can often be removed as an intact mass. Ultrasonic aspiration is used to "clean up" the tumor bed to ensure as much gross tumor is removed as possible.

Lateral Approach to The Cerebellum in Cats [8]

When approaching the lateral and dorsal aspects of the cerebellum in cats, an approach has been described that considers the consistent and predictable anatomy unique to felines. The tentorium osseum is attached further rostrally in cats compared to dogs and thus contributes to a more rostral extent of the caudal fossa. This provides the cat with an area rostral to the nuchal crest but caudal to the attachment of the osseous tentorium where surgical access to the lateral and dorsal aspects of the cerebellum is possible. On the external skull, the point of transition from the widest part of the cranial convexity to the flat plain of the temporal fossa delineates accurately the rostral limit of the caudal fossa (Figure 24.14). To access this area, the approach is begun with a skin incision extending from 1 cm caudal to the bregma to the level of C1 on dorsal midline. Subcutaneous tissues and superficial muscles are sharply incised along the external sagittal crest and continued ventrally following the nuchal crest. The temporalis muscle fascia is then incised along its attachment to the nuchal crest and the muscle partially elevated from the caudal third of the skull exposing the temporal fossa. The temporalis muscle is retracted cranially with Gelpi retractors. A distinct line running in a caudodistal to rostroventral direction is identified on the parietal bone at the juncture of the cranial convexity with temporal fossa. A drill is used to create the craniectomy defect using this line as the rostral boundary. The approach allows good visualization into the cerebellar fossa and lesions affecting the dorsolateral aspect of the cerebellum and/or the ventral aspect of the osseus tentorium are more easily and safely accessed over occlusion of the transverse sinus. The midline occipital approach may also be used in cats for lesion affecting the caudal aspect of the cerebellum (Figure 24.15).

Closing and Reconstruction

After completing the goals of surgery, small dural defects may be sutured closed; in dural defects with inadequate available dura, duraplasty is performed using commercially available porcine intestinal submucosa (Vetrix® BioSiS). The material is cut to size to cover any exposed neural tissue and tacked in place to adjacent meninges with 5-0 or

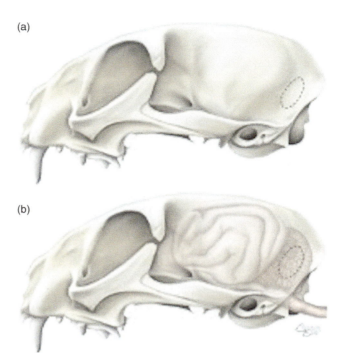

Figure 24.14 Feline caudal fossa anatomy and lateral surgical approach. Cranial bone anatomy is consistent and predictable in felines. On the lateral aspect of the skull, the point of transition from the widest part of the cranial convexity to the flat plain of the temporal fossa delineates the tentorium and rostral limit of the caudal fossa. A distinct line running in a caudodorsal to rostroventral direction is identified on the parietal bone at the juncture and surgical access is safely performed to the lateral and dorsal aspects of the cerebellum.

6-0 monofilament suture material. If meninges have been widely resected due to tumor invasion, the material may be tacked to other soft tissues outside the bony defect. The duraplasty serves as an effective protective barrier, preventing adhesions to overlying fat or muscle and providing a durable scaffold promoting bony ingrowth. Reconstruction of the occipital bone is largely based on the size of the defect and to a lesser degree on the pathology being treated. Larger craniectomies that include most of the caudal occipital bone and nuchal crest may be reconstructed using titanium mesh and screws (Synthes® MatrixNEURO™ cranial plating system) or polymethylmethacrylate (PMMA) may be used [9]. In the case of forming a PMMA plate, sterile compressed gelatin sponge is initially placed over the entire defect to protect it during the process. Liquid PMMA can be handled manually at about four minutes into the curing process. It is first flattened into an appropriate-sized piece of 1–3 mm thick, shaped into a size slightly larger than the craniectomy, and laid it over the absorbable gelatin compressed sponge and edges of the craniectomy. This PMMA "blanket" can then be gently pressed against the outer edge of bone to form a natural contour that prevents slippage and obviates the need for mesh, screws, or suture to hold

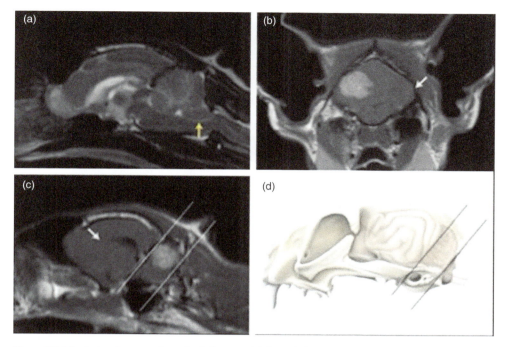

Figure 24.15 Lateral approach to the feline caudal fossa. MR images from an 8yo FS DSH. (a) Clinical signs of acute herniation were consistent in this cat at the time of presentation. This can be seen on T2W MR images performed shortly thereafter (yellow arrow). (b and c) Parasagittal and transverse T1W post contrast MR images revealing a contrast-enhancing mass on the left cerebellar hemisphere (white arrows). Marked displacement of the fourth ventricle is also seen (black arrow). (d) A lateral approach to the cerebellum was used to excise the mass, diagnosed as a cryptococcoma. The cat recovered well and neurologically normal two years later.

in place. At about six minutes into the cure, while it is still cool and handleable, the PMMA plate can be removed and placed in saline during the exothermic part of the cure reaction. The protective absorbable gelatin compressed sponge is discarded and the PMMA plate is set in place. The apposition of muscles over the plate holds it in position. The deep cervical musculature is closed on midline using a simple continuous pattern with monofilament absorbable suture. If necessary, muscular attachments of the biventer cervicis can be sutured rostrally to remaining muscle attachments or to the temporalis fascia. The superficial muscle layer, subcutaneous tissues and skin are closed in routine fashion. The incision site is covered with a sterile waterproof bandage.

Surgical Notes:

1) The cerebellum may be retracted dorsally, ventrally, and laterolaterally with extreme care. It is helpful to have an assistant assigned to this task during mass resection to limit over-retraction as well as repeated insults to the cerebellum. Avoiding excessive retraction on the cerebellar peduncles is critical since this may result in (worsening of) vestibular signs that are usually transient but, however, may take some time to resolve.
2) Even very small amounts of hemorrhage or exudation of blood into the fourth ventricle after removal of ventricular masses may cause hematoma to form that can lead to CSF outflow obstruction. Hematoma will be visualized on postoperative imaging and immediate attempts to evacuate and control any ongoing hemorrhage are recommended.
3) Ultrasonic aspiration is useful for tumor removal. This may be especially important when removing masses within the fourth ventricle to reduce small vessel disruption.
4) Intraoperative ultrasound may be used to identify the location and limits of a mass, especially those arising in the cerebellum. This is helpful when resecting masses that do not have strict delineation grossly (e.g. glioma, infectious disease).

Postoperative Care

A relatively rapid recovery from anesthesia is usually desired to facilitate timely postoperative neurological evaluation. Delayed extubation may be considered in some circumstances:

a) Marked caudal brainstem dysfunction or respiratory compromise such that the patient may not be unable to maintain a protected airway post-extubation.

b) Primary traumatic injury to the brainstem or surgery related trauma.
c) Hemorrhage or hematoma formation within the fourth ventricle.

Postoperatively, MR imaging prior to recovery is recommended to assess surgery-related complications that may lead to hypoventilation and intracranial hypertension. Specifically, it allows for visualization of forming hematoma in the fourth ventricle, excessive cerebellar swelling, and potential CSF outflow obstruction; it also allows an evaluation of the extent of surgical resection. Patients generally recover from anesthesia and surgery in the intensive care unit to allow serial neurologic examination and rapid response to abnormalities/complications that may develop. In addition, postop intensive care allows continuous, strict monitoring of blood pressure, intracranial pressure, aspiration pneumonia, and consistent pain control.

Medications commonly used:

a) Anti-emetic drugs: prophylaxis for postop vomiting with ondansetron or maripotent is recommended with the proximity of the vomiting center to the area of surgical manipulation.
b) Corticosteroids: dexamethasone sodium phosphate is used perioperatively to treat surgical-related swelling and inflammation.
c) Pain control: short-acting opioids, such as fentanyl, are titrated to effect to in the individual patient and may be used as a continuous rate infusion in the immediate postop period; dexmedetomidine in combination with opioids is often used to provide sufficient pain control and sedation.
d) Gastrointestinal protectants and pro-motility drugs: to minimize the occurrence and effects of aspiration.
e) Antibiotics: IV antibiotics are used throughout the operative period and at least 24 hours into the postoperative period.

Complications

Neurosurgical procedures involving caudal fossa pathology carry a higher incidence of neurologic complications when compared with supratentorial procedures. Most commonly, these include the following:

a) Lacerations of sinuses causing loss of visualization and potentially significant blood loss if not addressed quickly. When tamponading sinus bleeding, care must be taken not to occlude past the level of the confluens sinuum as this could lead to venous outflow obstruction and acute cerebral edema.
b) Hematoma formation. Postop hematoma usually occurs with inadequate hemostasis of the tumor bed and/or ongoing sinus hemorrhage. Initial clinical signs indicative of an expanding hematoma causing brainstem compression and/or outflow obstruction of CSF include deteriorating consciousness and focal neurologic deficit. Postop imaging and surgical evacuation are critical for effective treatment (Figure 24.16).
c) Excessive manipulation or retraction of the cerebellum can lead to cerebellar swelling and/or injury to the cerebellar peduncles.

Injury to cranial nerves is a potential complication that appears to occur very rarely in dogs with the current surgical approaches used. This is likely because in trying to get to more ventral locations in brainstem, one will often encounter robust hemorrhage thus limiting surgical resection and impact on CNs. As future caudal fossa surgical techniques and corridors are improved, it is likely this could become a larger consideration.

Video clips to accompany this book can be found on the companion website at:
www.wiley.com/go/shores/advanced

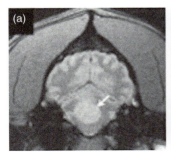 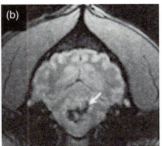

Figure 24.16 Postoperative complication. Multiple echo recombined gradient echo (MERGE) MR image obtained on an 8 yo FS Golden Retriever undergoing resection of an intraventricular mass. (a) Intraventricular mass seen on preop imaging showing no hemorrhage associated with it. (b) Postoperative images show intraventricular hemorrhage is occurring within the fourth ventricle. Concern for outflow obstruction and poor outcome merited return to surgery to attempt evacuation of hematoma and improved hemostasis. The patient died 24 hours later from poor recovery of neurologic function and aspiration pneumonia.

References

1. Evans, H.E. (1993). The muscular system. In: *Miller's Anatomy of the Dog*, 3e. Philadelphia, PA: WB Saunders.
2. Evans, H.E. (1993). Veins of the central nervous system. In: *Miller's Anatomy of the Dog*, 3e. Philadelphia, PA: WB Saunders.
3. Oliver, J.E. (1968). Surgical approaches to the canine brain. *Am. J. Vet. Res.* 29: 353–378.
4. Vermeersch, K., Ham, L.V., Caemaert, J. et al. (2004). Suboccipital craniectomy, dorsal laminectomy of C1, durotomy and dural graft placement as a treatment for syringohydromyelia with cerebellar tonsil herniation in Cavalier King Charles Spaniels. *Vet. Surg.* 33: 355–360.
5. Dewey, C.W., Berg, J.M., Barone, G. et al. (2005). Foramen magnum decompression for treatment of caudal occipital malformation syndrome in dogs. *JAVMA* 227: 1270–1275.
6. Bagley, R.S., Harrington, M.L., Pluhar, G.E. et al. (1997). Acute, unilateral transverse sinus occlusion during craniectomy in seven dogs with space-occupying intracranial disease. *Vet. Surg.* 26 (3): 195–201.
7. McAnulty, J.F., Budgeon, C., and Waller, K.R. (2019). Catheter occlusion of the dorsal sagittal sinus – confluens sinuum to enable resection of lateral occipital multilobular osteochondrosarcoma in two dogs. *JAVMA* 254: 843–851.
8. Kent, M., Glass, E.N., and Schachar, J. (2020). A lateral approach to the feline cerebellar fossa: case report and identification of an external landmark for the tentorium ossium. *J. Feline Med. Surg.* 22 (4): 358–365.
9. Moissonnier, P., Devauchell, P., and Delisle, F. (1997). Cranioplasty after en bloc resection of calvarial chondroma rodens in two dogs. *J. Small Anim. Pract.* 38: 358–363.

25

Transzygomatic Approach to Ventrolateral Craniotomy/Craniectomy

Martin Young and Sandy Chen

Bush Veterinary Neurology Service, Leesburg, VA, USA

Introduction

The transzygomatic approach to intracranial surgery has been advanced and frequently modified over the last three decades in human medicine [1]. This technique provides excellent access to the middle fossa and the cavernous sinus [2]. Similarly, in veterinary medicine, this approach has been described by several authors with a variety of adaptations most commonly involving removal of a portion of the zygomatic arch [3–6]. The most common indication for this approach is neoplasia, such as a trigeminal nerve sheath tumor or piriform lobe glioma (Figure 25.1) [7, 8]. Both diagnostic biopsy and complete resection can be achieved through this corridor. Without the use of neuro-navigational or intraoperative ultrasound equipment, knowledge and understanding of the regional anatomy is imperative.

Patient Positioning/Preparation

The patient is shaved from the orbit to the level of the atlas vertebra on the appropriate half of the head. A headframe built by the authors as seen in Figure 25.2 was used to secure the patient's head by the maxilla with the mandible hung open to move the ramus rostrally. The headframe is then rotated to a 45° angle until the central structure of the zygomatic arch is parallel to the surgery table (Figures 25.3). This improves the surgeon's line of sight of the piriform lobe. The surgical site is then scrubbed and disinfected per normal standards of care. If a Styrofoam bead vacuum bag is used to position the head, a mouth gag should be used to help direct the ramus of the mandible rostrally. Care should be taken in cats as persistent use of a mouth gag has been associated with cortical blindness [9].

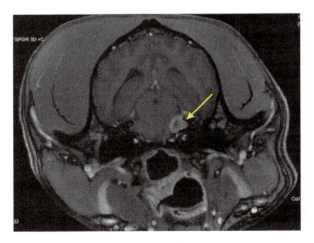

Figure 25.1 A T1+C transverse MRI image of a dog with a trigeminal nerve sheath tumor (arrow).

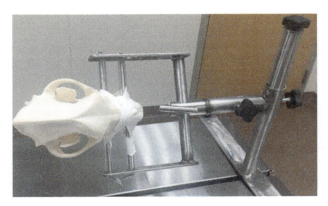

Figure 25.2 A stainless-steel headframe made that allows rotation of the head for this procedure and secures the head in this position for the duration of the procedure.

Advanced Techniques in Canine and Feline Neurosurgery, First Edition. Edited by Andy Shores and Brigitte A. Brisson.
© 2023 John Wiley & Sons, Inc. Published 2023 by John Wiley & Sons, Inc.
Companion site: www.wiley.com/go/shores/advanced

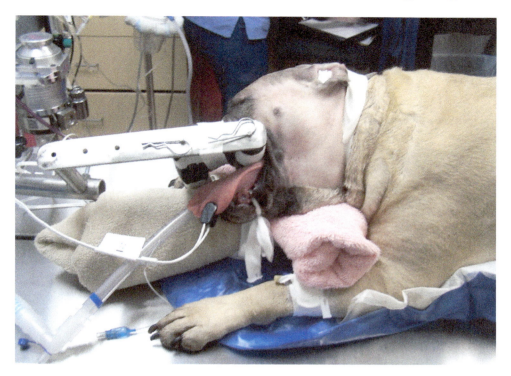

Figure 25.3 A headstand designed to securely position the patient for the transzygomatic approach. This patient is in sternal recumbency, and the head is positioned in a headstand with an approximate 45° rotation to the right to facilitate this approach to the left side.

Surgical Procedure

An incision is made between the lateral canthus and the tragus at the level of the dorsal aspect of the zygomatic arch (Figure 25.4). Caution must be taken at this level as the auriculopalpebral branches of the facial nerve (cranial nerve VII) and the auriculotemporalis nerve branches of the trigeminal nerve (cranial nerve V) are directly superficial to the dermis and transection can occur. The auriculopalpebral nerve crosses the zygomatic arch and continues to the orbit,

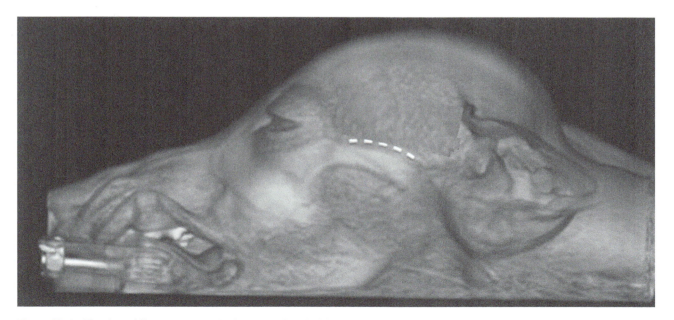

Figure 25.4 The dotted line represents the location of an incision made between the lateral canthus and the tragus at the level of the dorsal aspect of the zygomatic arch.

and the auriculotemporalis nerve runs perpendicularly to the caudal aspect of the zygomatic arch and emerges between the masseter muscles [10]. Once identified, they can be gently dissected from the platysma and fascia to allow for light retraction and to avoid postoperative facial paralysis [6].

Prior to dissection, the zygomatic arch, lateral rim of the orbit, and temporomandibular joint are identified by gentle palpation. The zygomatic arch has three parts: the zygomatic process of the maxilla, the zygomatic bone, and the zygomatic process of the temporal bone (Figure 25.5). Rostrally, the zygomatic arch supports the orbit structure by forming the ventral and lateral rim. The central structure runs lateral to the ramus of the mandible and provides lateral contour to the face. The caudal part serves as an origin for the masseter muscle. The muscular attachments along the dorsal and ventral edges of the zygomatic arch are incised, and a freer/elevator can then be used to clear the muscle away from the portion of the zygomatic arch to be removed. A high-speed pneumatic drill is used to remove the caudal up to 3/4 of the zygomatic arch, which includes the caudal portion of the frontal process and the rostral portion of the temporal process. A maximum of ¾ of the arch can be removed without disruption of the orbit and causing collapse (Figure 25.6) [11]. Alternatively, this portion of bone can be removed using an osteotome, mallet, and Kerrison rongeurs [11, 12].

The temporalis muscle is dissected from the zygomatic arch to a level proximal to the temporomandibular joint. A mix of sharp and digital dissection is made through the temporalis muscle to the level of the skull. Right angle Gelpi's are used to retract the tissues (Figure 25.7). Landmarks for craniectomy are identified by palpation and visualization. The convergence of the frontoparietal and parietotemporal sutures form a horizontal T (Figure 25.8) that is roughly the dorsal margin of the craniectomy window. The craniectomy is performed with a high-speed pneumatic drill and rongeurs. The dimensions of craniectomy window can be adjusted based on tumor location to the parietal/temporal suture, and the temporomandibular joint [1].

The ventral margin is at the junction of the temporal bone and the zygomatic process of the temporal bone or the ventromedial curvature of the frontal bone which forms the caudal aspect of the orbit (Figure 25.9). Use caution at this level as the optic canal (CN II), orbital fissure (CN III, CN IV Ophthalmic branch of CN V and CN VII), and the rostral alar foramen (Maxillary branch CN V) are located several millimeters medial to the window being created. There is variability between breeds, but in a

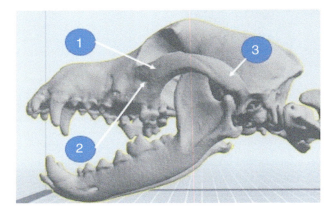

Figure 25.5 The zygomatic arch has three parts: the zygomatic bone (1), the zygomatic process of the maxilla (2), and the zygomatic process of the temporal bone (3).

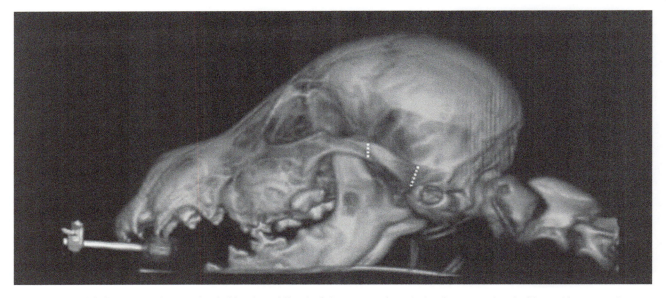

Figure 25.6 This illustrates the margins (white dotted lines) of the zygomatic arch that is removed to facilitate this approach.

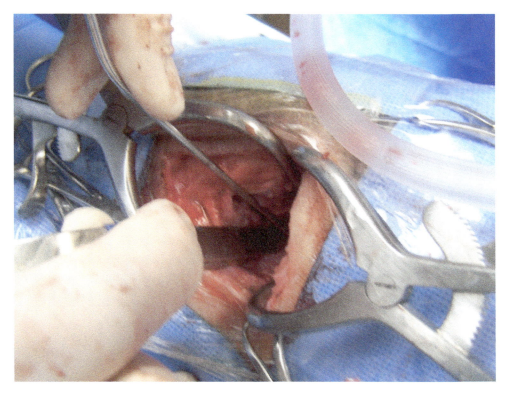

Figure 25.7 Intraoperative view showing placement of the right angle Gelpi retractors.

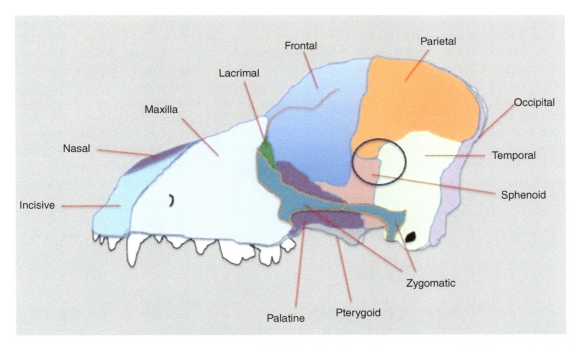

Figure 25.8 In this illustration, the area located within the circle shows the convergence of the frontoparietal and parietotemporal sutures that form a horizontal T and represent the dorsal margin of the craniectomy window.

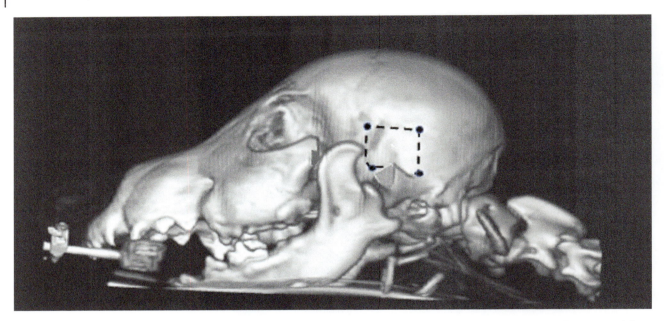

Figure 25.9 The ventral margin of the craniectomy begins at the junction of the temporal bone and the zygomatic process of the temporal bone. In this illustration a portion of the zygomatic bone has been removed and the area shown by the dashed lines is the approximate dimensions of the craniectomy.

medium to large dog a window of 2 cm in height by 2 cm in length is reasonable.

The middle meningeal artery is identified and skeletonized (dissected and preserved) to prevent bleeding. Alternatively, it can be ligated and transected. The dura can be completely removed at this stage or a flap can be made to replace once surgery is complete. Dural bleeding can be controlled with bipolar cautery, chilled saline, and absorbable hemostatic gelatin sponge or other hemostatic agents. The pseudosylvian sulcus and the lateral rhinal sulcus intersect and are visualized as a reversed capital letter T. The sylvan, caudal composite, and caudal portion of the ectosylvan gyrus form a U shape around the ectosylvan sulcus. Ventral and medial to the lateral rhinal sulcus lies the piriform lobe. Kerrison rongeurs can be used to extend the craniectomy window ventral as needed to expose the trigeminal nerve, the lateral margins of the cavernous sinus, or ventral piriform lobe. It may be necessary to elevate the piriform lobe or caudal composite gyrus to improve access to a primary tumor. If traction is used allow a period of rest every three to five minutes.

Prior to closure, complete hemostasis should be achieved with a combination of chilled saline, hemostatic agents, and foam sponges. Prior to a routine closure the brain can be covered with the original dura, a synthetic dural replacement such as SIS or gelatin sponge. At this level the author has not created a replacement for the bony window as there is enough muscle and bone protection; however, a titanium or polypropylene mesh can be used and secured with small titanium screws. After removal of all blood clots, the craniectomy site is lavaged copiously with saline solution. The muscle, fascia, and dermis are closed in routine fashion.

 Video clips to accompany this book can be found on the companion website at: www.wiley.com/go/shores/advanced

References

1. Campero, A., Ajler, P., Emmerich, J. et al. (2014). Brain sulci and gyri: a practical anatomical review. *J. Clin. Neurosci.* 21 (12): 2219–2225.
2. Chotai, S., Kshettry, V.R., Petrak, A., and Ammirati, M. (2015). Lateral transzygomatic middle fossa approach and its extensions: surgical technique and 3D anatomy. *Clin. Neurol. Neurosurg.* 130: 33–41.
3. Forward, A.K., Volk, H.A., and De Decker, S. (2018). Postoperative survival and early complications after intracranial surgery in dogs. *Vet. Surg.* 2018 (47): 549–554.
4. Fossum, T.W. (2012). *Small Animal Surgery: Surgery of the Brain*, 1438–1448. Maryland Heights, MO: Mosby.

5. Shihab, N., Summers, B.A., Benigni, L. et al. (2014). Novel approach to temporal lobectomy for removal of a cavernous hemangioma in a dog. *Vet. Surg.* 43 (7): 877–881.

6. Forterre, F., Jaggy, A., Rohrbach, H. et al. (2009). Modified temporal approach for a rostro-temporal basal meningioma in a cat. *J. Feline Med. Surg.* 11 (6): 510–513.

7. Bagley, R., Wheeler, S., Klopp, L. et al. (1998). Clinical features of trigeminal nerve-sheath tumor in 10 dogs. *J. Am. Anim. Hosp. Assoc.* 34 (1): 19–25.

8. Slatter, D.H. (2003). *Textbook of Small Animal Surgery: Brain*, 1163–1172. St. Louis, MO: Elsevier Health Sciences.

9. Stiles, J., Weil, A.B., Packer, R.A., and Lantz, G.C. (2012). Post-anesthetic cortical blindness in cats: twenty cases. *Vet. J.* 193 (2): 367–373.

10. Evans, H.E. and Lahunta, A.D. (2013). *Guide to the Dissection of the Dog: The Head*, 208–262. St. Louis, MO: Elsevier Health Sciences.

11. Boudrieau, R.J. and Kudisch, M.M. (1996). Miniplate fixation for repair of mandibular and axillary fractures in 15 dogs and 3 cats. *Vet. Surg.* 25 (4): 277–291.

12. Johnson, A.L., Houlton, J.E., and Vannini, R. (2005). *AO Principles of Fracture Management in the Dog and Cat: Fractures of the Maxilla*, 116–128. Germany, Stuttgart: Thieme.

Index

a

acrylonitrile butadiene styrene (ABS) 17
additive modeling (AM). *see* 3D printing (3DP)
anal sac balloon catheter 245
arterial blood gas analysis 94
aspiration pneumonia 203
atlantoaxial instability/ subluxation (AIS) 6

b

bio-printing 23
blade fenestration 73
brachycephalic dogs 229
brain biopsy techniques 179

c

cauda equina syndrome. *see* degenerative lumbosacral stenosis (DLSS)
caudal fossa
  anatomy 249–250
  cerebellum in cats 258
  complications 260
  extended lateral approach 255–258
  indications 250
  midline occipital approach 252–255
  postoperative care 259–260
  preoperative assessment and anesthetic management 251
  reconstruction 258–259
  surgical positioning 251–252
  venous system 250
caudal vertebral malformation-malarticulation syndrome (CVMMS) 7

CCJ. *see* craniocervical junction (CCJ) anomalies
cellulose eye spear 246
central diabetes insipidus (CDI) 200
Cerebral Salt Wasting Syndrome (CSWS) 202
cervical disk disease 5–8
cervical fractures, and dislocations 7
cervical hemilaminectomy 149–150
cervical IVD syndrome
  advanced imaging 49–50
  clinical signs 47–48
  history 47
  radiographic signs 48
  surgical indication 50
cervical spine cord
  perioperative and postoperative care 58
  ventral approach to 50–54
  ventral slot method 54–57
cervical vertebral column
  anatomical considerations 96–97
  complications 106–107
  diskectomy 99
  distraction 98–99
  implant selection 97
  indications 96, 101
  intervertebral spacer 99–100
  monocortical screw/PMMA fixation 101–102
  multiple spaces 105
  positioning and approach 97–98
  postoperative assessment 105–106
  preoperative planning 96
  surgical stabilization 101–105
  vertebral body plates 102–104
cervicothoracic spine
  clinical results 165–166

pathological conditions 161
surgical anatomy 161–163
surgical technique 163–165
choroid plexus tumors 35
Clinical Target Volume (CTV) 27
computed tomography (CT) 49
  canine patient 92
  degenerative lumbosacral stenosis 132–133
  3D reconstruction 92
computer aided design (CAD) 19
conformity index (CI) 33
congenital spinal anomalies 124
  diagnostics 124–125
  prognosis 126–127
  treatment 125–126
cranial thoracic compressive spinal lesions
  indications 86–87
  patient positioning 87–88
  postoperative care 89
  surgical anatomy 87
  surgical technique 88–89
craniocervical junction (CCJ) anomalies
  definition 153
  medical and surgical management 154
  MRI 153
  outcomes 159
  patient preparation and positioning 155–156
  surgical anatomy 154–155
  surgical technique 156–158
cranioplasty 23, 220–221
craniotomy anesthesia drug protocol 43
Cyberknife® 31

Advanced Techniques in Canine and Feline Neurosurgery, First Edition. Edited by Andy Shores and Brigitte A. Brisson.
© 2023 John Wiley & Sons, Inc. Published 2023 by John Wiley & Sons, Inc.
Companion site: www.wiley.com/go/shores/advanced

d

degenerative lumbosacral stenosis (DLSS)
- clinical signs   130
- computed tomography   132–133
- diagnosis   130–134
- electromyography   134
- force plate analysis   134
- L7–S1 foramina anatomy   129–130
- magnetic resonance imaging   133–134
- myelography   132
- neurologic examination   131
- orthopedic examination   130
- pathophysiology   129
- physical examination   130
- postoperative management   139
- radiography   131–132
- surgery   134–139
- treatment   134

DICOM formatted images   181
diskectomy   99
DLSS. *see* degenerative lumbosacral stenosis (DLSS)
dorsal laminectomy   3
- degenerative lumbosacral stenosis   135–136

dorsal sagittal sinus (DSS)   217–218, 229–230
dose-painting technique   28
durotomy   67, 157

e

early-delayed effect   26
electroencephalogram (EEG)   42
electromyography (EMG)   134
endoscopic third ventriculostomy (ETV)   241
erector spinae plane block (ESPB)   43
ETV. *see* endoscopic third ventriculostomy (ETV)

f

facetectomy   137
falcine strip procedure   230
fenestration. *see* thoracolumbar disk fenestration
foraminotomy   136–137
force plate analysis (FPA)   134
frame-based stereotactic brain biopsy (SBBfb)   179–181

frameless stereotactic brain biopsy (SBBfl)   185
- fiducial markers   185–186
- magnetic resonance images   186
- registration   186–187
- sample processing   187
- trajectory planning   187

fused deposition modeling (FDM)   17

g

Gelpi retractors   57
glial tumors   34–35
gradient index (GI)   33
gross-total resection (GTR)   223

h

hemilaminectomy   65–66
- closure   67
- complications   67–68
- disk material removal   66–67
- indications   59
- oblique patient positioning   60
- partial pediculectomy technique   59
- postoperative care   68
- surgical approach   64–65

Hoerlein, B.F., 3
hyperadrenocorticism   203
hypercoagulability   203
hypoadrenocorticism   202
hypoglycemia   202–203
hypophysectomy   190–192
hypothyroidism   202

i

intensity-modulated radiotherapy (IMRT)   28, 29
intervertebral disk herniation (IVDH)   78
intracranial pressure (ICP)
- during anesthesia   41
- cerebral perfusion   40
- clinical signs   39
- contrast myelography   42
- Cushing reflex   40
- dynamics   39–40
- hydrocephalus   42

intracranial surgery   8–11, 43
intracranial tumors
- choroid plexus tumors   35
- glial tumors   34–35
- meningioma   33–34

outcome   25
radiation therapy   25
- DNA   25–26
- fractionation   26–28
- normal tissue injury   26

spinal tumors   35–36
stereotactic radiosurgery and stereotactic radiation therapy   36
treatment planning
- beam energy selection   28
- delivery systems   31–32
- dose calculations   28–29
- evaluation   32–33
- target localization strategies   29–31

intraoperative ultrasound
- accuracy   173
- appearance of tumor   175–176
- artifacts   172–173
- diagnostic imaging   171
- guided procedures   177
- scanning procedure and equipment   173–175

j

James, C.W., 3

k

Keratoconjunctivitis Sicca (KCS)   204

l

laminectomy   157
laser ablation   78–79
lateral ventricular fenestration   242
- cerebrospinal fluid   242
- complications   243
- polypropylene mesh   242
- ventriculostomy   242

locked cervical facets
- clinical presentation   91–92
- description   91
- in humans   91
- postoperative care   94, 95
- surgical techniques   92–94

longus coli muscle   55
lumbosacral compression. *see* degenerative lumbosacral stenosis (DLSS)
lumbosacral spine
- aftercare   122

anatomy   118
complications   120–122
implant selection   119–120
positioning and approach   118
postoperative imaging   120
reduction   119

m

magnetic resonance imaging
(MRI)   18
craniocervical junction
anomalies   153
degenerative lumbosacral
stenosis   133–134
frameless stereotactic brain
biopsy   186
skull tumors   216–217
meningiomas   11, 33–34
anatomy   223–225
clinical presentations   143
combined rostrotentorial–
transfrontal approach
234–235
cytology/histology   147
resection and instrumentation
236–237
rostrotentorial craniectomy/
craniotomy   231–234
Simpson classification of   235
suboccipital craniectomy   235–236
transfrontal craniotomy   225–231
vascular supply   223
middle meningeal artery   266
mini-hemilaminectomy   63–64
complications   67–68
dorsolateral approach   60–61
indications   59
oblique patient positioning   60
partial pediculectomy technique   59
postoperative care   68
surgical approach   60
variation   61–63
minimally-invasive transilial vertebral
(MTV) blocking   138–139
mitotic death   26
multilobular osteochrondrosarcoma
(MLO)   211–212. see also
skull tumors

n

neuroanesthesia   39–43
neurologic monitoring   42

neuroradiographic techniques   2
nociception monitoring   42–43
nuclear magnetic resonance (NMR)   2

o

osteosarcoma   211–212

p

pedicle screw and rod fixation
(PSRF)   138
pediculectomy. see mini-
hemilaminectomy
percutaneous laser disk ablation
(PLDA)   78
candidate selection   79
complications and
recurrence   82–83
criteria   79
description   80–82
diagnostic evaluation   83–84
laser ablation   78–79
peripheral nerve sheath tumors (PNST)
clinical presentations   143
cytology/histology   147–148
MRI   144–147
pin placement techniques   137
Planning Target Volume (PTV)   27
PLDA. see percutaneous laser disk
ablation (PLDA)
pneumatic bur drill   55
point-to-point forceps   93
polyetheretherketone (PEEK)   17
polylactic acid (PLA)   17
port films   30
power fenestration   73–75
pulmonary thromboembolism   203
Purdue diamond modification
228–229

r

radiation therapy (RT)
choroid plexus tumors   35
glial tumors   34–35
intracranial tumors   25
DNA   25–26
fractionation   26–28
normal tissue injury   26
meningioma   33–34
spinal nerve root tumors   151
spinal tumors   35–36
radiographic techniques   1
Redding, R.W., 3

rostrotentorial craniectomy/
craniotomy   231–234

s

SBB. see stereotactic brain biopsy (SBB)
techniques
SBBfl. see frameless stereotactic brain
biopsy (SBBfl)
sculpting programs   19
segmentation   18
sensory-evoked responses (SERs)   42
skull tumors   22
complications and risks   219–220
cranioplasty   220–221
diagnosis and characterization   212
dorsal sagittal sinus   217–218
extension   218
MRI   216–217
multilobular osteochrondrosarcoma,
211–212
osteosarcoma   211–212
resection   214–216
surgical planning and
treatment   212–214
zygomatic arch and ramus of the
mandible   218–219
Soft Palate Dehiscence   205
somatosensory-evoked potentials
(SSEPs)   42
SOP plating   93, 137–138
spinal nerve root tumors
cervical approach   148
clinical presentations   143–144
cytology/histology   147–148
diagnosis   144
dorsal surgical approach   149–150
imaging   144–147
lateral surgical approach   148–149
L7–S1 foramen   150
lumbar approach   150
postoperative care   150–151
prognosis   151
radiation therapy   151
surgery   148
spinal stabilization
cervical vertebral column
96–107
of thoracolumbar spine   109–122
spinal tumors   35–36
Standard Triangle Language   19
stereolithography (STL)   17–18

stereotactic brain biopsy (SBB)
techniques
  contraindications 179
  headframe placement and
    acquisition 181
  indications 179
  planning 181–183
  postoperative care and adverse
    events 184
  preoperative evaluation 181
  procedure 183–184
  specimens 184
stereotactic radiosurgery (SRS) 28
stereotactic radiotherapy (SRT) 28
sternohyoideus muscles 52
suboccipital craniectomy 235–236
Swaim, S.F., 3

t

tentorial meningiomas 225
thoracolumbar 2–5
  decompression 59–68
thoracolumbar disk fenestration
  blade fenestration 73
  complications 75–76
  diathermy 72
  indications 70–71
  lateral annulus 72
  postoperative care 76
  power fenestration 73–75
  surgical approach 71–72
thoracolumbar spine

decompression with
  stabilization 111
implant selection 111–114, 114–116
positioning and approach 114
pre-drilling 111
preoperative planning 109–110
spinal stapling/segmental
  fixation 116–117
three-dimensional conformal
  radiotherapy (3DCRT) 28, 29
3D printing (3DP) 17
  acquisition 18
  anatomic additive model 19
  anatomic modeling 19
  current brain applications 21–23
  current spinal applications 20
  customized tools 20–21
  file format creation 19
  fused deposition modeling 17
  future applications 23
  manifold manipulation 19
  segmentation 18
  stereolithography 17–18
  thresholding 18
tissue density 18
transarticular implants 20–21
transfrontal craniotomy 225–231
transsphenoidal hypophysectomy
  (TSH) 190
  case selection for 191–192
  hospital care 200
  long term follow up 205

neurologic exam 192–193
postoperative complications 200–205
preoperative testing and
  diagnostics 193–196
surgery 196–200

u

unilateral locked cervical facets
  (ULCF) 91
unilateral transfrontal
  craniotomy 229

v

ventral approach 6
ventral midline incision 51
ventral slot method 54–57
ventriculoperitoneal (VP)
  shunting 241
ventrolateral craniotomy/craniectomy
  patient positioning/preparation
    262–263
  surgical procedure 263–266
veterinary neurosurgery
  cervical disk disease 5–8
  imaging techniques 1–2
  intracranial surgery 8–11
  thoracolumbar 2–5
  3D printing in 17–23
veterinary radiology 1

w

Wobbler Syndrome 7